Deutsches Krebsforschungszentrum

Current Cancer Research

1998

Springer-Verlag
Berlin Heidelberg GmbH

Cover illustration:

Tumor cells invade into surrounding tissue. This process is simulated in a model with a human lung tumor cell outside the organism. Forty individual consecutive images through the cell were made by confocal microscopy. These images were recombined by a computer program to obtain an image of the whole cell with 3-D impression (Dr. Torsten Porwol and Prof. Dr. Helmut Acker, Max-Planck-Institut für Molekulare Physiologie, Dr. Anja-Rose Strohmaier and Prof. Dr. Eberhard Spiess, Deutsches Krebsforschungszentrum)

ISBN 978-3-7985-1122-4
ISBN 978-3-642-95995-0 (eBook)
DOI 10.1007/978-3-642-95995-0

ISSN 0940-0745

Additional material to this book can be downloaded from http://extras.springer.com

Coordination:

Elisabeth Hohensee, M.A.

Co-workers:

Dipl.-Biol. Dagmar Anders
Ulrike Hafner
Christine Hesse
Dipl.-Biol. Dr. Sibylle Kohlstädt
Dipl.-Biol. Ulrike Nell
Dipl.-Biol. Renate Ries
Dipl.-Biol. Dr. Claudia Walther

Translation:

Stefanie von Kalckreuth, akad. gepr. Übers., Heidelberg
Angela Lahee, PhD, Gaiberg
Scitech Communications GmbH, Heidelberg

Layout:

Heidi Hnatek
Stefan Bieck, Büro für Öffentlichkeitsarbeit, Köln

Photos:

Josef Wiegand

Photos in the research reports by the authors or by their co-workers

Fig. 10 copyright Kindler Verlag, Zürich 1968; fig. 11 with kind permission of Daniel Stoffler, Biozentrum Basel; fig. 12 Monika Brettel, Division of Cell Biology; fig. 13 Cäcilia Kuhn, Division of Cell Biology; figs. 14, 15 Dr. Herbert Spring, Biomedical Structure Analysis Group; fig. 16 with kind permission of Dr. J. Faber, from: Normal Table of Xenopus Laevis (Daudin), edited by P. D. Nieuwkoop and J. Faber, North-Holland Publishing Company, Amsterdam, reprint by Garland Publishing Inc., New York; Fig. 26 with kind permission of Heidelberg University Dermatology Clinic; fig. 27 with kind permission of BASF Aktiengesellschaft, Ludwigshafen; fig. 28 with kind permission of Boehringer Ingelheim GmbH; figs. 32, 33, 34 with kind permission of evi, Arbeitskreis Ernährungs- und Vitamininformation e.V., Frankfurt; figs. 52, 53 Dr. Claus-Wilhelm von der Lieth, Central Spectroscopy; Figs. 71, 72 Dr. Sibylle Kohlstädt, Office of Press and Public Relations; fig. 77 with kind permission of Doros Panayi, European Molecular Laboratory, Heidelberg; fig. 78 with kind permission of Priv.-Doz. Dr. Peter R. Galle, Medical University Clinic, Gastroenterology Department, Heidelberg; fig. 82 with kind permission of Dr. Michael Schwarz, Heidelberg; fig. 120 with kind permission of Foto Studio Gärtner, Heidelberg; fig. 137 Brigitte Engelhardt, Arbeitsgruppe Foto; Abb. S. 245 Luftbild Krug, Heidelberg

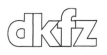

Chapter		Page

Chapter			Page

Chapter		Page

The Fight Against Cancer in Germany – A Critical Review

by Harald zur Hausen

Each year in Germany there are more than 300 000 new cases of cancer, a figure which we expect to rise annually by 6000. More than 210 000 cancer deaths per year in this one country justify not only the high level of attention which this disease arouses in the public, but also the enormous efforts that are undertaken worldwide in order to prevent its occurrence and its consequences, and at least to alleviate the latter.

Let us first consider the current state of affairs: I believe that Germany possesses a very good foundation for basic cancer research. Together with the national cancer research center, the Deutsches Krebsforschungszentrum, we have a large number of university and non-university facilities which carry out a significant amount of efficient cancer research. Particular points of focus can be identified in cell and tumor biology, in tumor immunology, and in tumor virology; these activities are also held in high regard abroad. Molecular biology has come to play an important role in cancer research and will have a lasting influence on its further development.

Despite a whole series of promising beginnings, cancer genetics – by which I mean here less the functional molecular-biological analysis of modifications in the genetic material of cancer cells and more the molecular epidemiology and the mapping of cancer genes – has been slower getting started here than elsewhere, particularly in the United States, a fact which also holds for epidemiological research in general. One may seek the reasons for this not only in the chequered history of genetics in this country, but also in the absence of a consistent concept for human genome research. It is to be welcomed that the Federal Ministry for Education, Science, Research, and Technology has given a clear signal by financing a German Genome Program and that the first positive effects of this are already perceptible in cancer research.

Worrying, on the other hand, are the developments in the German pharmaceutical industry, which has relocated essential elements of its application-related genetic engineering work abroad, such that our young scientists, mostly with an excellent training in basic research, have hardly any hope of finding a job in this country. The single positive effect of this development is undoubtedly the enormous competition for academic positions in this area; simultaneously, however, the large majority of talented young scientists have no chance here to develop their careers further. Today we are already able to see that the most agile and talented brains are seeking long-term positions abroad, again predominantly in the United States.

All this, despite the fact that the frequently mentioned technology transfer from basic research to the applications area took place in German cancer research to a significant degree already in the past: one of the most important chemotherapy drugs, Endoxan, was invented in Germany; diagnostic markers for a whole range of cancers using re-expressed fetal antigens, or through the detection of soluble keratins or other components of the cytoskeleton were developed here and are now applied on a routine basis throughout the world; tumor viruses, which today are thought to be involved in 10 % of all cancer cases worldwide, were discovered in Germany and the mechanism of their tumor-inducing properties at least par-

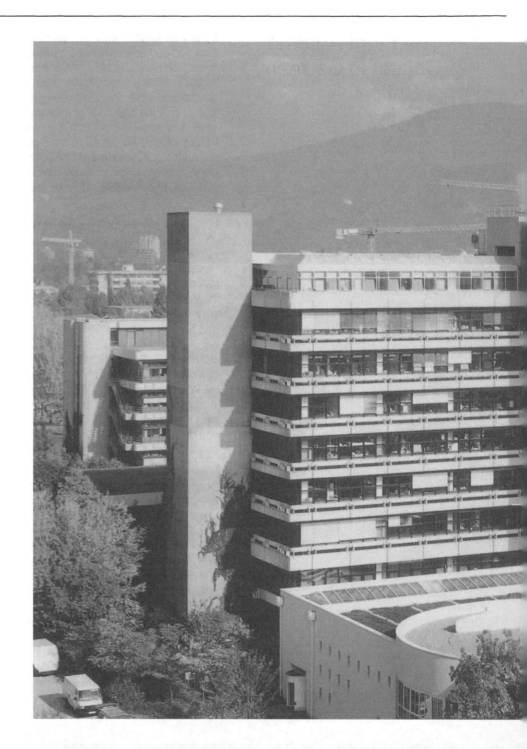

Fig. 1
The Deutsches Krebsforschungszentrum and its communication center for conferences, conventions and exhibitions are shown in the foreground. In late 1997 an eighth floor was completed, which expanded the building. The laboratory building for applied tumor virology which was placed into operation in 1992 is located behind the main building. The Center is located in the middle of the university campus and is in direct proximity to clinics and institutes in the biological and natural sciences as well as the technology park of the city of Heidelberg

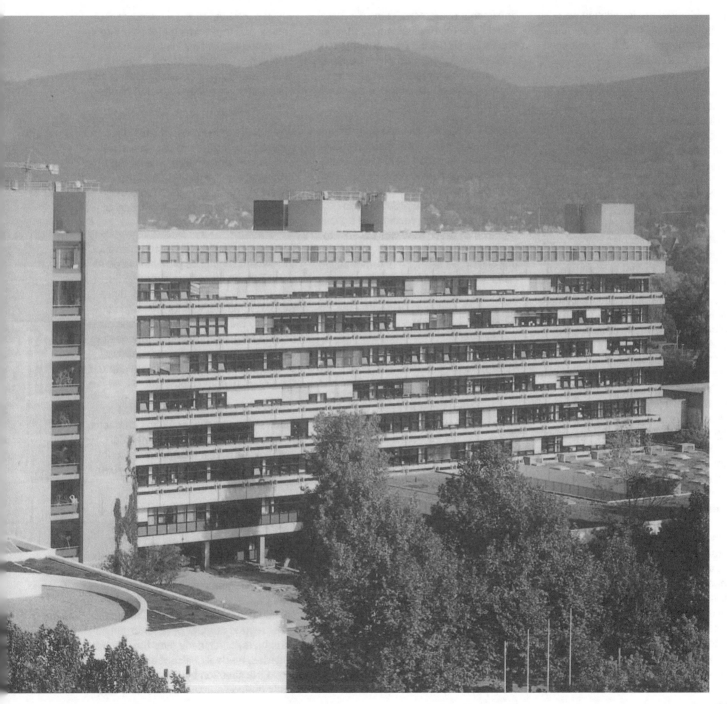

tially explained; the foundation was subsequently laid for the major immunization programs that are now beginning or in preparation.

An outstanding role today is played by the development of new concepts of tumor therapy and by preventive approaches. Even though the area of gene therapy and what it can and can't achieve is the favorite topic of public discussion, it is not this sector that is predominantly offering new prospects in cancer research today. Our knowledge of the molecular structure of proteins and other molecules whose modification contributes to the growth of certain types of cancer is increasingly allowing us, with the help of the computer, to design tailor-made inhibiting or activating substances whose chemical synthesis should make possible their application in cancer treatment in the future. The combination of immunological and gene-therapeutic procedures is a fascinating topic at present, even though the existing results do not yet give cause for any great optimism. The early discussions of gene therapy as a possible cancer treatment were certainly premature and remain so as long as essential questions remain unanswered – e.g., the development of suitable carrier systems for genes, the cell specificity of the carrier molecules, gene persistence, and the regulation of gene expression. Finally, our knowledge of suitable target systems, i.e., of target genes, is far more fragmentary than one might think when reading the relevant specialist literature. Thus, a large amount of fundamental research still has to be carried out, research for which we in Germany possess a good basis. It is my belief that we should largely ignore both the exaggerated op-

timism that characterized the first attempts and the disillusionment that has subsequently set in. The concepts remain promising; it is simply necessary to do the proper groundwork and this, without question, will still need quite some time.

A decisive matter, as I see it, is the prevention of cancer: Here there is a need for immediate action. In the field of the development of vaccines against virally induced forms of cancer there have certainly been some promising advances, e.g., in the vaccination against hepatitis B, which may well be able to prevent the occurrence of liver cell cancer. Since this is a type of tumor which does not play a dominant role here, the preventive character of this program will serve largely as a model for the fundamental concept of a cancer vaccine.

In the case of cervical cancer, of which there are about 15 000 new cases each year, the situation is different: now that the role of specific papillomaviruses in the development of this cancer has been confirmed, experiments on animal papillomavirus infections have shown that these can be effectively prevented by vaccination. At present, efforts are underway in a number of countries to produce vaccines against human papillomavirus infections; the first clinical tests are already in progress. If these are successful, we can look forward, not only to an effective prevention of cervical cancer, but also to a means of preventing the earlier pre-cancerous stages of the disease, which themselves also require treatment.

Chemopreventive measures are today still very much in their infancy. For example, we still know far too little about the exact components of our diets

which contribute to the development of cancer and those which can offer direct protection against the disease. However, a series of clinical studies have produced promising first results and should encourage intensified research efforts in this area.

What, then, is the present situation with regard to clinical research, particularly clinical cancer research, in Germany? And what are the projects and programs that can really contribute to changing the prospects, especially of cancer sufferers?

Clinical research is research on and for the patient as well as patient-related research in the laboratory aimed at improving prevention, diagnostics, therapy, and rehabilitation. Its role is to contribute to the avoidance of disease, to enable early and accurate diagnoses to be made, to optimize therapy, and to shorten the course of the disease and the period of convalescence.

Today's clinical reasearch has lost much of its previous empirical character and now demands of many medical professions a high level of basic knowledge of natural science and molecular biology.

Seen from this viewpoint, one might ask whether clinical research in Germany can match the level set by the English speaking countries. The German Research Association (Deutsche Forschungsgemeinschaft, DFG), the Max Planck Society, the German Cancer Aid (Deutsche Krebshilfe) and certainly a good number of other organizations have, particularly over the last two decades, made significant efforts to improve the situation by offering grants for study periods abroad, by initiating clinical research groups, and by sponsoring selected clinical research projects. These efforts have undoubtedly had a measurable success, but by international standards one that lags behind other countries.

Can we attribute this overall unsatisfactory situation to particular structures of the German research environment? It is my belief that we can, and in the following I will try to give what I see as the most important arguments. For a young medical student, Germany offers no wide-ranging course of study with the possibility of finally gaining a Dr. rer. nat. (Doctor of natural sciences), equivalent to the English or American M.D. and Ph.D. programs (Medical Doctor, Doctor of Philosophy). It has only been very recently that some efforts to introduce such a program have been made. Once the status of post-doctorate has been achieved, it is very difficult to make up for the lack of a basic grounding in natural science and molecular biology. This deficiency cannot be alleviated by employing natural scientists in the hospitals, because the scientists usually are not given direct access to the patients, are on a lower salary scale than the doctors, and frequently pursue their research in the host hospital in "splendid isolation", thus, being spatially integrated but lacking the desired interaction when it comes to research content.

If the German universities were called upon to develop carefully devised interdisciplinary courses of study leading to a doctorate in natural sciences for interested students of medicine, this would create a new basis for clinical research in this country and would probably also have the beneficial side effect of counteracting the currently

falling numbers of students of physics and chemistry.

The graduate-support programs of the German Research Association are certainly a step in the right direction, but in my view do not go far enough. Here a joint initiative needs to come from the Conference of Arts and Education Ministers of the German States.

Much has been said and written about the routine burden on German university hospitals, and also about the significant teaching duties, which together leave very little time for concrete research projects. Even though the structure of the university hospitals is currently being fundamentally changed, such that expenditure for research and teaching is being separated from the funds needed for treating patients, are these measures that are likely to give increased impetus to clinical research?

In one sense they are. The reduction in the number of beds and the shortening of hospital stays can both make more time available for scientific endeavors. But the parallel efforts to reduce staff and save money, the lower number of patients available, and the decreased opportunity to carry out careful long-term controls are all likely to have the opposite effect.

Training, on the one hand, and time and opportunity for research, on the other, can be identified as important factors underlying the problems in clinical research. But beyond these, what are the prospects for the scientifically oriented physician?

A considerable number of doctors who work in the university hopitals carry out scientific research with the short-term aim of gaining the qualification "Habili-

tation", prerequisite for a university professorship in Germany; they then look to acquire an externally funded professorship so as to have a good basis for eventually being appointed to a well-paid post as hospital director or head of department, at which point they give up all scientific activities.

All in all this often leads to a thesis for the „Habilitation" which is produced under great pressure of time and without sufficient experience in supervising doctoral students, or more rarely postdoctoral scientists. The competition for suitable thesis topics and for the support of hospital directors is enormous and this occasionally leads to the publication of poorly founded predictions and, in the worst case, even to the fiddling of results.

These, of course, are extreme examples. Many of the senior physicians and externally funded professors who leave their jobs are people who would like to have continued their scientific activities, but are not given any long-term opportunity at the teaching hospitals, remain unsuccessful on the appointments carousel, and are forced by their contracts with the insurance institutions and the state, regional, or municipal hospitals to give up their scientific work.

It is clear that the best people should be selected to head our university hospitals. But in the process, many talents are possibly left by the wayside, talents that are not directly suited for leading our perhaps rather too conventional university hospital structures. These people may see the move into practical medicine as one alternative and the somewhat rougher road of a career abroad as another. When one nowadays visits hospitals, especially research-oriented hospitals, in the USA,

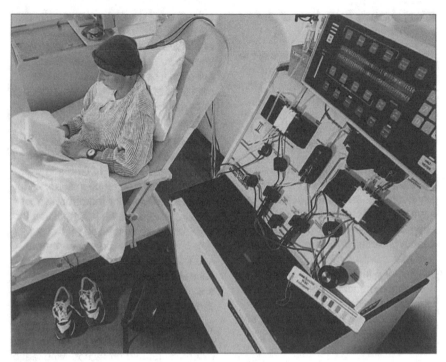

Fig. 2
The new ward of the Clinical Cooperation Unit for Molecular Hematology/Oncology in the medical clinic and polyclinic was established in 1996 so that researchers and physicians could cooperate closely at the patient's bedside to rapidly introduce the latest research developments into practice

in England, or in Canada, why is it that one encounters so many German doctors among the senior physicians and even among the hospital directors?

I am convinced that this is a reflection of another, particularly important, structural problem: the comparatively poor opportunities for clinicians to do research at non-university hospitals.

Even in today's economic climate with its lack of positions, talented academics in the areas of natural science and technology can still hope to find suitable employment at a number of research facilities besides the univer-

sities: the Max Planck Institutes, the National Research Centers of the Helmholtz Association, the research institutes of the Fraunhofer Society or the Science Association "Blaue Liste" (WBL), the departmental research of the Federal Government, industrial research, and a number of institutes of the individual states.

This is not the case for the clinically oriented medical doctors, much as they may be envied by some natural scientists. They can of course seek employment in a research position at a number of the above-mentioned institutes, but

for the clinical research which is their main concern there are very few opportunities outside the universities: the Max Planck Society only pursues clinical research as a somewhat peripheral activity; the Max Delbrück Center in Berlin and the Deutsches Krebsforschungszentrum engage in a certain amount of clinical research; a few institutes of the WBL, e.g., in Magdeburg, Hamburg, and Düsseldorf, make some significant efforts in this direction; and beyond these, there are just a handful of further institutions (e.g., in Freiburg, Mannheim, and Berlin) that are financed from other sources.

The shortcoming here is easy to define: in Germany there is no form of organization in the non-university clinical sector which represents the cause of clinical research. I believe that the creation of an umbrella organization for clinical research, in the sense of a "Medical Research Council", with particularly stringent quality criteria, would be a structural change that would give our clinical research decisive, new momentum in the long term. But this must not be a measure that works to the disadvantage of university research – it must supplement, support, and stimulate the latter. It must provide the additional scope, lacking due to the restricted number of positions at our universities, to give talented young people the opportunity to develop their potential in clinical research as well.

I am convinced that such a structural measure – provided it receives the necessary political support – can be realized with little or no immediate additional costs: an "Association for Clinical-Biomedical Research" (Verbund Klinisch-Biomedizinische Forschung, KBF) has already been founded and this could

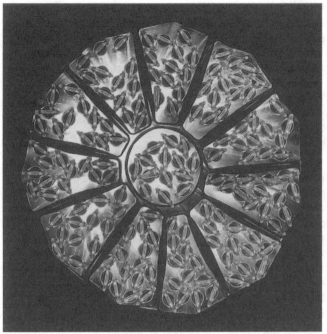

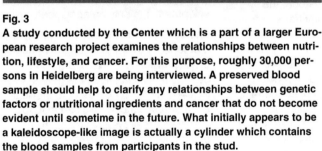

Fig. 3
A study conducted by the Center which is a part of a larger European research project examines the relationships between nutrition, lifestyle, and cancer. For this purpose, roughly 30,000 persons in Heidelberg are being interviewed. A preserved blood sample should help to clarify any relationships between genetic factors or nutritional ingredients and cancer that do not become evident until sometime in the future. What initially appears to be a kaleidoscope-like image is actually a cylinder which contains the blood samples from participants in the stud.

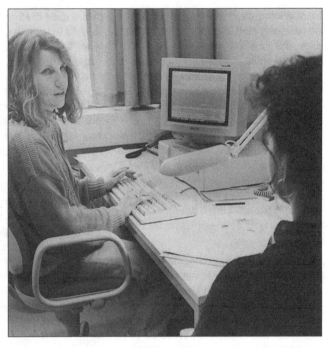

Fig. 4
Persons who have completed a questionnaire about their eating habits will subsequently be interviewed concerning their lifestyles. The responses are immediately entered into the computer. Afterwards, as a token of appreciation, the study participants receive an analysis of the composition of their daily nutritional intake with recommendations for any necessary changes in their eating habits

surely serve as the seed for the development projected here.

A minimal solution, so to speak, would be the creation of interactive structures between clinical university and non-university research. But anyone who has been practically involved in such schemes knows the amount of difficulties they entail.

The Deutsches Krebsforschungszentrum, for example, jointly with the University Hospitals of Heidelberg/Mannheim has created clinical cooperation units, of which the fifth comes into being in 1997. These are temporary research units, which operate like a department of a National Research Center under the leadership of an appointed clinician within the university hospitals. Three of these units are equipped with their own beds. They are simultaneously provided with well-equipped laboratories in research centers. A cooperation agreement regulates the funding of the units. These units are structures that are integrated into the normal running of the hospital; without question, they suffered from a number of teething problems and necessitated a considerable learning process for both parties in the agreement.

The difficulties encountered in the initial phase included the status of the head of the unit in relation to the clinic director, the integration of the specially funded research staff into the clinical activities – for example, night shifts and weekend shifts -, also the recognition of the work done in such units for the specialist medical qualifications, as well as many other details. The difficulties were compounded by the different mode of funding and by legal problems concerning sideline activities. Nonetheless, with good will on both sides, most of these questions could be solved and negotiations over several years led to the first units being established, the oldest of which has now been operating for three years.

The existing cooperation units are led, if in some cases only temporarily, by young and talented physicians who have also demonstrated their scientific enterprise. As a result, following a good two years in this position, the head of the first unit has now been appointed to a university professorship. This is of course a gratifying and desirable development, even though it clearly hampers the coherent building up of the units. The lability of such structures, which can be additionally burdened by a change in the leadership of the corresponding university hospitals, becomes particularly evident here.

Clinical cooperation units are nonetheless an element that can to some extent compensate for the structural weaknesses of clinical research in Germany – in the same way as the clinical research groups of the Max Planck Society and the German Research Association.

The opposite approach, namely the creation of research opportunities for university clinical groups in the non-university research sector, is also being pursued to an increasing extent and

has shown itself to be thoroughly successful in certain cases. It is my experience that the day-to-day availability of the clinical partner is often a problem here. Experiments that are set up in a spare moment in the evening are not always the best conceived results are not always followed up to the necessary depth and in a few cases are too rapidly and uncritically accepted.

The discussion so far has been restricted to aspects of the interaction between university and non-university structures and has not touched upon the clearly very important interaction between clinical and fundamental research within the universities themselves. This is indeed a matter that is relevant to the founding of new and highly regarded interdisciplinary university centers for clinical research.

Today one hears much about the improvement of technology transfer from research into practice, and also from research into the hospital. Only recently, the Federal Ministry for Education, Science, Research, and Technology has developed a series of structural initiatives: the „Bio-Regio" program has proved to be a great success and has led in many places to intensified cooperation between scientific research facilities and industry and to the creation of new small companies. Special spearhead projects are intended to give additional impetus to these developments, and further support is provided by an aggressive patenting policy and publicity designed to attract venture capital.

What is the present situation regarding the transfer of results from biomedical research into clinical practice? Is this occurring with the necessary efficiency to satisfy the justified concern of the tax-payer and the patient that what

they see as high research expenditure is also accompanied by progress in prevention, diagnostics, and treatment of disease? Here I believe that further efforts are necessary to modify and improve existing structures.

In one channel the transfer is almost too fast: the practical implementation of new diagnostic tools. Monoclonal antibodies, the polymerase chain reaction (PCR), hybridization kits, and enzymatic reactions often find their way into routine diagnostics faster than would be justified by a thorough prior evaluation. The reasons for this are as obvious as they are simple: the introduction of new testing procedures quickly leads to results, is frequently lucrative, and raises the reputation of the clinical laboratory involved. When this leads to an impoved early diagnosis and a shorter and simpler treatment then such a development can only be applauded.

The other side of the coin, however, is a potentially over-hasty judgment about predisposition to disease, e.g., concerning modifications of the genes BRCA-1 and BRCA-2 that are implicated in breast cancer. This can lead to unnecessary preventive measures being taken and to patients being scared by test results whose prognostic significance is insufficiently determined. In isolated instances so-called "modern procedures" are even used to support unscientific and inaccurate statements – as is the case when it is claimed that such procedures enable a general cancer diagnosis to be made from a blood sample.

In contrast, the transfer of methods for disease prevention and therapy frequently occurs in a rather sluggish and lethargic manner. Here, too, the reasons are easy to identify: the introduction of a suitable vaccine for disease prevention requires a prior period of clinical testing in order to prove that it is both effective and harmless, and also conditions for its production that are far above normal laboratory standards. The costs for manufacture and clinical testing are enormous, frequently reaching eight- or nine-figure sums, and have to be carefully calculated and balanced against the expected profit. Here the transfer into practice can only take place via the pharmaceutical industry. The time required is often alarmingly long; a vaccine against certain papillomavirus types, which has good prospects of preventing the occurrence of a high proportion of modifications of the cervix and cervical cancer itself, will probably only be introduced at the beginning of the next century, even though the underlying discoveries were made about 20 years earlier.

A similar situation pertains in the transfer of new therapeutic approaches into clinical use, although here the time schedules are not always as long as for the above-mentioned vaccines. Nonetheless, the manufacturing requirements, quality control, and preclinical and clinical testing still swallow time and money in amounts that state-funded scientific institutes can scarcely afford, such that here too a collaboration with the pharmaceutical industry is essential.

This collaboration has undergone a visible change in the recent past; alongside the previously described government initiatives, the reorganization of many industrial companies with its concomitant reduction in staff and cutting back of research activities has more or less forced industry to intensify its involvement in state-funded research in universities and non-university facilities. At present this is undoubtedly a particularly invigorating element in the transfer of results from clinically oriented fundamental research into clinical practice.

Since the pharmaceutical industry is reliant on patents to protect its products, this collaboration requires a change in the protection of inventions policy of the scientific institutes involved. In particular the universities have often offered their professors the opportunity to patent their ideas and subsequently utilize the patents themselves. But due to the rapidly growing patent fees and legal costs, particularly for international patent applications, and often in the absence of suitable contacts to potential industrial partners, the personal resources of the inventor are very quickly exhausted. In view of the inevitable additional delay in the publication of scientific results that is entailed, these circumstances have led to a widespread lack of interest in patenting.

This also has a lasting influence on the development of clinical research and can only be corrected by a change in the patenting policy of the institutes concerned. It is in my view absolutely essential not only that technology-transfer positions be created in the universities, but also that the universities take advantage of patents themselves, thereby also accepting the risk of the patent registration and later giving the inventor an appropriate share in any profits. A possible model would be that employed by the Max Planck Society and other non-university institutes, whereby the institute, the department, and the inventor each receive one-third of the earnings from a patent.

In the past, the main need for action was perceived as being a need to change our clinical structures. Although this is still the case, there are other matters now of even greater urgency: to change our system of higher education, to expand the spectrum of clinically oriented research opportunities, and to achieve significant changes in patenting policy and in the transfer of results, in particular from the universities, into clinical and industrial practice. I believe that this medium- to long-term aim urgently requires the support of individuals who are aware of the present deficits – people from the teaching, research, and hospital professions, and from legislative and executive sectors. However, this must not distract us from that fact that, particularly in relation to fighting cancer, other political measures could today already prevent many thousands of cases of premature illness and death.

Our greatest and at the same time most tragic failure must be acknowledged here: it is the failure of our efforts to check the consumption of tobacco in our country. About 70 000 people die each year in Germany from cancers caused by tobacco smoke. The World Health Organization estimates the total number of deaths in Germany due to tobacco smoking, including those from diseases of the heart and respiratory tract, at 112 000 per year. This is 0.14 percent of the German population! One really has to stop and think about these numbers in order to comprehend the extent of the tragedy. The British epidemiologist Richard Peto has calculated that, on average, each of these people loses more than eight years of life.

That Germany is one of the few European countries holding out against a European ban on tobacco advertising can surely only be understood in the

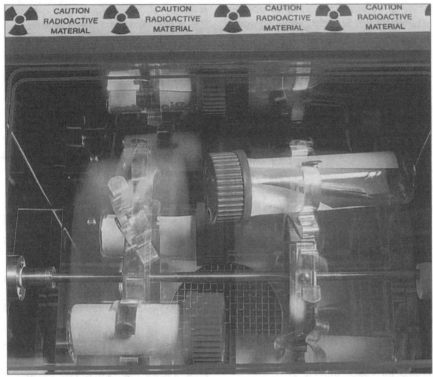

lack effective political and communication strategies for avoiding the most important known cancer risk factor.

Prof. Dr. Dr. h.c.mult. Harald zur Hausen
Chairman and Scientific Member
of the Management Board of the
Deutsches Krebsforschungszentrum

Fig. 5
In the future, an important new research area of the Center will be cancer prevention. Among other objectives, specific goals will include the identification of substances in food that both promote and provide protection against cancer, as well as the treatment of cancer precursors so that these will not develop into a tumor. Following chemopreventive treatment, this particular arrangement of equipment can, for example, detect the activity of genes that indicate the effectiveness of the administered therapy (hybridization experiments)

light of the bizarre fact that the annual tax revenue from the tobacco industry reaches the fantastic sum of DM 20 billion in this country. Thus each tobacco-related death corresponds to earnings of DM 180 000 per year – a calculation which we should emphasize to those holding the political responsibility. This sum should also be held up against the burdens due to tobacco-related diseases, which must be carried by the health insurances, other welfare facilities, the families, and the victims themselves.

Fundamental cancer research in Germany is undoubtedly flourishing, even though weaknesses can still be identified. In order to strengthen clinical cancer research, changes in the research environment are necessary and must be initiated in the next few years. In the area of prevention, progress has only been made in some sectors – we still

Conditions and Structures in Research

by Josef Puchta

Over the past few years, the Deutsches Krebsforschungszentrum has continuously strengthened its international reputation as a center of competence in the field of cancer research. This is evidenced by the increase in the number of publications, the vast majority of which appear in high-ranking journals, and by the high citation index of these

publications. Furthermore, a number of prizes have been awarded to scientists from the Deutsches Krebsforschungszentrum, including the Leibniz Prize of the German Research Association (DFG), the Karl Heinz Beckurts Prize for Technology Transfer, and the Behring-Kitasato Prize. Moreover, in the years since 1990, more than 25 young

Fig. 6
The above graph relates the number of journal articles published by scientists at the Center; the graph below indicates the number of citations in scientific journals (from: Institutional Citation Report of the Deutsches Krebsforschungszentrum, Heidelberg 1996)

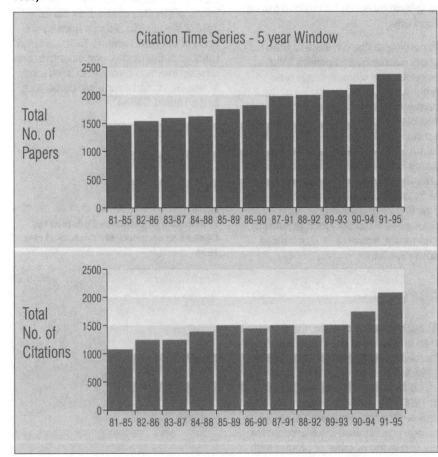

scientists from the Deutsches Krebsforschungszentrum have been appointed to professorships at other research institutes.

Since the early 1990s, for the first time in this century, a decline in cancer mortality has been registered in Germany. The new edition of the *Atlas of Cancer Mortality in the Federal Republic of Germany* (published in fall 1997) gives more detailed information about this remarkable trend. Although one can hardly credit individual research facilities with such achievements, this decline clearly serves to demonstrate how long-term research can lead to the desired end.

According to opinion leaders from science, economy, and politics alike, biosciences and biotechnology rank among the key technologies of the 21st century. Here, experts predict the creation of high-profile jobs in science and economy and see an investment in the future. One would expect that this combination of scientific achievements, decrease in cancer mortality, and key technological position would mean the dawning of „a golden age" for the Deutsches Krebsforschungszentrum. The reality, however, is much more down-to-earth.

Staff Situation

At the beginning of 1998, the number of staff employed at the Deutsches Krebsforschungszentrum was equivalent to 1385 full-time positions. There are 727.5 regular positions – 34.5 less than in 1995. The Federal Ministry for Education, Science, Research, and Technology has dictated a 1.5 percent reduction in the number of regular staff at

all research facilities belonging to the Hermann von Helmholtz Association of National Research Centers (HGF). For the Deutsches Krebsforschungszentrum this means a loss of about 60 such positions between the years of 1995 and 1999, equivalent to more than 8 percent of the existing number. In addition, due to the significant cuts in staff funding from the University Special Program for the Deutsches Krebsforschungszentrum, about 50 positions for young scientists can no longer be filled in future. The career prospects for the up-and-coming generation of scientists have been reduced by this development, which also contradicts the concept of bioscience being a leading science of the next century. Today, a large number of the best young scientists are already leaving Germany to seek jobs in non-European countries, particularly in the United States.

Fig. 7
The number of permanent posts at the Center has continuously decreased since 1994

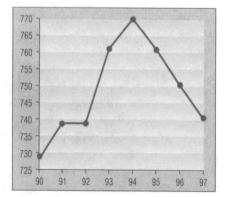

In the past, the Deutsches Krebsforschungszentrum has endeavored to retain as much flexibility as possible in the filling of established posts for scientists, i.e., to have a significant percentage of temporary contracts. Tenured positions are only awarded after many years of proven excellence and a stringent evaluation of the candidate's performance by a „Tenure Commission". The existing legal regulations for temporary employment contracts and the current employment protection legislation certainly do not facilitate a flexible management of staffing plans. Moreover, conflicts with the staff representatives are predestined.

In order to comply with the staff cutbacks foreseen by the Center's sponsors, any posts that become vacant have to be abolished. As a result, the flexibility of the staff plan is being reduced.

The great significance of human resources for a research center is evident and does not need to be discussed here. Despite the expected restrictions, the Deutsches Krebsforschungszentrum will continue its efforts to attract top scientists and to retain the best performers at the Center. In view of the conditions mentioned above, i.e. the reduction in personnel and flexibility, the task of attracting and retaining excellent scientists, and the establishment of new divisions, we are really facing a classical business optimization problem.

Financial Situation

Over the past few years, the Center's budget has suffered a reduction in real terms. Inflationary adjustment and in-

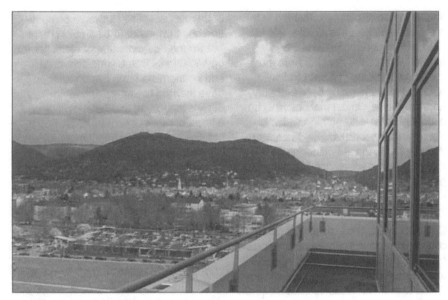

Fig. 8
The view from the eighth floor of the Center, in which all the administrative divisions have been combined, shows Heidelberg and the Neckar river valley

creases in pay rates are no longer allocated to the budget, but instead have to be earned by the Center. To compensate for the budget cuts and to be able to maintain the Center's research program, the Deutsches Krebsforschungszentrum has to intensify its efforts to obtain funding from external sources and expand its cooperations with industry. In 1997, more than 300 research projects with a financial volume of more than DM 34 million were carried out at the Deutsches Krebsforschungszentrum, the main sponsors being the German Research Association (DFG), the European Union, the German Research Ministry, and industry. The amount of external funding received is a result of hard scientific work and high-quality proposals – a remarkable achievement considering the increasing competition for external funding. Equally gratifying

is the significant increase in scientific cooperations with industry – a fact which also manifests itself in the financial volume stemming from such cooperations: in 1997 it reached about DM 5 million.

Apart from these intensive efforts to win independent funding, an increasingly important role in compensating somewhat for the stagnant situation in basic funding is also played by private donations and estates dedicated to cancer research. As part of the Center's growing endeavors to prevent cancer, it has launched the initiative „Unternehmer für Gesundheit" (Enterprises for Health), which aims to bring the concept of prevention into private-sector organizations with the hope that these, in turn, will support the setting up of a new research focus on cancer prevention at

the Deutsches Krebsforschungszentrum.

Patent Situation

Alongside fundamental research, the Deutsches Krebsforschungszentrum also attaches growing importance to the exploitation of research results. In this context, the 1996 patent initiative of the Research Ministry has clearly set the right course. Technology transfer bridges the gap between research and commercial application. Hopefully, the increasing collaboration between science and industry will encourage synergy effects that will help preserve the innovative resources and competitiveness of the German economy and create new jobs. In the light of this argumentation, technology transfer can be seen as a management task and thus represents an important part of the policy of a research center.

In spring 1997, the Center began to reestablish its unit for technology transfer, which reports directly to the Management Board. In the start-up phase, this office endeavors to increase the scientists' awareness of the value of the protection of rights; inform them about the possibilities of, and legal framework for, patent applications; identify at an early stage know-how and inventions that are worthy of protection; and establish the necessary contacts with industrial enterprises. Indeed, the ultimate aim behind patenting special know-how and inventions is their exploitation, normally in the form of a license agreement.

The fact that today it is possible to both publish and patent an idea within a short space of time leaves little room for argument against such an application. This means, patenting does not exclude publishing. A registration can be carried out within just a few days, and thus the proprietary rights are secured – whether or not a patent is later awarded.

Following the Center's decision in 1992 to take advantage of itself, in principle, all inventions of its employees, it has experienced a significant increase in the number of patent registrations. The Center bears all patent application and maintenance costs. In 1997, these amounted to more than 1 million DM. In 1998, the revenues will exceed the costs. For companies working in biotechnology, a field marked by global connections, it is particulary important to have licensed not only a national, but also an international patent. For the Deutsches Krebsforschungszentrum this means that patent application and maintenance costs will probably increase over the next few years.

The Deutsches Krebsforschungszentrum grants inventors a share of 30 percent of the license revenues from an invention. A further 30 percent are assigned to the inventor's division, and the remaining 40 percent to the Center. The decision taken by the Federal Ministry for Education, Science, Research, and Technology in spring 1997 to place 100 percent of the revenues from the economic exploitation of patents at the disposal of the research center (instead of 60 percent as in the past) is a positive and welcome incentive to utilize patents.

I am pleased to be able to report that at the beginning of 1998, the total number of patents awarded or pending at the Deutsches Krebsforschungszentrum amounted to about 200 and that a con-

tinuing increase can be observed in the number of applications. In the field of biosciences, it often takes a long time before the material benefits from the licensing of patents can start to flow back, because in many cases lengthy and expensive clinical trials have to be conducted first – something which is not necessary, for example, in an area such as mechanical engineering. As a rule, several years elapse between the granting of a patent license to a company and the introduction of a corresponding product onto the market.

One obstacle to the licensing of patents continues to be the stipulation in appendix IV of the financial statute of the HGF facilities, according to which it is not permitted to grant an exclusive license (the latter requiring an individual application for permission from the sponsor , i. e., the Research Ministry). In view of the long amortization period of the development and patenting costs, this is a matter that calls for action.

To avoid misinterpretation I should like to stress once again that the Deutsches Krebsforschungszentrum continues to be a facility engaged in application oriented fundamental research. It is not intended to restrict these activities in any way. What we do intend, however, is to facilitate an economic exploitation of the Center's scientific potential.

BioRegio

In fall 1996, the Rhein-Neckar triangle was chosen as one of the three winning regions (out of 17 entries) of a competition organized by the German Research Ministry. The Deutsches Krebsforschungszentrum made a crucial contribution to the entry of the region and has strongly supported the realization

of the concept. The BioRegio competition has turned out to be a strong catalyst for the advancement of biotechnology. Within its framework, scientists and economists have come together, have learned to understand each other's language, and have conceived a large number of joint projects. Federal funding now goes into these projects with the industrial partner bearing up to 60 percent of the overall project costs. Several new companies offering dozens of highly-qualified jobs have already been established and we expect further foundations of new companies from existing organizations, including the Deutsches Krebsforschungszentrum. Alongside providing advice to potential founders of new companies, the Center supports them in every possible way, e.g., by granting leave, making research results available, and permitting external activities.

The BioRegio concept rests on three pillars: a non-profit organization („BioRegion Rhein-Neckar-Dreieck e.V."), a profit organization („Heidelberg Innovation GmbH"), and a seed-capital fund („Seed Capital Rhein -Neckar GmbH & Co. KG"). These three components are meanwhile well established, and the first projects have been granted support. The next few years will tell whether this interaction of science and economy fulfills its promises and whether the perceptible new trend towards the creation of a sound basis for biotechnology in Germany will persist and continue to create new jobs.

Guidelines of the Federal Research Ministry

The guidelines for a strategic reorientation of the existing research structures in Germany issued in summer 1996 by the Research Minister have initiated a discussion which has also influenced the HGF research facilities. The central idea of the Ministry's policy is to encourage increased competition between the research facilities and increased competition also for the funds made available to them. Of a total budget of almost DM 3 billion for the 16 member institutes of the HGF it is planned to gradually withdraw up to DM 150 million from the facilities' budgets and assign them to a strategy fund. The institutes are then given the opportunity to apply for these funds on a competitive basis by submitting project applications. For the Deutsches Krebsforschungszentrum this means that funds of several million are not initially assigned to the budget, but have to be applied for on a competitive basis. The additional burden that the application procedures entail is evident. Whether the new strategy fund will really promote a shift of focus towards the key technologies of the 21st century remains to be seen. However, one critical remark seems appropriate here: the promise of linking the strategy fund – i. e., the withdrawal of budget funds – with the granting of more flexibility in budget matters has yet to be fulfilled. The tools for achieving more flexibility in the management of budgets as provided by the Research Ministry fail to meet the expectations of the research institutes. Essential demands, e.g., for global budgets, abolition of fixed staffing plans, and the possibility of transferring funds into the next fiscal year, have not been met sufficiently. These measures, however, will become essential in order to be able to cope with the above-mentioned budget and personnel restrictions expected in the coming

years. Here we must intensify our endeavors to convince the politicians that these are necessary instruments for flexibility.

The main demands for the coming years will be to further improve the administrative and scientific framework and structure of the Deutsches Krebsforschungszentrum:

– Analogous to private-sector organizations, the freedom of action concerning policy decisions of research facilities should be significantly expanded. The control of these facilities should lie in the hands of the boards (board of directors, board of trustees), instead of being subject to the restrictive interpretation of various regulations.

– Within global budgets the research institutes should be given the opportunity to decide for themselves how to use their budget funds.

– The basic structure of the salary levels for employees of the federal government (BAT) is not really suitable for a research facility. Attention should be given to the development of a specific salary agreement for research.

– Procedures for the appointment of professors working jointly at research centers and universities take too long. Vacancy periods of up to 2 years – frequently needed for the appointment negotiations to be concluded – should be dramatically reduced to an appropriate period of a few months.

– A temporary employment, in particular of young scientists, for more than 5 years should be made possible. In many cases this would facilitate a sensible conclusion of research work

and enable a further qualification (such as a „Habilitation") to be gained and it would also make it easier for the scientists to move into the private sector or found a company of their own.

Over the next few years, the Deutsches Krebsforschungszentrum will have to walk a fine line between maintaining and further raising its high level of scientific performance on the one hand and coping with a difficult administrative environment on the other. Furthermore, the Deutsches Krebsforschungszentrum will have to answer the question of whether the positive developments becoming apparent in the prevention and therapy of cancer will have the predicted effects and thus be of benefit to mankind.

Dr. Josef Puchta
Administrative Member
of the Management Board of the
Deutsches Krebsforschungszentrum

Mission and Structure of the Deutsches Krebsforschungszentrum

The Deutsches Krebsforschungszentrum (DKFZ) was founded in 1964 on the initiative of the Heidelberg surgeon Prof. Dr. Dr. h.c. K. H. Bauer, who died in 1978 at the age of 86. By decision of the government of the State of Baden-Württemberg, it was set up as a foundation of public law. Since 1975, it has been one of Germany's Major Research Centers. It is financed to 90% by the Federal Government (Federal Ministry for Education, Science, Research, and Technology) and to 10% by the State of Baden-Württemberg (Ministry for Science, Research, and Art) on the basis of § 91b of the German Constitution.

According to its statutes, it is the task of the Center to „pursue cancer research". In view of this very general formulation, it is evident that the question of whether all the research projects pursued at the Krebsforschungszentrum actually entail „cancer research" - a term defined differently by every discipline - will have to be posed again and again. This means that in a center with a multidisciplinary structure, the discussion about the research content never ceases and the „balance of forces" has to be continually sought anew. This process is sustained by new discoveries, the significance and weighting of which has to be determined against the background of the Center's statutory mission. It involves considering the interests of scientists who approach the problem of cancer from different methodological angles and assigning them different priorities in the competition for financial resources. On the other hand, the potential benefits to be gained by the scientists in solving their research problems from the discussion and collaboration with a large number of experts from all fields relevant to cancer research gathered together in one research institution are enormous and cannot be provided by any other form of organization.

Since 1991, the Deutsches Krebsforschungszentrum has been operating with a new organizational structure. The former institutes have been replaced by subject-oriented Research Programs (Forschungsschwerpunkte), which are represented by coordinators and as a rule are limited to a working life of six years. This period can be extended depending on the results achieved. Alongside the existing permanent divisions, temporary divisions operating under a time limit of, as a rule, five years have also been established. This concept is designed to give young scientists between the ages of 30 and 35 the opportunity, at an early age, to take on responsibility for running an independent research unit. This makes it possible to better respond to the rapid developments in cancer research. If a division's line of research becomes an essential part of the respective Research Program, the divisional head can be appointed on a permanent basis.

The flexible structure of the Deutsches Krebsforschungszentrum also fosters the exchange of experiences between scientists from a wide range of disciplines. In addition, it facilitates the rapid changeover to new tasks once a working program is considered as fulfilled.

The complex problems of cancer research and the fight against cancer touch upon a large number of disciplines from the biosciences, natural sciences, as well as the social sciences. The only way to tackle them with some prospect of success is a close national and international collaboration of scien-

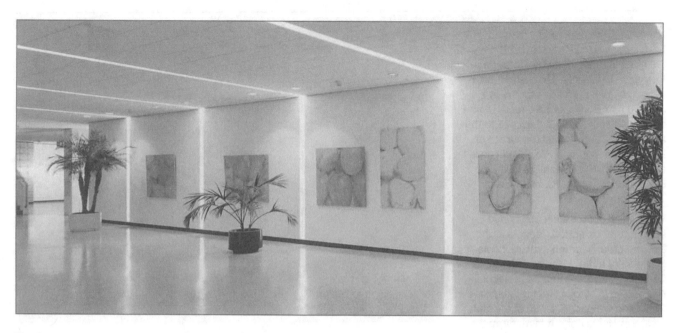

Fig. 9
The newly designed foyer with works by Brigitte Bergamotte

tists from all these disciplines and a concentration of existing research capacities.

The scientific mission of the Deutsches Krebsforschungszentrum is to make substantial contributions to the understanding of carcinogenesis, the identification of cancer risk facts, and also the prevention, diagnosis, and therapy of cancer.

The sheer number of different types of cancer that can affect man gives a clue to the complexity of the problems faced in scientific analysis.

The Center's research endeavors since 1994 have been pursued within eight multidisciplinary Research Programs:

1. Cell Differentiation and Carcinogenesis
2. Tumor Cell Regulation
3. Cancer Risk Factors and Prevention
4. Diagnostics and Experimental Therapy
5. Radiological Diagnostics and Therapy
6. Applied Tumor Virology
7. Tumor Immunology
8. Bioinformatics

In 1996, the Research Program „Bioinformatics" was extended to include aspects of genome research and was consequently renamed „Genome Research and Bioinformatics".

In the future, the identification of genes showing modifications or functional defects that lead to a dysregulation of cell growth will play a special role in the Center's research. The thematically oriented research program reflects a general shift towards molecular-biological approaches in cancer research and indicates a new focus on the analysis of human tumors. In 1996, a resource center of the German Genome Project was set up in Heidelberg and Berlin simultaneously; the Heidelberg project is led by Dr. Annemarie Poustka, head of the Division of Molecular Genome Analysis of the Deutsches Krebsforschungszentrum, the Berlin project by Prof. Dr. Hans Lehrach from the Max Planck Institute for Molecular Genetics. The Heidelberg group is responsible for the creation and quality control of gene libraries, i.e., a comprehensive collection of genes conserved on special filters. They are made available to working groups, which can use them to search for specific genes. In addition, scientists from research institutes and industry are offered the opportunity to send DNA samples to Heidelberg and have the gene libraries searched for a gene they seek to identify. Thanks to the existence of joint resource centers in Heidelberg and Berlin, smaller research laboratories now also have access to the material and technology resources of the German Genome Project, which is supported by the Federal Ministry for Education, Science, Research, and Technology.

The clinical cooperation units have been further extended. Alongside the existing groups for Molecular Oncology/Pediatry at the University Pediatric Clinic in Heidelberg and for Molecular Hematology/Oncology at the Medical Clinic and Outpatient Clinic of the University of Heidelberg, a third, dermatological-oncological research unit in cooperation with Mannheim Hospitals has been established and a head of research appointed. The clinical research groups are established at the clinics for a period of five years each. In this concept, the Deutsches Krebsforschungszentrum provides the medical treatment, while the clinics provide the hospital beds and the clinical infrastructure. The Krebsforschungszentrum bears any costs that are not covered by the patients' health insurances. The aim of the clinical cooperation units is to facilitate a swift transfer of results from basic research into clinical practice. In 1996, the ward of the clinical cooperation unit „Molecular Hematology/Oncology" was inaugurated following a complete overhaul of the premises. This is the Center's first ward and it is equipped with eight beds for cancer patients.

Research

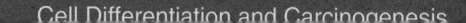
Cell Differentiation and Carcinogenesis

2

Cell Differentiation and Carcinogenesis

The confrontation of scientists in basic research with the problem of cancer has yielded a multitude of new findings and new approaches in theory and experimental research in recent years. While the selction of promising research approaches in the past tended to be somewhat fortuitous and accidental, i.e., was based on isolated observations of differences between normal and malignant cells, in recent years it has also become possible to investigate the origin, diagnosis as well as possible prevention and therapy of cancer diseases with well-defined aims, following basic principles of cell and molecular biology.

Changes in the gneome or in the expression of specific genes in somatic cells are in many cases reponsible for the early events of carcinogenesis, leading to fundamental disturbances in the social and growth behavior of cells. In functional terms, two different principles of tumorigenesis can be distinguished: 1) enhanced activity of oncogenes may lead to uncontrolled growth; 2) the failure of genes suppressing cell transformation, the tumor suppressor genes, may have the same effect. The research program Cell Differentiation and Carcinogenesis therefore directs special attention at finding and analyzing those genes and their products that might play a role in carcinogenesis. Cell biological and molecular biological methods are used to find genetic probes for specific chromosome changes, for gene mutations or for integrated viral genes which may be applied in tumor diagnostics as well as possibly in the prevention of cancer, such as the identification of patients at risk.

Another line research is directed at the examination of disturbances in gene expression and in the synthesis of certain gene products. Differences in gene expression between normal and transformed cells, between resting and proliferating cells, and between cells in various states of differentiation are detected using appropriate nucleic acid probes or monoclonal antibodies against specific gene products. "Cell typing" by the microscopic identification of marker molecules characteristic for the specific state of differentiation contributes to the correct diagnosis of tumors, and in many cases allows the detection of primary and metastatic tumors as well as the identification of the initial tumor from which a metastasis has spread. In addition, the research program examines the biological function of the proteins and hormones involved in the regulation of gene expression and the growth and metastatic spread of certain kinds of cancer.

Embryonic development of an organism including the controls of cell division and tissue formation provides the master plan for the normal and healthy correlations of cell proliferation and differentiation. An understanding of these elementary life process will therefore point the way for future experimental cancer research. Consequently, the division Molecular Embryology has recently been established in the research program to study fundamental processes in embryonic development.

Coordinator of the Research Program:
Prof. Dr. Werner W. Franke

Divisions and their heads:

Cell Biology:
Prof. Dr. Werner W. Franke

Molecular Biology of the Cell I:
Prof. Dr. Günther Schütz

Molecular Biology of the Cell II:
Prof. Dr. Ingrid Grummt

Development Genetics:
Prof. Dr. Bernard Mechler

Molecular Embryology:
Dr. Christof Niehrs

2.1 The Cytoskeleton: A Complex System of Dynamic Structural Elements

by Harald Herrmann-Lerdon

The Structure of the Cytoplasm

Single-cell animals, such as those in the subclass Radiolaria, can assume extremely complicated shapes by using their internal mineral skeletons. Other unicellular organisms lend shape to their cell by means of a hard shell. In contrast, amoebas appear to be missing any sort of framework. Their shape constantly changes. Nonetheless, they do not completely dissipate and can in individual cases become very large. Investigations employing the electron microscope have shown that a complex network of fibrillar and filament-forming proteins are responsible for this change in form. Research in cell and molecular biology during the past 20 years has shown that this network or cytoskeleton principally consists of the same molecules in all eukaryotic cells, the cells of higher organisms.

The Filamentous Components of the Cytoskeleton

The cytoskeleton mainly consists of three, different, independent filament systems: 1) microfilaments with a diameter of 7 nanometers (nm), 2) microtubules, tube-shaped filaments with a 25 nm external diameter, and 3) intermediate filaments that were so named, because their diameter at 10 nm lies between that of the microfilaments and microtubules. Every eukaryotic cell contains microfilaments and microtubules; both are essential for life, even for simple organisms such as yeast. In contrast, intermediate filaments have until now only been found in animal organisms, not in plants, protozoans or simple multicellular organisms.

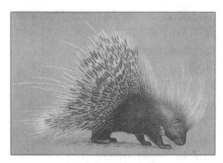

Fig. 10
The long quills of porcupines are an unusual creation of nature. They mainly consist of pseudo-crystalline, intermediate filament bundles that are interconnected and arranged in parallel. In the 1930s, research into the structure of proteins with x-rays began with their examination

In 1938 Wladimir Engelhardt clearly characterized the first cytoskeleton protein, myosin, and its function. It is a muscle protein and was designated the "contractile enzyme" by Dorothy Needham in 1972. An entire generation of biochemists was very surprised to discover that the searched for "motor protein" was not found in the "cellular fluid", but had instead always been thrown away in the form of insoluble structures that composed the centrifugation precipitate.

Muscular motion is caused by the myosin filaments "gliding along" the microfilaments that are made of actin. This "mechano-enzyme system" that was originally assumed to be limited to the muscles has during the past several years been detected in almost every cell. It is seen with increasing clarity that almost every cellular movement and all intracellular transport processes depend on filaments. Even cellular motion that employs flagella and cilia, the transport of vesicles or the distribution of chromosomes to the daughter cells during cell division is based on the interaction between ATP (adenosine triphosphate) splitting motor proteins and filaments. It is easy to imagine that such a state of complex mobility (external movement accompanied by simultaneously occurring diverse internal transport processes) can very rapidly degenerate into a state of complete chaos. Where are "points of stability" to be found?

Structure of the Intermediate Filament Proteins

The histochemical analysis of many cell types in the 1970s, especially in humans, yielded the finding that the tissues of the more developed vertebrates contain a third filament system. These so-called intermediate filaments are present in addition to the microfilaments and the microtubules in almost every cell. The intermediate filaments do not form any polar structures and cannot, therefore, be used by motor proteins for directed movements. Using immunological methods, one recognized that intermediate filaments are extremely heterogeneous in their composition although they cannot be externally distinguished from one another, not even with the electron microscope. A human being possesses approximately 50 different intermediate filament proteins; these are comparable in their composition and similar in biological structure. However, their primary sequence, the genetically determined order of the amino acids in the different intermediate filament proteins, varies greatly. Scientists conclude from this that filaments formed from such pro-

teins can possess very different properties and can, therefore, usually not form any mixed complexes. This is also the reason why two different intermediate filament systems may exist independently of one another in a single cell.

All kinds of different proteins belong to the family of intermediate filament proteins: lamins are transported into the cell nucleus where they stabilize the nuclear membrane and the nuclear pores; neurofilament proteins fill out the long axonal processes in nerve cells; vimentin is found in connective tissue cells and the lens of the eye; and the cytokeratins (CK) that pervade the cytoplasm of internal epithelial cells and covering tissues, ranging from the external nuclear envelope to the plasma membrane; they are the main protein in the epidermis. Along with interconnecting proteins, the cytokeratins, after the cells that produce them have died, form scales, hair, feathers and nails. The long quills of the porcupine are an unusual creation of nature that consist of interconnected, quasi-crystalline, intermediate filament bundles arranged in parallel order.

Such a diversity of proteins may confuse non-specialists and may appear insignificant to them. However, for histologists and pathologists this has proven to be extremely useful since malignant cells usually retain "their" intermediate filament protein. Because of this, it is possible to determine the histogenetic origin of a tumor by immunologically ascertaining the type of intermediate filament protein. Thanks to their intermediate filament protein profile, very small tumors and micrometastases can also be quickly identified. This procedure has in the meantime become a main technique in tumor diagnosis.

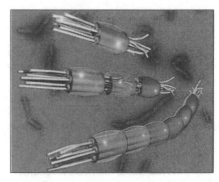

Fig. 11
The computer model depicts how the long "filaments" of the intermediate filaments are formed. Initially, standardized and uniform minifilaments (above) are created. These subsequently combine, one after another, to form long cords as shown in the center and below

At the Deutsches Krebsforschungszentrum more than 50 different monoclonal antibodies have been produced that are routinely used throughout the world to diagnose tumors according to the expression catalog for cytokeratins compiled by Roland Moll and Werner W. Franke in the Division of Cell Biology. Detailed knowledge of the protein recognized by the antibody with respect to its biochemical properties as well as its tissue-specific expression is a necessary prerequisite for using the cytokeratins in diagnostic procedures. This means that closely related intermediate filaments must also be distinguished from one another. Often this proves difficult since several of the identified cytokeratins were originally viewed by many scientists as being degradation products of a frequently occurring cytokeratin of the skin. In our laboratory, Christine Collin was, for example, able to demonstrate that CK2e and CK2p are indeed distinct cytokeratins. The late "cloning" of the gene for cytokeratin 20 was surprising since this occurred at a time at which one generally thought that all the human cytokeratins were known. This cytokeratin is only synthesized in very few cell types, but is invaluable in tumor diagnostics. In combination with antibodies directed against other cytokeratins, antibodies specific for CK20 are employed in the differential diagnosis of adenocarcinomas.

Significant progress resulted from realizing that intermediate filament proteins release relatively stable fragments (the (-helix coiled coils) during the decomposition of tumor cells. These fragments are in turn easily detectable with immunological methods even when present only in very small quantities. In the early stages of certain types of lung tumors, fragments from cytokeratin 19 (CK19; cloned by Bernhard Bader in our laboratory) can be detected in the blood. In this case, an early detection of cancer is possible by simply drawing blood and employing serodiagnosis. This "CYFRA21-1 test" is in the meantime being used worldwide to detect non-small cell lung tumors.

Function of the Intermediate Filament Proteins

What are the advantages for a multicellular organism consisting of organs and tissues in synthesizing such a large number of different proteins and regulating them in such a complex diversity that is specific for each cell type? Why is this necessary? In the end, only a single system of apparently similar filaments is maintained in the cells. What happens when the synthesis of these

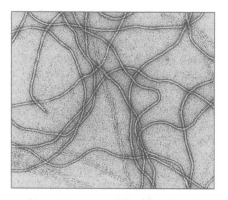

Fig. 12
Bacterial vimentin, the "standard representative" of the intermediate filaments, combines to form long protein filaments (image taken with an electron microscope; 160,000 x enlargement)

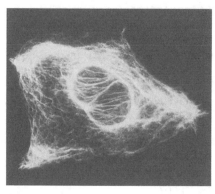

Fig. 13
The network of intermediate filaments composed of vimentin in a human cell made visible by antibodies

filaments is disturbed or the proteins contain genetically caused "errors"?

The organizational structures in the cells find their counterpart in the form of a complex structure outside of the cells that is not lacking in diversity when compared to the internal structures. This so-called extracellular matrix that is located near the cells is, for example, mainly excreted by fibroblasts in epithelial tissues. In a "self-associating" process, they form a system of insoluble fibrils that consist of several filaments. Transmembrane proteins, of the integrin type among others, bind the extracellular matrix to the internal cytoskeleton by means of specific protein complexes. Other transmembrane proteins, the cadherins, assume the task of coupling the cytoskeletons between individual cells. In this manner, a transcellular cytoskeleton pervades the entire tissue. Cytoskeleton and matrix proteins have a unique quality that distin-

guishes them from many other cell proteins: they already form gels in relatively small quantities. While many globular proteins hardly "thicken" a solution even in high concentrations, fibrillar proteins such as the intermediate filaments make solutions highly viscous when they are present in only one part per thousand.

Biophysical examinations of the three filament systems have shown that they are fundamentally different in one parameter, namely in their viscoelasticity. For example, under torsional stress the ability of the intermediate filaments to react elastically increases.

A redistribution of the molecules in the filament is probably responsible for this. In contrast, microfilaments and microtubules break under such conditions. This means that intermediate filaments elastically "buffer" shear forces in an ideal manner. Among the intermediate filament proteins there are relatively large differences with respect to their viscoelastic properties that are additionally influenced by the proteins, with which they are associated. Therefore, the specific "cellular elasticity" depends on the types of intermediate filaments that are present in the cell.

These findings from experiments conducted on tissue cultures readily led to the assumption that intermediate filaments may also have something to do with stabilizing cells against tensile stress in the living organism. Clarifying the cause of a certain genetically-based skin disease (epidermolysis bullosa simplex) has confirmed this in an impressive manner. In patients so affected the basal cell layer of the epidermis breaks away upon the slightest pressure, thereby, forming blisters. These patients are missing an extensive intermediate filament system in the basal cell layer. Intermediate filaments are instead found in aggregates near the cell nucleus. The cause of this clumping is a mutation that leads to the exchange of an amino acid at a certain location in cytokeratin 5 or 14. How can such an apparently slight change have such drastic effects? Similar to the dynamic filament systems of the microfilaments and microtubules the actual elements of the cytoskeleton, the intermediate filaments, are not static, rigid cell components. They form extremely rapidly from their soluble components through fusion of short "standard filaments". Already slight variations in the molecule can lead to the formation of flat or clump-like aggregates instead of the desired filaments.

From this the question arises: what are the possible consequences of such malformations in a filament system for

the cells and the tissue in a living organism? Important answers came from "transgenic" animals, named so because they are made to express an experimentally introduced foreign gene. In the nerve cells of the mouse, human neurofilament proteins lead to the aggregation of neurofilaments in the cell body and a decrease in their numbers within the axon, the "process" of the nerve cell. Thereafter, the nerve cells die. In contrast, the additional, quantitatively comparable synthesis of appropriate mouse neurofilaments is tolerated by the mouse nerve cells without any recognizable problems. Since the two proteins from man and mouse are very similar, it follows that even very slight differences may bring about the completely opposite behavior of the respective proteins in the nerve cells. The appearance of "incorrectly" folded proteins may result in soluble proteins that are important for cell functions being captured in such aggregates. Thereby, the feedback loops in the cell can be affected.

"Improper" environment for a protein may mean that it is transported into a completely different cell compartment than is usually the case. As in the case of synthesizing frog vimentin in mammalian tissue cultures, such errors in topogenesis ("location") may not have any serious consequences. This protein is deposited in band-shaped aggregates in the cytoplasm. However, a slightly altered version of this protein is transported into the cell nucleus and, after lowering the temperature from 37 °C to 28 °C (because of the temperature sensitivity of amphibian proteins), forms extensive intermediate filament bundles in this location. In contrast, the synthesis of an epidermal cytokeratin in

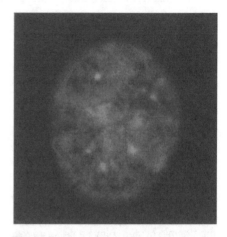

Fig. 14
Vimentin – artificially introduced into a cell nucleus – glows red. Using this method, it was possible for the first time to visualize the spaces in the cell nucleus into which the vimentin had spread

the pancreatic islet cells of a transgenic mouse proved to be fatal. In this case, solely the synthesis in the "wrong" cell meant that a cytoplasmatic protein typical in the skin was transported into the cell nucleus. Within a few weeks after birth, the mice developed a severe case of diabetes since the islet cells died. Under certain conditions, ectopic synthesis (occurring "at the wrong location") may have more serious consequences than the complete absence of an intermediate filament protein.

This latter finding was made by using gene "knockout" experiments. By employing techniques from genetic engineering a certain gene in the germ plasma of a mouse can specifically be switched off. As a consequence of this, the corresponding protein is no longer synthesized in this „knockout" mouse. For example, the inactivation of vimentin apparently had no visible effect on the embryonic development of this mouse. This proved to be puzzling, because scientists had previously assumed that this protein plays a central role in the mesoderm development of the mouse. In contrast, the inactivation of the gene responsible for the sister molecule of vimentin, called desmin, that is exclusively synthesized in the muscle resulted in severe damage to the heart muscle. Contractions of the heart could only be inadequately (elastically/mechanically) absorbed. Thus, the desmin system plays a decisive role in the mechanical stability of this organ.

The original assumption that intermediate filament proteins are found with pronounced complexity only in higher vertebrates can no longer be defended. Even a small roundworm such as *Caenorhabditis elegans,* one of the model organisms used in cell differentiation studies, contains a multitude of intermediate filament proteins that partially possess a high degree of sequence similarity to the corresponding mammalian proteins. One can assume that research using this "model" will, in the future, also deliver interesting information concerning the function of intermediate filaments in human beings.

Integration of the Filaments in the Cytoskeleton

In the approximately 200 different types of cells found in human beings, the three filament systems are always found together with a multitude of associated proteins that are usually also synthesized in a tissue-specific manner. For example, this includes the proteins of the desmoplakin family, elongated æ-helical proteins, that form molecular

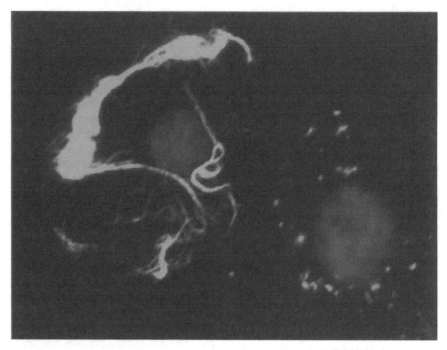

Fig. 15
Colcemid, a substance related to colchicine from the meadow saffron, destroys the arrangement of the vimentin filaments, components of the cellular skeleton. The genetic material in the cell nuclei is colored red; the "clumped" vimentin filaments are green. The image is produced with a laser scanning microscope using an immunofluorescence technique

chains and can bridge larger distances in the cell. Desmoplakins may partially be extracted with nonionic detergents and, therefore, do not strictly fulfill the criteria of a cytoskeleton protein. However, since these molecules coordinate the filament systems and are a part of the cytomatrix, this shows that the concept "cytoskeleton" is an operational term that merely describes the stability of several cytoplasmic components in the cell with respect to certain extraction methods. It does not describe the functional, dynamic entity of the interacting systems. One of these molecules is plectin. This giant protein consists of approximately 5,000 amino acids and, depending on cell type, is capable of binding intermediate filaments with microtubules, microfilaments or with fodrin (a fibrillar protein of the plasma membrane skeleton). Cell poisons such as colchicine that dissolve microtubules and bring about a drastic reorganization of the vimentin intermediate filament system mainly leave the plectin network undisturbed. However, a certain portion of the plectin become displaced by the intermediate filaments. From this, it follows that different posttranslationally modified plectins are functionally present in a cell.

Another protein from the desmoplakin family, BPAG1n, connects neurofilaments with microfilaments in nerve cells and is an additional cross-linking protein for the cellular filament systems. Desmoplakin, which lends its name to this family of proteins, is almost exclusively found on the interior side of the cell at desmosomes, special cell-to-cell binding structures. Either alone or with the assistance of additional components and mainly in epithelial cells, but also in the heart muscle, it recruits intermediate filaments onto the cell membrane. In this manner, the cell-to-cell binding complexes join the intermediate filament systems of individual cells in a single epithelium or organ into an elastic support system that pervades the entire tissue. The multitude of these protein/protein interactions is not permanently fixed, but can be regulated in a variety of ways. Only this enables cells to move out of or through organized tissue.

The latter fact is of decisive importance in the formation of tumors and their dissemination throughout the body in the process of metastasis. The mechanisms wich involved in the migration of cells out of an epithelium and which require, among other things, that the desmosomes which bind the cells dissolve are still unexplained. However, scientists were recently able to demonstrate that proteins located in the cell-to-cell binding structures are components of signal chains or are themselves transported into the cell nucleus where they may possibly participate in the control of gene activity. Thereby, it appears feasible to examine the direct influence of the cytoskeletal components on the regulation of gene activity. These studies may in the future permit a focused intervention in the molecular mechanisms that enable cells in primary tumors to break free and form metastases in other tissues.

Priv.-Doz. Dr. Harald Herrmann-Lerdon
Division of Cell Biology

Participating staff

Monika Brettel
Prof. Dr. Werner W. Franke
Christine Grund
Dr. Ilse Hofmann
Cäcilia Kuhn
Dr. Kevin R. Rogers
Dr. Herbert Spring

In collaboration with

Dr. Joanna Bridger
Priv.-Doz. Dr. Peter Lichter
Division of Organization
of Complex Genomes,
Deutsches Krebsforschungszentrum

Prof. Dr. Jörg Langowski
Division of Biophysics
of Macromolecules,
Deutsches Krebsforschungszentrum

Prof. Dr. Ueli Aebi
Biocenter, University of Basel,
Switzerland

Prof. Dr. Jürgen Markl
Institute of Zoology,
University of Mainz

Prof. Dr. Manfred Schliwa
Institute of Cell Biology,
University of Munich

Selected publications

Moll, R.: Cytokeratine als Differenzierungsmarker. Expressionsprofile von Epithelien und epithelialen Tumoren. Gustav Fischer Verlag, Stuttgart, Jena, New York, 1–197 (1993)

Herrmann, H., Eckelt, A., Brettel, M., Grund, C., Franke, W.W.: Temperature-sensitive intermediate filament assembly: Alternative structures of Xenopus laevis vimentin in vitro and in vivo. J. Mol. Biol. 234, 99–113 (1993)

Schmidt, A., Heid, H.W., Schäfer, S., Nuber, U.A., Zimbelmann, R., Franke, W.W.: Cell type-specific desmosomal components and epithelial differentiation. Eur. J. Cell Biol. 65, 229–245 (1994)

Herrmann, H., Häner, M., Brettel, M., Müller, S.A., Goldie, K.N., Fedtke, B., Lustig, A., Franke, W.W., Aebi, U.: Structure and assembly properties of the intermediate filament protein vimentin: the role of its head, rod and tail domains. J. Mol. Biol. 264, 933–953 (1996)

Herrmann, H., Münick, M.D., Brettel, M., Fouquet, B., Markl, J.: Vimentin in a coldwater fish, the rainbow trout: Highly conserv-ed primary structure but unique assembly properties. J. Cell Sci. 109, 569–578 (1996)

Leube, R.E., Kartenbeck, J.: Molekulare Komponenten der Intermediärfilamente und ihrer Verankerungsstrukturen in Epithelzellen: Differenzierungsmarker in der Gewebe- und Tumordiagnostik. In: Onkologie. Hrsg.: Zeller, W.J., zur Hausen, H., Ecomed Verlagsgesellschaft 1995, Supplement II–1, 1–32 (1996)

2.2 Developmental Control Genes – Identification and Function

by Christof Niehrs

The understanding of the molecular basis of cancer requires first of all insight into the mechanism of regulation of growth and differentiation of normal cells. Precisely this is the aim of molecular embryology, which asks which genetic mechanisms regulate the development of the fertilized egg into adult. We now know that there are specific genes that control particular processes during embryogenesis. It turns out that these developmental control genes not only regulate embryonic processes but can also play important roles in cancer. Moreover, developmental control genes have been modified very little during evolution and are used in many different processes. For example, the ras gene regulates eye development in the fruit fly, while it is important for the development of muscle and blood in the frog. Yet, in adult man and mouse a defective ras gene can lead to cancer. Thus, the medical significance of developmental control genes is that they often represent potential cancer – or oncogenes. Due to the importance of these genes one major goal of current molecular embryology is, therefore, to identify new developmental control genes and to study their roles.

The evolutionary conservation of developmental control genes allows one to use lower species as model organisms to study them. Our division of molecular embryology uses the South African clawed frog, Xenopus laevis, a traditional subject for embryologists. These frogs are bred specifically for scientific research. They are particularly well suited for the analysis of early embryonic development, since hundreds of embryos are obtained from a single frog, which develop outside the mother in the pretri dish. Identification of developmental control genes is easier in the frog than in mouse or man and their function can often be tested more directly. Therefore, the frog embryo serves as a model system for man to study developmental control genes.

In contrast to Central European frogs, Xenopus can be induced to lay eggs throughout the year by hormone treatment. The eggs are fertilized in vitro and develop synchronously. Embryogenesis from the fertilized egg to the swimming tadpole takes only two days, and the larvae begin feeding after one week.

Function of Developmental Control Genes

There are many developmental control genes known that function at different stages and in different tissues. These genes encode proteins with diverse biochemical roles. They may be hormones, hormone receptors or direct regulators of gene activity. Often a developmental control gene is only active in a few regions of the embryo. The brachyury gene, for example, regulates the differentiation of mesodermal cells, which give rise to blood, connective tissue, and muscle. Such selective expression is probably an important factor regulating the activity of developmental control genes.

In the frog, the function of a developmental control gene is tested by activating the gene in regions of the embryo which normally do not express it. To do this, the genetic information of the gene which has been isolated by cloning, is translated into so called messenger ribonucleic acid (mRNA) in the test tube. A tiny amount of the gene is incubated

Fig. 16
Stages in the embryogenesis of the South African clawed frog

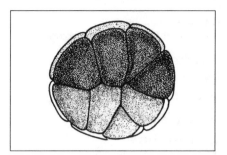
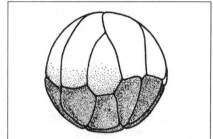
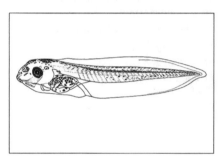
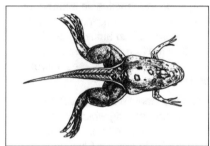

in the presence of a special enzyme together with the four nucleic acid bases that make up mRNA to yield artificial mRNA. This synthetic mRNA can be introduced into the embryo by microinjecting it into a desired region with a fine glass needle. This then leads to the artificial activation of the gene. The developing embryo can subsequently be analyzed for the formation of unusual tissues at the injected site, which would give an important hint towards the function of the gene in regulating cell differentiation.

Dozens of developmental control genes have been indentified in this manner. There are developmental control genes whose micoinjection leads to the formation of siamese twins, which have two heads and trunks. These genes are way up in the hierarchy of embryonic development and serve as main switches, initiating and organizing embryogenesis. The later a gene acts during development the more restricted its regulative properties typically are. While early expressed developmental control genes can induce whole siamese twins, the late genes will only be able to induce for example muscle tissue. Embryogenesis is thus controlled by a series of hierarchically ordered developmental control genes, which serve progressively more specialized functions during development.

Identification of New Developmental Control Genes

Many developmental control genes were discovered in the fruit fly, where mutants were isolated, which show distinct embryonic malformations. The affected genes have been meanwhile cloned and homologs of most of these have been isolated in vertebrate species.

To identify new developmental control genes that may not yet have been found in the fly, we have devised a novel screen in our laboratory. In this project hundrets of genes are presently isolated in the frog embryo to discover novel genes among them. If one were to do this screen with mice, about 600 pregnant females would have to be sacrificed. In the frog only 60 females are needed, since every animal lays hundreds of eggs. Furthermore, the frogs need not be sacrificed since they lay the eggs into the aquarium.

To discover novel developmental control genes, genes are taken randomly from a gene library and the distribution of their gene products, their mRNA, is analyzed in the whole embryo using a special staining procedure. Genes showing a particularly interesting staining pattern are then selected and analyzed more carefully. In cooperation with Dr. Hajo Delius the sequence of the deoxyribonucleic acid (DNA) of these genes is determined and compared to the sequence of known genes that are compiled in databases. Often genes are found that already have a human homolog which was identified in the worldwide efforts to sequence the human genome. Frequently, nothing but the DNA sequence is known for the gene. The staining of the homologous frog gene yields valuable information about a potential function in human. This allows one to analyze specifically whether the human gene may be involved in inherited diseases and/or cancer.

We have identified 200 novel genes in this manner among which are many developmental control genes. The next step will be to test the function of the developmental control genes by micro-injection and to study selected genes more closely. This screen yields an abundance of data, photos of staining patterns of the genes as well as DNA sequences. We will make these data available to the public by releasing them on the internet in form of a gene expression database. In cooperation with Dr. Hans Lehrach at the Max Planck Institute in Berlin we plan to continue this screen on an even larger basis, to systematically study embryonal gene expression, and to discover new developmental control genes.

Dr. Christof Niehrs
Division of Molecular Embryology

Participating scientists

Dr. Volker Gawantka
Rebecca Nitsch

In collaboration with

Dr. Hajo Delius
Oligo-Nucleotide Synthesis and Sequencing Group,
Deutsches Krebsforschungszentrum

Dr. Hans Lehrach
Max Planck Institute of Molecular Genetics,
Berlin

Selected publications

Niehrs, C., De Robertis, E. M.: Vertebrate axis formation. Curr Opin Genet Dev 2, 550–555 (1992)

Gawantka, V., Delius, H., Hirschfeld, K., Blumenstock, C., Niehrs, C.: Antagonizing the Spemann organizer: role of the homeobox gene Xvent-1. Embo J 14, 6268–6279 (1995)

Niehrs, C.: Mad connection to the nucleus. Nature 381, 561–562 (1996)

Onichtchouk, D., Gawantka, V., Dosch, R., Delius, H., Hirschfeld, K., Blumenstock, C., Niehrs, C.: The Xvent-2 homeobox gene is part of the BMP-4 signalling pathway controlling dorsoventral patterning of Xenopus mesoderm. Development 122, 3045–3053 (1996)

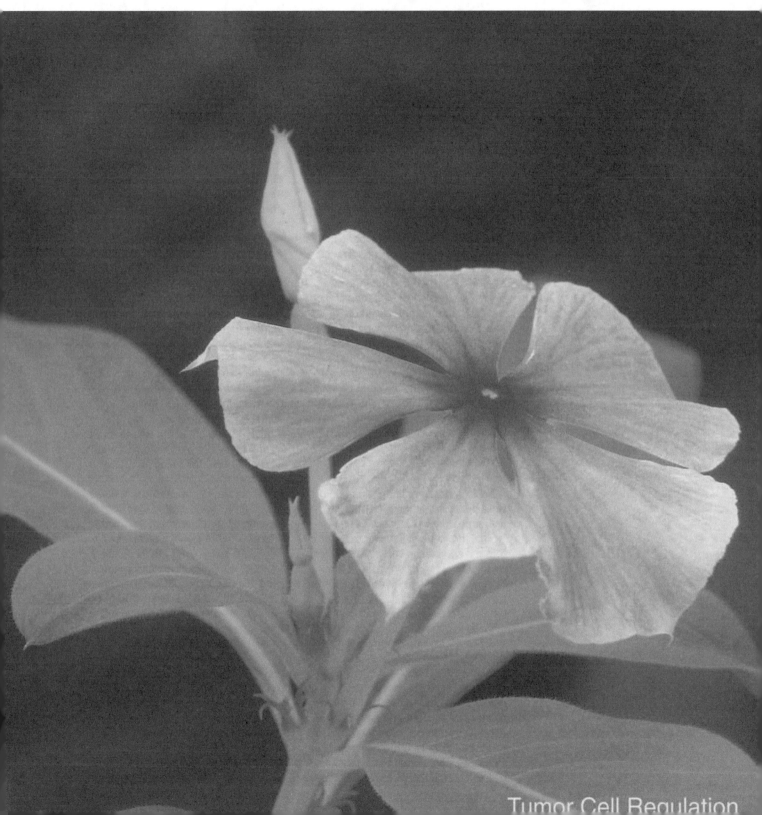

Tumor Cell Regulation

3

Tumor Cell Regulation

Cancer is a disease in which the body's communication system ceases to function properly. Both the communication between cells and that between tumor tissue and the whole organism are disrupted. This is due to a constellation of genetic defects that occur either by chance or as a result of external influences and is expressed in the chaotic and destructive proliferation and inappropriate functioning of cells. The communication between cells relies, generally, on a continuous exchange of chemical signals which, depending on their source and target location, are known variously as hormones, neurotransmitters, cytokines, mediators, or growth factors. Every cell of our bodies is able to send and receive such signals and in this way maintains continuous contact to all other cells. This communication system guarantees that the different components of the body behave in a coherent and cooperative fashion, much as if they were following a pre-arranged plan.

A basic principle of intercellular communication is that the medium and the message are not identical. In other words, the same signal can provoke different responses in different cells (for example, reproduction, special functions, movement, or death). Thus, recipient cells attribute their own specific meaning to every signal. This job of interpretation is carried out by a highly complex system of interactions between protein molecules. It is accompanied by the creation of specific molecular activity patterns, for example, of genes and enzymes, which enable the cell to give an adequate response to external influences. In its mode of operation, this „cognitive" network can most closely be compared to the nervous system, hence the corresponding meta-phor „brain of the cells". When trying to understand disease, it is important to know that the cognitive apparatus of a cell reacts not only to the body's own signal molecules, but also to stress factors from the environment, including micro organisms, radiation, and also carcinogenic and other toxic substances. These protective and emergency reactions are also linked with a well-defined pattern of modulation of the activity of certain genes and enzymes. In view of the fact that communication and cognition are fundamental life processes, it is easy to understand why cellular signal processing is the subject of intense research efforts, especially when one considers that the genetic defects leading to cancer, and also many other diseases, manifest themselves as a malfunctioning of this system.

Here lies the main emphasis of the research carried out in the Research Program Tumor Cell Regulation. Several of its groups are attempting to identify how the pathological changes occurring in the cellular signal processing correspond to the various stages of progressive tumor development. Of particular interest are the signal molecules with which the tumor cells can stimulate themselves, thereby, achieving a degree of independence from the organism. The substances concerned are various growth factors and also a group of compounds called eicosanoids, which include prostaglandins, thromboxanes, leucotrienes, and lipoxins and many other short-lived but highly active molecules. These are involved in the regulation of nearly all tissue and bodily functions and their role in disease processes, including cancer, is becoming increasingly evident.

A key role in the signal processing mechanism within the cell is played by the biochemical process of protein phosphorylation together with its participating enzymes (protein kinases and phosphatases). This reaction actually represents - analogous to the electrochemical impulse in the nervous system - a universal binary code for cellular data processing. Within the Research Program several groups are working to isolate and characterize this type of enzyme and to discover their exact role in physiological and pathophysiological processes.

Protein phosphorylation is also the means by which the genes are regulated. Indeed, the adjustment of the gene activity, and hence protein synthesis, to suit external circumstances plays a central role in the behavior of cells. The regulatory proteins that are necessary for this, for example the transcription factors, are components of the cognitive network of the cell. The regulation of their function - among other things by phosphorylation -, how this regulation is influenced by carcinogenic factors, and the consequences of this for the cell are all being studied in detail using the example of the transcription factor AP1.

In addition to the phosphorylation enzymes, the cellular signal processing and the formation of activity patterns also require a molecular switching element which is provided by molecules known as G proteins. A pathological overactivation of the G protein Ras is amongst the most common disturbances associated with cancer. Another topic of study within the Research Program are the Ran proteins, which belong to the same family and are responsible for controlling the exchange of material between the cell nucleus and the cytoplasm. This is a process of vital significance for the cell, essential among other things for cell division or

mitosis. A better understanding of cell division is also the major aim of the investigations of the proteins of the mitotic apparatus and the chromosomes.

The communication between cells and the protection against poisonous substances are two processes in which transport proteins play an important role by facilitating the export of substances. When such transport processes are overactivated this can lead, among other things, to the dreaded resistance to anticancer drugs (chemotherapy resistance). These interrelations, which are clearly of vital importance in cancer therapy, are being studied by several of the groups of the Research Program.

In view of the complexity of the topics, the work carried out in this Research Program demands the combined use of microscopic, cell-biological, biochemical, and molecular biological methods and, thus, a close collaboration between the individual divisions and also with other programs within the Center. Furthermore, affiliated with this Research Program is a highly sophisticated spectroscopy department which employs the most modern analytical methods. The common aim of all these endeavors is to extend our knowledge about the molecular „data-processing apparatus" of cells so as to open up new avenues in the prevention and cure of cancer and to improve existing methods. An approach that holds great potential is chemoprevention. The idea of this is that suitable substances can inhibit the occurrence of cancer or cause existing tumors to stop growing or even shrink before they reach the stage of malignancy. A prerequisite for this, however, is a knowledge of the molecular processes that one wants to

manipulate. A drug that is frequently discussed in relation to chemoprevention is aspirin and also its relatives. These substances are found to inhibit the development of intestinal cancer in humans. They selectively influence the communication between cells by inhibiting the formation of certain signal molecules, namely the previously mentioned prostaglandins. With the emphasis more on treatment than prevention, cell poisons are currently being tried out. Almost all of these have serious side effects which, in combination with the problem of resistance, means that their applicability is quite limited. But there are good prospects of better controlling the side effects, again by selectively influencing the intercellular signal transmission. Hence there is reason to hope that existing cancer treatments can become more successful.

Coordinator of the Research Program:
Prof. Dr. Friedrich Marks

Divisions and their heads:
Pathochemistry:
Prof. Dr. Volker Kinzel

Biochemistry of the Cell:
Prof. Dr. Dieter Werner

Biochemistry of
Tissue-Specific Regulation:
Prof. Dr. Friedrich Marks

Differentiation and
Carcinogenesis in vitro:
Prof. Dr. Norbert Fusenig

Tumor Biochemistry:
Prof. Dr. Dietrich Keppler

Molecular Biology of Mitosis:
Prof. Dr. Herwig Ponstingl

Signal Transduction
and Growth Control:
Dr. Peter Angel

3.1 Research without Animal Experiments: The Development of a Cell Culture Test for Chemicals that Irritate the Skin

by Karin Müller-Decker and Friedrich Marks

Alternative methods for animal experiments are earnestly demanded both by the public and the legislature. We have developed a cell culture test which evaluates skin-irritating chemicals by measuring a central trigger mechanism in skin inflammations. Specifically, we focus on the release of the primary mediators of inflammation, interleukin-1α and arachidonic acid from human keratinocytes. This reaction represents a general cellular response to the effect of substances that irritate the skin. The validity of the test was confirmed in experiments on humans. Clinical symptoms of inflammation such as erythema and a disturbance in the barrier characteristics of the skin, as well as the local release of arachidonic acid and its resulting products, correlate well with the data measured in the cell culture.

On the basis of these findings, it appears that this procedure may be a suitable alternative method for certain animal experiments. It is possible to further develop this test to detect certain aspects of carcinogenic effects.

From Animal Experiment to Cell Culture Test

Thousands of new chemicals are developed every year in the pharmaceutical, cosmetic, food, and chemical industries. Before such substances can be used, they must be tested for harmful effects, such as whether or not they cause inflammations, have caustic effects, are associated with deformities, or are carcinogenic. The legislature requires various animal experiments for this very purpose. Although we cannot yet do without such experiments in light of the current state of scientific knowledge, their value is being examined in

an increasingly critical manner. Not only do strong public feelings with respect to animal protection and animal rights play a role here, but also economic and scientific arguments are being openly discussed. Testing certain chemicals for their skin-irritating properties can serve as an example. For this purpose, the procedure developed by John Draize in 1944 is still being used to this very day. In this method test substances are placed on the skin or on the eye of a rabbit; the symptoms of an acute irritation are observed over the course of several days and are classified according to their degree of severity. Such symptoms include the reddening of the skin (erythema), which can be traced to an increased blood flow in the superficial vessels and swelling (edema) that occurs when the blood vessel walls become permeable and blood plasma passes into the tissue. Although these symptoms are evaluated according to a standardized key and the test satisfies the requirements of governmental authorities throughout the world, doubts exist about its reliability. For example, the reproducibility of results obtained in different laboratories and their transferability to humans has been questioned. Furthermore, the measured inflammatory reactions can prove to be very burdensome for the experimental animal since they are usually accompanied by pain. Therefore, the Draize Test stands under fire both from the public and from animal protection organizations. In particular, many people no longer understand the need to test products for personal hygiene in animal experiments. The European Union has yielded to this public pressure in its sixth amendment to the EU Cosmetic Guidelines. As of January 1, 1998, animal experiments are to be generally prohibited for testing the ingredients of cosmetic substances. However, there is reservation; scientifically valid alternate methods must be available. The legislature will only recognize such alternate methods if they are equivalent to the "gold standard" as defined by the Draize Test.

The development of alternate methods is complicated by the fact that the inflammatory process is a complex reaction in the human body. Many types of cells work together and its course also depends on the nature of the irritant. Such a process, in all its details, cannot be mimicked in cell and tissue culture. A possible means of avoiding this dilemma is to seek out biochemical reactions that are common to all inflammatory processes and that can to a certain degree be measured "in the test tube." This requires a clarification of the molecular mechanisms of action. We believe that we have identified such fundamental processes specifically for the inflammatory reaction of the skin. On this basis, we have developed a cell culture test for chemicals that irritate the skin; it should at least partially replace conventional animal experiments. Since inflammatory processes in the skin and in other tissues can promote, although not cause, cancer such a test should also be able to detect certain aspects of carcinogenic effects. In fact, the idea for the test arose out of many years of research that focused on the development of skin cancer.

The Response of the Skin to Irritants

As the protective organ of the body, the skin responds very sensitively to harmful influences in the environment. An effective barrier is found in the horny layer at the surface of the skin; it is formed from dead epidermal cells or keratinocytes and is sealed with fat-like substances. Irritants that pass through this barrier cause the deeper lying skin cells to respond with reactions that not only strengthen the protective function of the skin, but also awaken the body's defenses. In this scenario many types of cells cooperate: the keratinocytes in the epidermis and the Langerhans' and mast cells (which preferentially react to substances that cause allergies); the fibroblasts from the connective tissue of the subcutis as well as the cells of the blood vessels. In the next step, white blood cells (leukocytes) and defense cells of the immune system are attracted. They all communicate by means of hormone-like signal molecules that are called mediators of inflammation. Thereby, the characteristic symptoms of inflammation result: erythema, edema, a feeling of heat, pain, and possibly pyogenesis. Additionally, the epidermis is strengthened through accelerated cell production and cornification (hyperplasia). The keratinocytes in the epidermis appear to play a key role in triggering this cascade of reactions. As a kind of interface between the body and the environment, these cells are specialized to respond to stimuli by releasing mediators of inflammation and, thereby, to set in motion the protective and defense functions. Several of these signal substances are released within a few seconds, others with some delay. The immediately released, "primary" mediators of inflammation include the cytokine interleukin-1α and arachidonic acid (AA), a fatty acid, which is the starting product for a large number of active substances called eicosanoids. For example, members of the eicosanoid family include prostaglandins, leukotrienes and the hydroxy-eicosatetraenoic acids. Common to all primary mediators of inflammation is their storage within the cell so that they can be immediately released as needed. It is also typical that they appear either alone or together with other active substances in all phases of the inflammatory process. Their role is one of stimulating keratinocytes and other types of cells to synthesize and release additional mediators so that the cascade of protective and defensive reactions is set in motion.

The Release of Inflammation Mediators in Cell Cultures is a Measure of the Skin-Irritating Effect

The release of interleukin-1α and arachidonic acid from keratinocytes is a process that plays a central role in the inflammatory reaction of the skin. Furthermore, it can easily be measured in tissue culture. Is it possible to assess the skin-irritating effect of chemicals in this manner? In order to answer this question, one first had to prove that treating cell cultures with skin-irritating substances led to the release of the named mediators. In order to avoid problems associated with the differences between humans and animals from the very beginning, we chose human keratinocytes (HPKII cells) for these experiments. These cells in fact respond to 15 structurally different test substances by releasing interleukin-1α, arachidonic acid and eicosanoids. Arachidonic acid and eicosanoids were determined by using radioactively marked substances. Before the test, we grew cells in the presence of (14C) arachidonic acid which was taken up and incorporated into the lipids comprising the cell membranes. After treating the cells with the test chemicals, the arachidonic acid (and the eicosanoids) released into the nutritive solution was extracted using organic solvents, subsequently separated by thin layer chromatography, and finally quantified with respect to its radioactivity. At the same time, the release of interleukin-1α was measured with an immunological enzymatic test: an enzyme coupled to a specific antibody catalyzed a color reaction that was a measure for the quantity of interleukin. A vitality test was used to evaluate a cell-damaging effect. The test was based on the principle that only living cells can convert the colorless substance MTT to an insoluble, purple-black dye (formazan). The quantity of the dye corresponds to the proportion of living cells.

The release of interleukin-1α and arachidonic acid depends on the type and quantity of the test substance. The greater the irritating effect and the dose of a chemical, the greater was the quantity of inflammation mediators released by the cells. Clear differences were observed in the time course of the reactions: depending on the substance, the release of mediators either occurred quickly, delayed or late. A quick arachidonic acid response was not always coupled with a quick interleukin-1α response. Those substances that produced a quick cell response were not always the most effective irritants. Therefore, it was important to measure the release of mediators over a longer time period in order to be certain of detecting the irritating effect of a chemical.

It is usual to report the effectiveness of a test substance by indicating the quantity at which half the maximal response

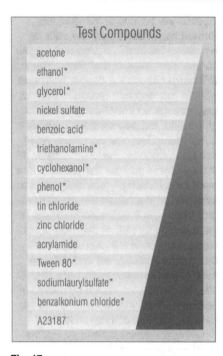

Fig. 17
Chemical substances that were examined in the "test tube" with the new technique. In testing on animals, the irritating effect of the chemicals increases from top to bottom. Those substances marked by a star were also tested on humans in order to evaluate the reliability of the results obtained with the new method

is elicited. In this context, we noticed that the cells reacted more sensitively to the release of arachidonic acid than to interleukin-1α. This is probably due to the fact that the cells must be quite significantly damaged before they release interleukin-1α while the arachidonic acid response requires significantly less irritation. Irrespective of this, both quantities taken together provided the most reliable information.

Confirming the Method in Humans

Are the results obtained with the cell culture an adequate measure of the effect of chemicals on the intact skin? At first glance, we thought that we would be able to answer this question with a "yes." However, a closer analysis of the relevant literature quickly demonstrated that the available data, predominantly originating from the Draize (rabbit) Test, were completely inadequate for an exact evaluation of this method. This was so even without considering the problem of data transferability from animals to humans. After receiving permission from an ethics commission and from governmental authorities and also in collaboration with the pharmacological division of Schering AG, we conducted a study to evaluate our results in humans. Since the sensitivity to skin-irritating chemicals varies greatly from person to person, a so-called patch test was used to determine the "individual irritant dose" for each test chemical. For this purpose, the specific substances were applied in various concentrations to the inner side of the lower arm and the treated skin areas were covered with special chambers for an entire day. For the next three days, a physician evaluated the visible symptoms of skin irritation, especially erythema and edema. Additionally, the extent of skin damage was measured. An especially sensitive measure for this is the permeability of the epidermis for tissue fluid, so-called transepidermal water loss. It was detected with a method that is described as the noninvasive measurement of evaporation among dermatologists. During a second round of treatment, the release of arachidonic acid, eicosanoids, and interleukin-1α in the skin were quantitatively analyzed. Randomly selected participants in the experiment had the test substances administered to their skin in quantities that corresponded to the previously determined individual doses for a given irritant. By applying negative pressure, skin blisters were produced above the test areas. The tissue fluid that collected in the blisters over time contained the mediators of inflammation that had been produced by the skin cells. The mediators were extracted from the blister fluid, were concentrated, and then chemically modified in such a manner so that they could be measured by gas chromatography/mass spectrometry, an especially sensitive method. This process quantitatively determined an entire spectrum of eicosanoids (PGD_2, PGE_2, $PGF_2\alpha$, 6-koto-$PGF_2\alpha$, LTB_4, 5-, 12, 15-HETE) in addition to the arachidonic acid. It was discovered that a skin-irritating effect caused by test chemicals always correlated with a clearly elevated eicosanoid level in the blister fluid. Barrier disturbances of the skin which are recognizable by increased water permeability were only caused by strong irritants. It is especially important that the irritating effect on the intact skin predominantly agreed with the data measured in the cell culture. This was demonstrated by a comparison of eight chemicals. However, the concentrations for interleukin-1α fluctuated so significantly from test person to test person that a statistically certain result could not be obtained.

Conclusion

We understand our studies to be a step towards developing a cell culture test to evaluate the inflammatory effect of

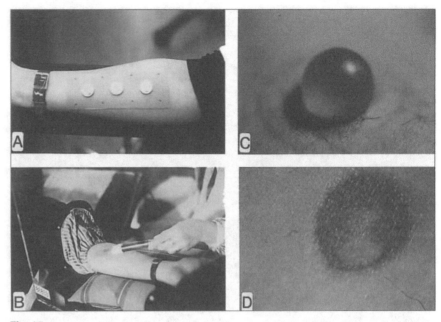

Fig. 18
Determination of the individual irritant dose for a particular test chemical in humans. Various test fields are applied to the underarm of a test subject (A). In order to detect damage to the skin barrier, the outflow of water from the cutis is measured (B). In the blister, which has been artificially created by suction on the cutis, messenger substances of inflammation collect as they are released by the skin cells (C). Sodium lauryl sulfate, which is contained in cleaning agents, causes a reddening of the skin (D)

chemical substances. In this context, we proceed from a more exact knowledge of the fundamental molecular mechanisms instead of measuring more or less unspecific symptoms as is done in conventional procedures.

The keratinocyte cell line (HPKII), which we used, can be easily kept in cell culture without any problems. The immunological enzymatic test and marking with isotopes are both standard procedures that can be conducted in any modern laboratory. However, both the economy and the ease of use of the test would still be significantly im-

proved if one could manage without radioactive substances by, for example, developing an immunological test for arachidonic acid.

If one bears in mind the complexity of the inflammatory process and the apparently very different mechanisms of action exhibited by inflammatory chemicals, the relatively high significance of such a simple test may at first glance prove surprising. However, one should consider that the release of primary inflammation mediators from a cell type that forms the outermost barrier of the body against the external world is a

Main uses of testcompounds in various products					
test compound	cosmetics	pharmaceuticals	food additives	cleaning/ desinfection/ household	other industries
ethanol	✓	✓	✓	✓	✓
glycerol	✓	✓	✓	✓	✓
cyclohexanol	✓		✓		✓
triethanolamine	✓		✓		✓
Tween 80	✓	✓	✓		✓
phenol	✓	✓		✓	✓
SLS sodiumlaurylsulfate	✓	✓		✓	✓
benzalkonium chloride	✓	✓		✓	✓

Fig. 19

Selected publications

Draize, J. H., Woodard, G., Calvery, H.O.: Methods for the study of irritation and toxicity of substances applied topically to the skin and mucous membranes. J. Pharmacol. Exp. Ther. 82, 377–390 (1944)

Barker, J.N., Mitra, R.S., Griffiths, C.E.M., Dixit, V.M., Nickoloff B.J.: Keratinocytes as initiators of inflammation. Lancet 337, 211–214 (1991)

Müller-Decker, K., Fürstenberger, G., Marks, F.: Keratinocyte-Derived Proinflammatory Mediators and Cell Viability as in Vitro Parameters of Irritancy: A Possible Alternative to the Draize Skin Irritation Test. Tox. Appl. Pharmacol. 127, 99–108 (1994)

Marks, F., Fürstenberger, G., Heinzelmann, T., Müller-Decker, K.: Mechanisms in tumor promotion: guidance for risk assessment and cancer chemoprevention. Toxicology Letters 82/83, 907–917 (1995)

Gruber, F.P., Spielmann, H.: Alternativen zu Tierversuchen. Wissenschaftliche Herausforderungen und Perspektiven. Spektrum Akademischer Verlag, Berlin-Heidelberg-Oxford (1996)

very general response to all sorts of external stimuli. Nevertheless, the cell culture test that we developed cannot by itself yet replace animal experiments, but should be included in a battery of additional tests.

Dr. Karin Müller-Decker
Prof. Dr. Friedrich Marks
Division of Biochemistry
of Tissue-Specific Regulation

Participating scientists

Dr. Gerhard Fürstenberger
Thomas Heinzelmann

In collaboration with

Prof. Dr. Werner Raff
Dr. Andrei Kecskes
Dr. Wolfgang Seibert
Ines Zimmer
Department of Clinical Pharmacology,
Schering AG, Berlin

Prof. Dr. Wolf-Dieter Lehmann
Central Spectroscopy,
Deutsches Krebsforschungszentrum

3.2 New Approaches to Counteract Multidrug Resistance in Cancer Chemotherapy

by Dietrich Keppler

The resistance of malignant tumors to anticancer drugs is a major problem in clinical oncology. Many malignant tumors initially respond to treatment with cytotoxic or cytostatic agents but develop subsequently a resistance to several, structurally diverse anticancer agents. This phenomenon is known as multidrug resistance of tumors. The molecular mechanisms underlying the multidrug resistance of malignant tumors and the development of drugs counteracting this resistance are intensively investigated by scientists in research institutions, clinical research laboratories, and in the pharmaceutical industry.

Different mechanisms lead to multidrug resistance of malignant tumor cells. An increasing number of molecular mechanisms causing multidrug resistance was recognized during the past ten years. These mechanisms include drug extrusion by adenosine 5'-triphosphate (ATP)-dependent membrane pumps, such as the P-glycoprotein encoded by the MDR1 gene or the multidrug resistance protein encoded by the MRP1 gene. These distinct membrane pumps function in the transport of different drugs across the plasma membrane of tumor cells into the extracellular space. The membrane pumps encoded by the MDR1 and MRP1 genes have different amino acid sequences and a different substrate specificity with respect to the compounds transported out of tumor cells. Additional mechanisms of drug resistance include those caused by an increased inactivation of cytotoxic drugs by binding to glutathione or the resistance of tumor cells to the signals causing programmed cell death (apoptosis).

Resistance to structurally diverse cytotoxic agents by ATP mediated export of

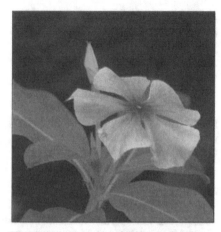

Fig. 20
Cancer drugs can be obtained from the Madagascan periwinkle, Catharanthus roseus, an evergreen plant from Madagascar. Vincristine is such a product. Along with ATP and glutathione, it can be transported out of the tumor cell by the multidrug resistance protein (MRP1)

drugs from tumor cells. It has been established that the MDR1 gene encoded P-glycoprotein, an export pump with a molecular mass of about 170 kilodalton, transports structurally diverse drugs including anthracycline-based cytostatic agents, vinca alkaloids, or the antimitotic drug taxol (paclitaxel). These anticancer drugs are widely used in the clinical treatment of hematological cancers, ovarian cancer, and mammary cancer. Effective concentrations of these anticancer agents may be prevented by the action of MDR1 P-glycoprotein. It has been recognized more recently that MDR1 P-glycoprotein transports not only exogenous cytotoxic drugs into the extracellular space but also a number of structurally different endogenous lipophilic compounds.

Another membrane protein with properties of an ATP dependent membrane pump causing resistance to a variety of cytotoxic agents has been cloned and sequenced from lung cancer cells in 1992 by a group of Canadian scientists. This membrane protein is often expressed in tumors which do not have increased levels of MDR1 P-glycoprotein and which are resistant to several anticancer drugs. This new pump has been termed multidrug resistance protein (MRP1). It is a glycoprotein with a molecular mass of 190 kilodalton and its amino acid sequence is only 15 % identical to the one of MDR1 P-glycoprotein.

The multidrug resistance protein (MRP1) functions as an ATP dependent export pump for conjugated substances. Intracellular formation of conjugates is observed when compounds poorly soluble in water are conjugated to a negatively charged substance, such as glutathione or glucuronate, yielding conjugates of better solubility. The function and substrate specificity of the multidrug resistance protein (MRP1) was recognized by our group in 1994 during the search for the membrane protein

Fig. 21
This diagram shows the localization and function of the conjugate export pumps known as multidrug resistance proteins 1 and 2. Cancer drugs, carcinogenic substances, and poisons that are taken up by the cell (right) can be coupled to internal cellular substances (conjugates) and transported out of the cell by ATP-dependent pumps

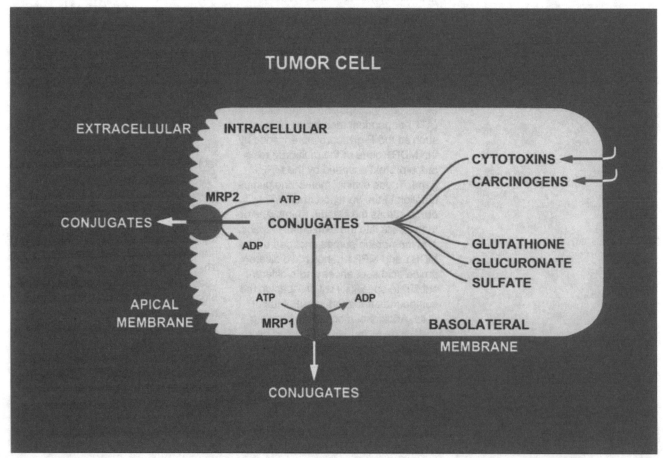

which mediates the ATP dependent transport of the glutathione conjugate leukotriene C4. MRP1 functions in ATP dependent membrane transport of negatively charged lipophilic compounds, such as glutathione conjugates and glucuronate conjugates of endogenous and foreign (xenobiotic) substances. Leukotriene C4 is an endogenous glutathione conjugate, which contributes to the development of human bronchial asthma and inflammation, and which is transported by MRP1 with high affinity. We have shown that conjugates of several cytotoxic agents with glutathione or glucuronate are substrates for MRP1 mediated transport across the plasma membrane of human tumor cells. An additional substrate of MRP1 is glutathione disulfide (GSSG) which is particularly formed under conditions of oxidative stress when GSSG must be transported into the extracellular space. Thus, MRP1 had been discovered and cloned as a membrane protein associated with multidrug resistance; however, only the elucidation of its function and substrate specificity has led to the molecular identification of the ATP dependent transport protein for glutathione conjugates and glucuronides. We have termed MRP1 a conjugate export pump in view of its capacity to transport many structurally diverse conjugates.

Cloning of a new ATP dependent export pump: The apical multidrug resistance protein (MRP2).

The cell surface of epithelial cells is characterized by specialized (apical) membrane domains which are oriented to the lumen of ducts and cavities. The ATP dependent transport of conjugates across apical membrane domains of epithelial cells had been known for a long time; however, the molecular identity of the corresponding transport protein was unknown. Our search for a MRP1 related transport protein in the apical membrane domain of liver cells (hepatocytes) identified a novel sequence that was related to MRP1, although the amino acid sequences of MRP1 and the novel MRP2 were only 49 % identical. The apical multidrug resistance protein has been termed MRP2 or canalicular multispecific organic anion transporter (cMOAT). The MRP2 gene-encoded conjugate export pump in humans is a glycoprotein with a molecular mass of about 190 kilodalton containing 1545 amino acids. The substrate specificities of MRP1 and MRP2 are rather similar in spite of the differences in the amino acid sequence of both transport proteins. The different localization of MRP1 and MRP2 in cells containing apical membrane domains indicates a difference in the functional specialization of both conjugate export pumps. MRP2 is predominantly found in the apical membrane of liver cells and cells of the kidney where it contributes to the transport of endogenous and xenobiotic conjugates into bile and urine, respectively. It is of considerable interest to establish that MRP2 contributes to multidrug resistance of primary liver cancer and renal cell carcinoma. Both types of cancer are very frequent world-wide and particularly resistant to anticancer drugs.

Multidrug resistance associated with drug conjugation to glutathione and ATP dependent export of conjugates from cancer cells. It has been known for some time that multidrug resistance of malignant tumors may be associated with enhanced cellular levels of glutathione and increased activities of glutathione-conjugating enzymes (i. e., glutathione S-transferases). Several clinical studies were conducted in an attempt to overcome the resistance to cytotoxic agents by lowering of the glutathione content of tumors and to counteract thereby the glutathione conjugation of cytotoxic agents. As a consequence of the elucidation of the function of MRP1 and MRP2 it has become apparent that an inhibition of the export of the cytotoxic drug conjugates with glutathione from the cell should be an additional target to enhance the antitumor action of drugs and to increase their intracellular concentration by inhibition of export. Susan Cole, Roger Deeley, and their collaborators in Canada recently showed that the cytotoxic agent vincristine, which is used in the therapy of leukemias and other types of cancer, is transported from tumor cells to the extracellular space as a complex with glutathione which is pumped out by MRP1. We observed that alkylating cytotoxic agents are transported out of tumor cells by MRP1 after their intracellular conjugation with glutathione. These results indicate that tumors expressing increased amounts of MRP1 in their plasma membrane may become resistant to a variety of structurally different cytotoxic agents if conjugation or complex formation of the drug with glutathione proceeds at a sufficient rate.

The conjugate export pumps MRP1 and MRP2 have important physiological functions, such as the biosynthetic release of the endogenous mediator leukotriene C4 and the excretion of bilirubin glucuronides and estradiol glucuronide. These conjugates with glucuronate are formed during the catabolism of hemoglobin and of the hormone estradiol, respectively. Moreover, the conjugate export pumps MRP1 and MRP2 play a role in the excretion of carcinogens since they pump carcinogen con-

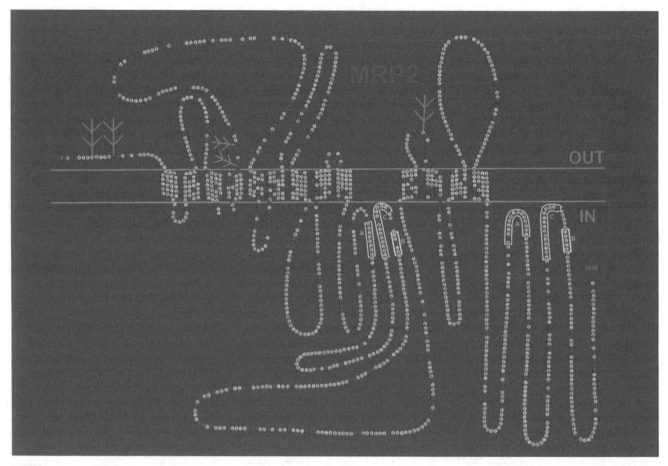

Fig. 22
MRP2 is a protein that facilitates the transport of substances through the cell membrane. The model shown here indicates that the amino acid chain penetrates the cell membrane 13 times. Amino acids that are identical in humans and rats are shown in yellow, while those that differ are shown in red. Extracellular oligosaccharide fragments are light blue, and intracellular ATP-binding regions (A, B, C) are presented in white

jugates out of cells before their intracellular mutagenic or carcinogenic action can take place. As an example, the carcinogen aflatoxin B1 is transported out of the cell as a conjugate with glutathione. Douglas Loe and his colleagues in Canada showed recently that the ATP dependent transport of the aflatoxin B1 conjugate with glutathione is mediated by MRP1. Thus, the detoxification of many foreign (xenobiotic) substances is not completed by conjugation with glutathione or glucuronate in liver and kidney but requires as a final and decisive step the ATP dependent export of the conjugate by MRP1 or MRP2.
New inhibitors of the conjugate export pumps MRP1 and MRP2 counteract multidrug resistance. The molecular identification and the characterization of the substrate specificity of the conjugate export pumps MRP1 and MRP2 has enabled studies on inhibitors of these transport proteins which counteract the multidrug resistance of tumors. Most of the inhibitors identified at present are negatively charged lipophil-

ic compounds that are structurally related to the endogenous leukotrienes C_4, D_4, and E_4. These inhibitory substances were originally developed as leukotriene receptor antagonists for the treatment of bronchial asthma and allergic disease. These substances overcome the multidrug resistance of tumor cells only at higher concentrations because of an insufficient uptake of these negatively charged compounds by tumor cells. Based on our studies of the substrate specificity of MRP1, indicating that estradiol-17b-glucuronide is a preferred substrate, Bryan Norman and his colleagues in the USA recently developed a compound which is structurally related to estradiol glucuronide. This compound, which is a derivative of the estrogen receptor modulator raloxifen, effectively counteracted the MRP1 mediated resistance of human tumor cells to anthracycline and vinca alkaloid drugs which are widely used in cancer chemotherapy. This development indicates that it has become a promising and realistic goal to overcome the multidrug resistance of some tumors overexpressing MRP1. Further advanced is the development of inhibitors of MDR1 P-glycoprotein which currently undergo clinical trials. Future studies should answer the question which ATP dependent export pumps decisively contribute to the multidrug resistance of a certain tumor type and which inhibitors are effective in patients to overcome multidrug resistance and to improve the results of clinical cancer chemotherapy.

Prof. Dr. Dietrich Keppler
Division of Tumor Biochemistry

Participating scientists

Dr. Inka Leier
Dr. Gabriele Jedlitschky
Dr. Markus Büchler
Dr. Jörg König
Dr. Thomas Schaub

Selected publications

Jedlitschky, G., Leier, I., Buchholz, U., Center, M., Keppler, D.: ATP-dependent transport of glutathione S-conjugates by the multidrug protein. Cancer Res. 54, 4833–4836 (1994)

Leier, I., Jedlitschky, G., Buchholz, U., Cole, S. P. C., Deeley, R. G., Keppler, D.: The MRP gene encodes an ATP-dependent export pump for leukotriene C_4 and structurally related conjugates. J. Biol. Chem. 269, 27807–27810 (1994)

Büchler, M., König, J., Brom, M., Kartenbeck, J., Spring, H., Horie, T., Keppler, D.: cDNA cloning of the hepatocyte canalicular isoform of the multidrug resistance protein, cMrp, reveals a novel conjugate export pump deficient in hyperbilirubinemic mutant rats. J. Biol. Chem. 271, 15091–15098 (1996)

Jedlitschky, G., Leier, I., Buchholz, U., Barnouin, K., Kurz, G., Keppler, D.: Transport of glutathione, glucuronate, and sulfate conjugates by the MRP gene-encoded conjugate export pump. Cancer Res. 56, 988–994 (1996)

Keppler, D., König, J.: Expression and localization of the conjugate export pump encoded by the MRP2 (cMRP/cMOAT) gene in liver. FASEB J. 11, 509–516 (1997)

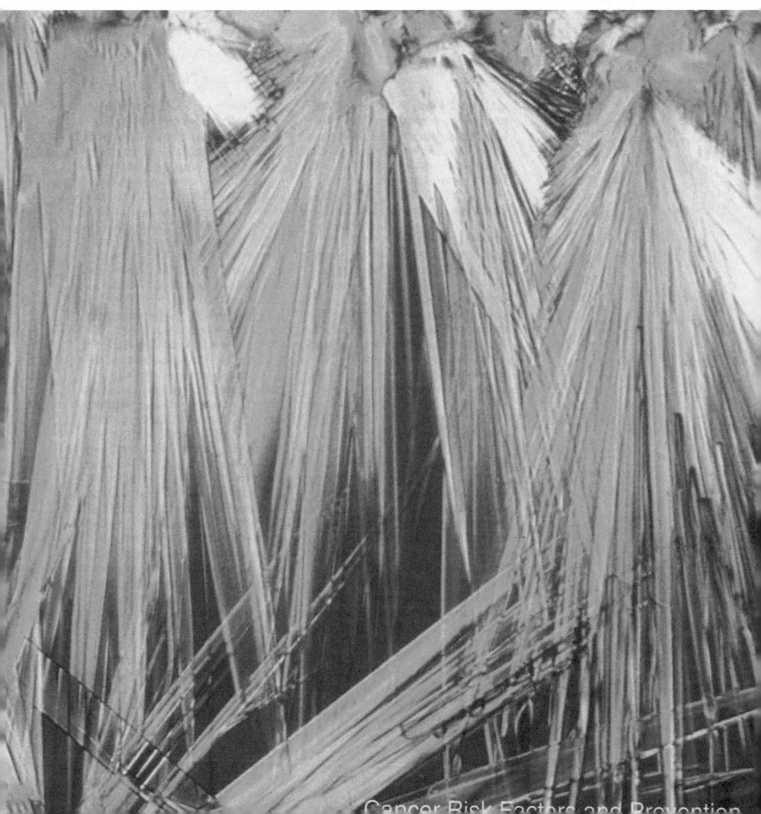

Cancer Risk Factors and Prevention

4

Cancer Risk Factors and Prevention

In view of the high cancer mortality figures and the unsatisfactory results of treatment, measures to prevent cancer are urgently needed. Prevention can be achieved both by the avoidance of risk factors (primary prevention) and by early diagnosis or halting the development of the disease (secondary prevention). But of course a prerequisite for targeted prevention is that the main causes of the disease and the mechanism by which it develops are understood. For many forms of cancer this is not the case. The Research Program Cancer Risk Factors and Prevention is investigating selected problems which are regarded as crucial for understanding the development of cancer and which promise to improve cancer prevention. The recognition and determination of risk factors and the investigation of their mechanisms are important prerequisites for preventive medical measures. Points of focus include: to identify and estimate the activity of exogenous and endogenous cancer risk factors and also protective factors by means of epidemiological, pathological, and toxocological methods; investigations of hereditary genetic modifications that contribute to the development of cancer; study of the carginogen-induced mechanisms that cause damage to the DNA or genes; identification and analysis of the preliminary stages of cancer; and chemoprevention and the development of anticancer drugs. With our growing knowledge of the causes and mechanisms, genuine possibilities for prevention are coming within reach. Their useful exploitation and further refinement are seen by this Research Program as its primary objective.

International epidemiological studies have shown that up to 80 percent of cancer cases are due, in the broadest sense, to environmental factors. Tobacco alone is responsible for 30 percent. Since dietary factors play a similarly important role, although the exact mechanisms of their influence are not yet known, the nutrition epidemiological research of the Epidemiology Division is seen as particularly significant. Another main area involves research into environmental carcinogens in the air we breathe and in our drinking water and the quantification of the associated risks. For a few environmental carcinogens the previous epidemiological research has already allowed a quantitative risk analysis. This in turn has led to legal measures being adopted and the risk factors themselves remaining objects of close scrutiny. Likewise, a large proportion of cancer deaths related to exposure at work can also be avoided by translating the results of epidemiological research into measures to protect workers. For this reason, the topic of occupation related cancer epidemiology represents another focal point. Genetic factors can also have a significant influence on an individual's likelihood of contracting certain cancers, for example, breast cancer. The investigation of these factors and the identification of high risk groups is a new and important field within the division with strong ties to molecular biology.

The Division Toxicology and Cancer Risk Factors undertakes studies of environmental risk factors and the interaction of carcinogenic substances with host factors (genetic disposition) in human carcinogenesis. An essential element here is the development of new methods and biomarkers which can be used in cancer epidemiology and intervention studies. It has been possible to develop and validate DNA markers which can indicate high levels of certain harmful substances (for example, polycyclic hydrocarbons) and also oxidative stress, caused in part by dietary factors. These markers have been successfully applied in human pilot studies. Such approaches are currently being employed to identify groups within the population that are particularly susceptible to cancer and to investigate the detailed etiology of cancers related to dietary factors. Another prominent area is the study of the molecular mechanisms by which chronic inflammation might cause or aggrevate carcinogenesis in humans. The examination of substances with regard to their carcinogenic properties is mainly carried out using the methods of genetic toxicology, often with molecular characterization of genetic damage in transgenic test systems. Data on the mutation spectrum or, as it is frequently called, the genetic fingerprints often include modifications that are attributable to carcinogens. These data are studied with the aim of identifying the effects of previous exposure, thereby allowing a retrospective determination of substances that can cause cancer in humans. A further area of interest is the isolation of cancer-inhibiting substances and the investigation of the principles underlying their properties, knowledge that can later enable them to be applied in chemoprevention. In clinical cooperation studies, investigations are being undertaken of a promising low-dose Sulindac therapy for the long-term treatment of adenomas in patients with familial adenomatous polyposis, and of the long-term effects of an anti-oxidant combination on the shrinking of dysplasias in the mucus membrane of the mouth.

The Division Interaction of Carcinogens with Biological Macromolecules studies both genes themselves and the products of DNA repair and replication in order to identify possible mutations and functional modifications. The work concentrates on DNA helicases and DNA polymerases. The metamorphosis from a normal cell into a cancer cell is strongly influenced by the number, type, and location of carcinogens or DNA adducts at the moment of DNA replication. In the process of DNA replication, the DNA adducts which are covalently anchored in the DNA matrix are converted - to an extent corresponding to the degree of possible base mispairing - into mutations. In this way, an exposure of the organism to carcinogens can rapidly lead to mutations even in the genes whose protein products are responsible for maintaining the integrity of the DNA, particularly in the genes of the DNA replication apparatus and of the repair enzymes. The modifications can lead, among other things, to a reduction in the accuracy of DNA copying so that in every cell-proliferation cycle further, carcinogen independent mutations are introduced into the genome (the „mutator hypothesis" of cancer causation). Investigations to date indicate that the DNA polymerases in cancer cells have an altered conformation and are particularly sensitive to inhibitory substances. A (selective) suppression of tumor growth thus seems to be a possibility.

The central objective of the Division Cell Pathology is to gain an understanding of the morphological, metabolic, and molecular changes occurring in the preliminary stages of cancer (precancerosis). The aim of these investigations is to improve the early diagnosis and prevention of cancer. The most important objects of study are various experimental models of the development of liver cancer, together with surgically removed human liver tissue from patients with severe chronic liver diseases that often lead to the development of liver cancer. In addition to studying the individual effects of chemical, hormonal, physical, and viral cancer risk factors, detailed investigations are attempting to unravel the interaction of a chronic virus infection with chemical carcinogens, in particular with the fungal poison aflatoxin B1. Furthermore, an industrial collaboration is testing a new model which removes the need for animal experiments when investigating the carcinogenic effects of chemical substances. Comparisons of the various models of the development of liver cancer with actual human liver tissue have recently demonstrated remarkable agreement in the cellular phenotype in the preliminary stages of cancer. The observed effects can be induced both by chemical and physical agents (e.g., x-rays or neutrons) or by cancer causing viruses and are also found to increase when these risk factors interact. These modifications to the cellular phenotype suggest a hormone-like action of the cancer causing agents, similar to that of insulin or thyroxin, which leads to the disruption of intracellular signal pathways. Its course is characterized by early-stage metabolic deviations and later switches in metabolism accompanied by a continuously increasing rate of cell replication. The molecular basis of these events remains a topic of study.

The research activities of the Division Molecular Toxicology can be divided into the areas toxicology and drug development. In the field of toxicology the main interest lies in detecting and elucidating the structure of DNA adducts so as to shed light on their mutagenic potential. Along with aristolochia acids and nitrophenols, studies will be looking at pyrrolicidine alkaloids. The detection of DNA adducts is achieved with the ^{32}P post-labeling procedure. In order to avoid the need to handle radioactive phosphorus, a method is being developed using a combination of capillary electrophoresis and laser-induced fluorescence. Also under active study is the synthesis of dendritic metal complexes for the marking of oligonucleotides, a system used for detecting hybridization with the electron microscope. In relation to drug development, work continues on the use of monosaccharide conjugates for the targeted introduction of therapeutic substances into tumors and into the brain. The aim here is to find efficient therapeutic methods with as little side effects as possible. A prototype compound, glucose ifosfamide mustard, has been undergoing clinical tests since July 1996. A further area of endeavor is the exploitation of the lectin-oligosaccharide interaction for the development of a drug targeting concept. Together with biochemical work on the characterization of tumor lectins, complex oligosaccharides are being employed as carrier molecules for therapeutic substances. Their sysnthesis is achieved using both chemical and enzymatic methods. Such chemical vectors based on branched oligosaccharides can also be used for the transport of oligonucleotides for antisense therapy.

The aims of this Research Program are supported by about 150 cooperations with 45 research centers in Germany and 60 research centers abroad.

Coordinator of the Research Program:
Prof. Dr. Helmut Bartsch

Cell Pathology:
Prof. Dr. Peter Bannasch

Toxicology and Cancer Risk Factors:
Prof. Dr. Helmut Bartsch

Molecular Toxicology:
Prof. Dr. Manfred Wießler

Interaction of Carcinogens with Biological Macromolecules:
Prof. Dr. Dr. Heinz W. Thielmann

Epidemiology:
Prof. Dr. Jürgen Wahrendorf

4.1 Evolution of Liver Cell Cancer – Interaction of Viruses and Chemicals

by Peter Bannasch

Liver cell cancer is one of the most frequent malignant neoplasms. Every year at least 250,000 and according to some estimates even as many as 1,000,000 human beings die from this hardly curable cancer, which is particularly widespread in Africa and South-East-Asia. Although liver cell cancer is less prevalent in Europe and North America, it nevertheless ranks tenth among the most frequent cancers in Germany.

Chronic infection with the hepatitis viruses B and C, ingestion of foodstuffs contaminated with aflatoxins, especially aflatoxin B1, and abuse of alcoholic beverages are considered major risk factors for the development of liver cell cancer. The importance of viruses as risk factors for liver cancer was only discovered during the last three decades by epidemiological and zoological observations. Today, we know that chronic carriers of the hepatitis B virus, which has originally been detected as the causative agent of infectious jaundice, have a more than 100-fold increased risk of developing liver cell cancer compared to uninfected individuals. This applies particularly to children who were already infected as newborns. It has been estimated that one in 200 infected newborns will contract liver cell cancer in the course of its life. As a rule, however, it takes several decades (30 to 50 years) until recognizable tumors appear in chronic carriers of the hepatitis B virus. During this long time period, the chronic carriers may be exposed to additional risk factors such as chemicals. In addition to the observations in humans, the discovery of a whole group of closely related viruses in different animal species was of utmost importance for the establishment of a causal relationship between viral infection and the evolution of cancer in the liver. These viruses resemble the human hepatitis B virus not only in their molecular structure containing DNA as genetic material (hepadnaviridae), but also in their ability to induce chronic hepatitis and liver cell cancer in their natural hosts, providing the basis for studying liver cancer development caused by viruses in animals. The animal models used were North American woodchucks infected with the woodchuck hepatitis virus (WHV) which is characteristic of this species. Nearly all chronic WHV-carriers infected as newborns develop liver cell cancer within two to three years. In addition, it has been discovered more recently that liver cell cancer regularly develops in transgenic mice containing genes or subgenomic fragments of the human hepatitis B virus, introduced by genetic engeneering. In experimental cancer research it has been known since the pioneering work of Takaoki Sasaki and Tomizo Yoshida in the thirties of this century that a large number of chemicals (carcinogens) produce liver cell cancer in laboratory animals, particularly in small rodents such as mice and rats. Similar to neoplastic development elicited by viruses, the development of liver cell cancer caused by chemicals has a long lag period. After exposure to weak chemical carcinogens or small amounts of strong carcinogens the lag period may approach (or theoretically) – even surpass the average life span of the respective species, so that during the life time only precursor lesions (preneoplasia) of cancer become evident. Due to this long period of cancer development the detection of carcinogenic agents is not only hampered in laboratory animals but also in man. In fact, in addition to poorly defined components

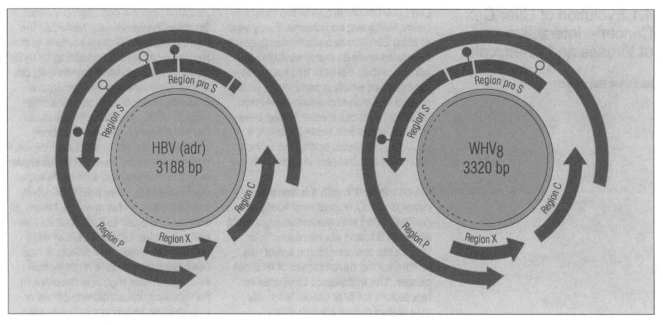

Fig. 23
The human hepatitis B virus (HBV) is shown on the left and the woodchuck hepatitis virus (WHV) on the right. The two viruses are closely related, as can be seen in the arrangement of their genomes. Both viruses cause chronic hepatitis and liver cancer in infected individuals. Because of this, it is possible to study the development of liver cancer in animals

of alcoholic beverages only a few chemicals have been established as causes of human liver cell cancer, namely the above mentioned aflatoxins, especially aflatoxin B_1, arsenic, and certain oral contraceptives of which the carcinogenic potential is relatively low. Most important are the aflatoxins which have been shown to be strong liver carcinogens in numerous species, including primates. The molds producing aflatoxins grow among other things on basic foodstuffs such as cereals and peanuts, particularly in regions with a moist climate which also show a high incidence of human liver cell cancer. A close relationship between the extent of the contamination of foodstuffs and the

frequency of liver cancer has been demonstrated in various high-risk areas, e.g., South China and Kenya. In addition, the excretion of metabolites of aflatoxins in the urine of affected persons, and characteristic alterations in certain genes (Codon 259 of the p53 gene) suggesting effects of aflatoxins were found in such regions.

Is human liver cell cancer mainly caused by hepatitis viruses or by aflatoxins? Or do these two risk factors act together (synergistically)? The answer to this intriguing question is complicated by the fact that geographic regions with viral epidemics largely overlap with the moisty climatic zones in which

molds grow particularly well. Under these conditions, an unequivocal assignment of the causation of human liver cell cancer to one of these two risk factors is hardly possible. As mentioned above, it is more likely that both risk factors act together.

In a model system we were able to verify this hypothesis for the woodchuck. Chronic carriers of the virus, which were infected with WHV as newborns and were administered low doses of aflatoxin B1 (injected in bananas) in their food, did not only develop liver cell cancer much faster but also more frequently than animals which were treated with the virus alone. In contrast, the administering of an intentionally low dose level of aflatoxin B1 never resulted in the appearance of liver cell cancer. Hence, under the conditions of this experiment the viral infection played a much stronger role in the induction of liver cell cancer than aflatoxin B1. Nevertheless, evidence for the independent carcinogenic potential of the aflatoxin has been provided by the finding of focal precursor lesions of liver cell cancer in half of the animals treated with this poison alone.

The establishment of a synergistic effect of chronic viral infection and poisoning with aflatoxin is a major step in the elucidation of the causes of liver cell cancer, but the mechanism of the interaction between these two risk factors at the cellular and molecular level remains to be clarified. In addition to differentiated liver cells (hepatocytes), undifferentiated liver stem cells (so called oval cells) have been considered as the site of origin of liver cell cancer by some authors. Although this concept has been supported by a number of observations, our own results indicate that at least the majority of liver cell cancers originate from differentiated hepatocytes, which gradually lose their differentiation (dedifferentiation) during transformation of the normal into the neoplastic cell.

Two major concepts have been proposed in order to explain the molecular mechanisms and the interaction of hepatitis viruses and aflatoxins. The first concept is based on the assumption of two different mechanisms of action of these risk factors: while one of the risk factors may induce specific mutations in the hepatocytes, the second risk factor may transform the mutated cell by unspecific effects such as the stimula-tion of reactive cell division following cell loss due to inflammatory or toxic tissue damage, or the inhibition of immunological defense against the propagation of the altered cells. Hepatitis viruses and aflatoxins were mutually considered to represent specific and unspecific factors, respectively, in this concept. The second concept requires that both viruses and aflatoxins induce multiple mutations the accumulation of which results in the gradual transformation of the normal hepatocytes into cancer cells. At present, neither concept has yet been sufficiently substantiated. The mutations in oncogenes of the myc family by insertion of WHV-DNA described by some groups in 50% of liver cell cancers in woodchucks were rare in our experimental material. In human liver cell cancer mutations by insertion of viral DNA were only found exceptionally. Conversely, the relatively frequent mutations of the p53-gene observed in human liver cell cancer, which were explained as effects of aflatoxins, were not detected in woodchucks exposed to aflatoxin B1.

In contrast to these discrepancies in alterations of the genetic equipment (genotype) of the cancer cells in different types of liver cell neoplasms caused by various carcinogenic agents, we discovered striking similarities in specific sequential changes of the hepatocellular phenotype in preneoplastic lesions, which are not only characteristic of different animal models of carcinogenesis, no matter whether this process is induced by viruses, chemicals or radiation, but occur also in chronic human liver diseases at high risk of developing liver cell cancer.

The sequence of structural and functional changes of the hepatocytes dur-ing neoplastic development follows two main cell lineages, which initially emerge in foci composed of well differentiated hepatocytes long before the definite cancer cells appear. The predominant sequence of hepatocellular changes commences with an excessive accumulation of the macromolecule glycogen (glycogenosis), a polymer of glucose, which stores energy and is involved in the regulation of the blood sugar level under normal conditions. Because of the focal character of the abnormal glycogen storage in early preneoplastic lesions, the analysis of biochemical changes associated with the appearance and further development of the preneoplastic phenotype is only possible with special methodological approaches such as enzyme histochemistry and microbiochemical analysis of focal lesions dissected under the microscope from freeze dried tissue sections by a laser beam. Using these approaches we were able to demonstrate that the excessive storage of glycogen is due to an inhibition of glycogen breakdown. The whole metabolic pattern of the preneoplastic glycogenotic foci suggests effects of carcinogenic agents resembling the action of insulin. This well known pancreatic hormone is involved via complex intracellular signal transduction pathways in the regulation of a large number of cellular functions, including the regulation of glucose homeostasis, cell differentiation, and cell proliferation.

In woodchucks both the chronic infection with the hepatitis virus and the poisoning with aflatoxin result in a focal hepatic glycogenosis, the intensity of which is significantly increased when both risk factors act together. This observation argues in favor of similar al-

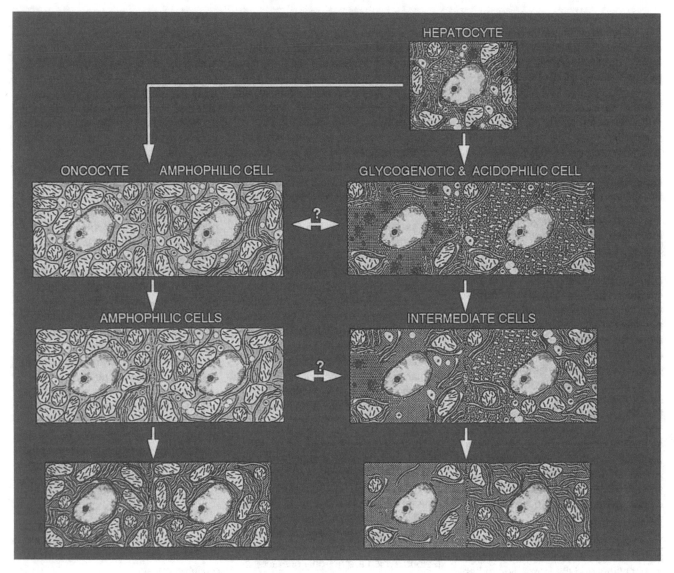

Fig. 24
During carcinogenesis, the functional and structural changes of the liver cells mainly follow two lines of development: Poisoning with most carcinogenic substances or infection with hepatitis viruses – as shown at the right – results in the excessive storage of glycogen (red points). In many cases, it is associated with the multiplication of a certain cell organelle (irregular light structures). During the transformation into cancer cells, glycogen decreases and the number of membrane-bound or free ribosomes increases (blue points). These are partially responsible for protein biosynthesis. In this manner, cancer cells that are poor in glycogen and rich in ribosomes develop from transitional cells that still contain glycogen. The effect of certain carcinogenic substances that do not directly interact with the genetic material of the cell as well as the infection with hepatitis viruses leads to the loss of stored glycogen, to a multiplication of mitochondria, and a progressive increase in the number of membrane-bound and free ribosomes (violet)

terations in signal transduction pathways by hepatitis viruses and aflatoxins, which may also be responsible for their synergistic effect. This interpretation is not limited to the woodchuck model since early metabolic changes of the same kind emerge during hepatocarcinogenesis in hepatitis B virus transgenic mice and in different species treated with various chemical carcinogens. Of particular interest is the finding of similar metabolic aberrations in preneoplastic focal hepatic lesions in explanted human livers (obtained from the Surgical Departments of University Hospitals in Heidelberg and Hannover) of a large number of patients suffering from chronic liver diseases, especially hepatitis B and C, abuse of alcoholic beverages, and inborn hepatic glycogenosis caused by a defect of the enzyme glucose-6-phosphatase, the activity of which is also frequently reduced in experimentally induced glycogenotic foci.

Light and electron microscopic observations in tissue sections of human livers infected by the hepatitis B virus revealed years ago that the viral surface antigen (HBsAg), which is usually secreted into the blood and has here diagnostic significance, may accumulate in large amounts in the smooth endoplasmic reticulum of hepatocytes, resulting in so called ground glass cells in chronic carriers of the virus. Although ground glass cells are characteristic of chronic carriers at high risk of liver cell cancer, they are usually lacking in the cancer tissue. A close connection between the appearance of ground glass cells and the development of hepatocellular neoplasms which are largely free from this cell type, has also been observed in the transgenic mouse

model of viral hepatocarcinogenesis established by Francis Chisari and in woodchucks which are chronic carriers of WHV. In both species we found that the expression of the viral surface antigen is usually lost early during the development of preneoplastic focal lesions. This applies particularly to the excessive accumulation of glycogen which is inversely correlated with a loss in the synthesis of the surface antigen. This observation is particularly remarkable in view of the metabolic aberrations in preneoplastic glycogenotic foci mentioned above, since Chen-Kung Chou and his coworkers have reported that cultivated human liver cancer cells which have maintained the ability of producing surface antigen lose this function completely when they are treated with insulin. This effect of insulin is also mediated by intracellular signal transduction cascades.

The most compelling evidence for a decisive role of this signal transduction cascade in hepatocarcinogenesis has been provided by recent results of cooperative investigations with Frank Dombrowski and Ulrich Pfeifer of the Institute of Pathology of the University of Bonn on an animal model established by these colleagues. Streptozotocin diabetic rats with markedly elevated level of blood glucose receive grafts of isolated pancreatic islet cells via the portal vein. The islet cell colonies settle in the liver, and may cure the diabetes by the secretion of insulin. However, when the number of grafted islet cells is insufficient, the blood sugar remains elevated compared to that of untreated controls. Under these conditions the production of insulin in the transplanted islet cells is strongly stimulated. As a consequence of this hyperinsulinism,

pronounced glycogenotic hepatocellular foci exhibiting marked cell proliferation and an increased rate of cell death emerge within a few days in the parenchyma immediately surrounding the islet cell colonies. Within one to two years a high incidence of benign and malignant hepatocellular neoplasms develop from these preneoplastic focal lesions. In this novel model of hormonal hepatocarcinogenesis the whole process of neoplastic development appears to be driven by the sustained secretion of the abnormally high amount of insulin.

In all models of hepatocarcinogenesis the phenotype of the early emerging glycogen storage foci is instable. During the course of carcinogenesis the glycogen initially stored in excess is gradually reduced, while the number of free and membrane-bound ribosomes increases, indicating an elevated protein synthesis. This process is associated with a fundamental shift in the cellular energy metabolism favoring alternative metabolic pathways such as glycolysis and the pentose phosphate pathway for the benefit of cell proliferation. The trigger for this metabolic shift has not been clarified, but we presume that an adaptation of the cellular metabolism to the early emerging aberrations in carbohydrate metabolism is responsible.

The second hepatocellular lineage in carcinogenesis has only been discovered in the last few years in certain animal models of chemical hepatocarcinogeneis and in hepadnaviral hepatocarcinogenesis in woodchucks. The chemicals eliciting this cell lineage include various „nongenotoxic" hypolipidemic drugs and the adrenal steroid hormone dehydroepiandrosterone the

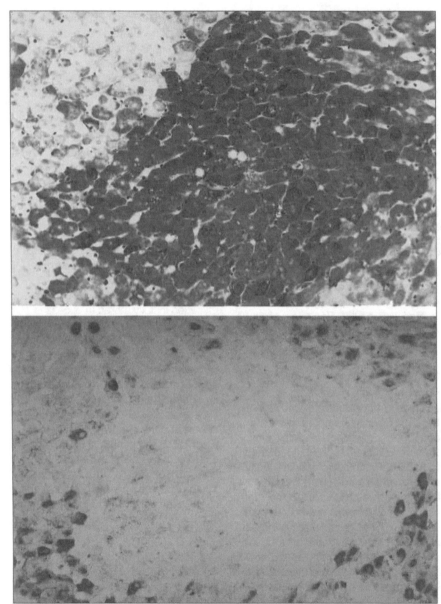

Fig. 25
Like the effect of carcinogenic chemical substances, a chronic infection with hepatitis
viruses results in an excessive, focal storage of the sugar molecule, glycogen. The
cells release a viral coating protein that is found in large quantities in many liver cells
during the early stages of the chronic hepatitis B virus infection and which is used
here as a diagnostic marker

hepatocarcinogenic effect of which has been studied in some detail in our laboratory. All of these compounds induce a marked proliferation of the peroxisomes, organelles rich in catalase and oxidases, and unlike „genotoxic" hepatocarcinogens do not react directly with DNA. Just as genotoxic chemicals, the nongenotoxic peroxisomal proliferators lead to early focal hepatocellular changes, but their phenotype differs essentially from that of glycogenotic foci, being mainly characterized from the very beginning by a depletion of glycogen and a striking increase in the number of mitochondria and a slight increase in rough endoplasmic reticulum. The mitochondrial proliferation is accompanied by various changes in mitochondrial enzymes, suggesting a disturbance of signal transduction pathways which are stimulated by thyroid hormones under physiological conditions. Similar structural and functional alterations of the mitochondria were observed in preneoplastic and neoplastic lesions occurring during hepadnaviral hepatocarcinogenesis in woodchucks. In both chemical and viral hepatocarcinogenesis there is circumstantial evidence for fluctuations between the hepatocytes rich in glycogen and mitochondria indicating possible cross-talk between different alterations in the complex network of intracellular signal transduction pathways.

The results reported do not only lead to new concepts of the mechanism of hepatocarcinogenesis induced by viruses and/or chemicals, but they also open new horizons for prevention and, perhaps, also for therapy of liver cell cancer. In primary prevention the systematic vaccination against the hepatitis B virus-infection already practiced in some countries, the extensive elimination of aflatoxins from foodstuffs, and the prevention of alcohol abuse retain priority and should be improved in the future. In addition, the maintenance of hormonal homeostasis by an appropriate diet and drugs may prove to be an effective preventive measure, especially since another research team has recently shown by an epidemiological approach that patients suffering from diabetes mellitus have a significantly increased risk of developing liver cell cancer compared to age-matched controls.

Specific inhibitors of overactive steps in disturbed signal transduction cascades might be used to correct functional and structural changes in preneoplastic and neoplastic liver lesions. However, the realization of this possible approach is hampered by the complexity of the intracellular regulatory networks. Theoretically, the recognition of preneoplastic lesions should improve secondary prevention by early detection of cancer development. However, in practical terms this aim can hardly be reached in an internal organ like the liver as long as the resolution of the imaging procedures available remains insufficient for the detection of the very small focal preneoplastic lesions the diameter of which is usually smaller than two micrometer.

Prof. Dr. Peter Bannasch
Division of Cytopathology

Participating scientists
Dr. Hans Jörg Hacker
Nasser Imani Khoshkhou
Uli-Rüdiger Jahn
Priv.-Doz. Dr. Doris Mayer
Christel Metzger
Dr. Svetlana Radaeva
Martina Schmitt
Dr. Qin Su
Dr. Ilia Toshkov

In cooperation with

Dr. Francis V. Chisari
Division of Experimental Pathology
Scripps Research Institute
La Jolla, Ca., U.S.A

Dr. Margund Mrozek
Dr. Uwe Zillmann
Central Animal Laboratory,
Deutsches Krebsforschungszentrum

Prof. Dr. Michael Roggendorf
Dr. Michael Elgas
Institute of Virology,
University of Essen

Dr. Annette Kopp-Schneider
Dr. Axel Benner
Central Biostatistics,
Deutsches Krebsforschungszentrum

Priv.-Doz. Dr. Uwe Haberkorn
Division of Oncological Diagnostics
and Therapy,
Deutsches Krebsforschungszentrum

Prof. Dr. Gerd Otto
Department of Surgery,
University Clinic Heidelberg

Prof. Dr. Rudolf Pichlmayr (†)
Department of Surgery,
University Clinic Hannover

Dr. Walter Hofmann
Pathological Institute,
University of Heidelberg

Dr. Frank Dombrowski
Prof. Dr. Ulrich Pfeifer
Pathological Institute,
University of Bonn

Selected publications

Toshkov, I., Chisari, F.V., Bannasch, P.: Hepatic preneoplasia in hepatitis B virus transgenic mice. Hepatology 20, 1162–1172 (1994)

Bannasch, P., Imani Khoshkhou, N., Hacker, H.J., Radaeva, S., Mrozek, M., Zillmann, U., Kopp-Schneider, A., Haberkorn, U., Tolle, T., Roggendorf, M., Toshkov, I.: Synergistic hepatocarcinogenic effect of hepadnaviral infection and dietary aflatoxin B_1 in woodchucks. Cancer Res. 55, 3318–3330 (1995)

Metzger, C., Mayer, D., Hoffmann, H., Bocker, T., Benner, A., Bannasch, P.: Sequential appearance and ultrastructure of amphophilic cell foci, adenomas and carcinomas in the liver of male and female rats treated with dehydroepiandrosterone (DHEA). Toxicol. Pathol. 23, 591–605 (1995)

Bannasch, P.: Pathogenesis of hepatocellular carcinoma: sequential cellular, molecular and metabolic changes. In: Prog. in Liv. Dis. Eds: Boyer, J.L., Ockner, R.K., Saunders, W.B., Philadelphia, 16, 161–197 (1996)

Radaeva, S., Bannasch, P.: Changes in catalase and glucose-6-phosphatase distribution patterns within oval cell compartment as possible differentiation markers during viral hepatocarcinogenese in woodchucks. Differentiation 60, 169–178 (1996)

Bannasch, P., Jahn, U.-R., Hacker, H.J., Su, Q., Hoffmann, W., Pichlmayr, R., Otto, G.: Focal hepatic glycogenosis: a putative preneoplastic lesion associated with neoplasia and cirrhosis in explanted human livers. International Journal of Oncology 10, 261–268 (1997)

Dombrowski, F., Bannasch, P., Pfeifer, U.: Hepatocellular neoplasms induced by low-number pancreatic islet transplants in streptozotocin diabetic rats. Am. J. Pathol. 150, 1071–1087 (1997)

4.2 Cancer Risk Due to Dioxin is Very Low in Germany – New Estimates

by Heiko Becher and Karen Steindorf

At least since the accident in Seveso (1976), the evaluation of health risks associated with dioxin has attracted great public interest. Often only a single chemical representative, so-called 2,3,7,8-tetrachlorodibenzo-p-dioxin (TCDD), of this entire class of substances is incorrectly understood to be dioxin. Although TCDD has clearly shown itself to be carcinogenic in animal experiments, the relevant epidemiological data is not as unambiguous as the public assumes. A new evaluation of dioxins by the International Agency for Research on Cancer was performed in the Spring of 1997. As a result of this, TCDD was classified as belonging to Group 1 (carcinogenic for humans) while it had previously been placed in Group 2B (potentially carcinogenic). Knowledge about effects in the low dose range is inadequate. During the past several years, therefore, epidemiological studies have been conducted at the Deutsches Krebsforschungszentrum to better evaluate the cancer risk associated with dioxin both in the world of work and the environment.

What is Dioxin?

Dioxins are molecules that consist of two benzene rings connected by two oxygen bridges to which up to eight chlorine atoms can be bound. Depending on the specific structure, 75 different dioxin molecules can be formed; dioxin serves as the collective term for this class of substances. The extremely poisonous and also the most examined congener is 2,3,7,8-tetrachlorodibenzo-p-dioxin (TCDD) in which chorine atoms are found at binding sites 2,3,7, and 8. This special molecule is biologically very stable. Dioxins are only slightly soluble in water, but are very soluble in fats. They accumulate in the body fat and are stored there for a long time. Dioxins and furans were never the desired products of a chemical reaction, but instead were produced as unwanted byproducts or impurities of the target substance. For example, they are created during the production of 2,4,5-trichlorophenol, an intermediate product used in the production of the herbicide, 2,4,5-trichlorophenoxy acetic acid (2,4,5-T). In the 1950s, this impurity was responsible for significant dioxin exposure among workers producing pesticides. However, this contaminant was reduced until the 1980s through improved procedures.

Today, dioxins and furans are found everywhere throughout the environment in which man finds himself. The most important sources for the introduction of dioxins and furans into our environment are:

- Combustion processes that involve garbage, coal, wood, cigarettes, leaded gasoline, and other substances,

- Chemical industry: certain production processes, use of impure chemicals, and

- Reservoirs in the environment such as contaminated earth or hazardous waste dumps.

Dioxins and furans can always be formed when carbon-containing substances are burned in the presence of chlorine. This can, for example, occur in several processes in chlorine chemistry.

For the past several years in Germany, a trend of decreasing dioxin exposure has been observed.

The behavior of the released substances in the environment is influenced by their poor decomposition with a half-life that is estimated to be approximately three to ten years, their poor solubility in water and a high absorption in the soil, sediment, and wind-borne dust. Dioxin can enter the human organism in four different ways: with food, with water, absorbtion through the skin, and with the inhaled air. Uptake through ingestion is the most significant route since more than 90 percent of dioxin enters the body in this manner.

To estimate the cancer risk associated with dioxins, however, all other dioxins (congeners) as well as the closely related class of substances, the furans, must also be considered. Furans differ from dioxins in that they have only one oxygen bridge between the two benzene rings. In order to be able to jointly evaluate the toxic potency so-called toxic equivalency factors (TEF) are employed. The factor 1 is assigned to 2,3,7,8-TCDD; other congeners have TEF values that range from 0.5 to 0.001. All dioxins or furans are, thereby, grouped together in so-called toxic equivalents.

Exposures in the environment are usually minimal; concentrations lie in the nanogram range. Studies enable one to estimate the background exposure for the population in Germany at approximately 4.3 ng of TCDD per kg of blood fat (median 3 ng/kg) or approximately 20 ng/kg TEQ. Defining the type and magnitude of the health risks associated with this level of exposure (especially with respect to the cancer risk in this low dose range,) is of great significance for reasons of health care.

Consequences for Human Health

As early as the 1950s, it was shown that dioxin can elicit strong, toxic ef-

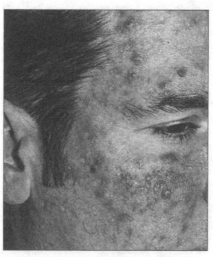

Fig. 26
Chlorinated hydrocarbons cause chloracne. Both the external contact with these substances and their ingestion in food causes dense blackheads that can become inflamed. Chloracne is recognized as an occupational disease

fects. An acute exposure (contact) to a significant quantity of dioxins is marked by the symptom of so-called chloracne, a persistent acnelike condition characterized by comedones, keratin cysts, and inflamed papules with hyperpigmentation. Additional accompanying symptoms may include headaches, muscle pains, difficulty concentrating, memory impairment, nausea, vomiting, as well as somnipathy.

It is known that the mechanism of action at the molecular level for dioxin that has entered the cell can involve its binding to the so-called Ah receptor (Ah stands for aromatic hydrocarbon). This complex then activates genes in the cell nucleus that are usually inactive and explains some of the effects caused by the dioxins. For example,

the binding of the dioxin/receptor complex to the hereditary substance causes an increased production of enzymes that oxidize foreign substances in the liver cells. In addition to intracellular processes, other mechanisms of action for dioxins are being discussed. Among other possibilities, these influence hormone metabolism as well as cell growth and differentiation. The same mechanism of action involving the Ah receptor has been observed both in humans and in laboratory animals. This fact significantly contributes to the plausibility of assuming that the carcinogenic effect of TCDD in animals may correspond to an analogous effect in human beings.

Knowledge concerning the causing of cancer by dioxin in human beings is based on different epidemiological studies that mainly concerned themselves with the effects of 2,3,7,8-TCDD in individuals exposed to significant quantities of this substance. For example, a cohort study of employees at the company, BASF, who in 1953 were exposed to dioxins as a result of an explosion that occurred in a facility used to produce (2,4,5,-trichlorophenoxy) acetic acid, provides important conclusions about the health effects of TCDD. Agent orange, a mixture of the herbicides 2,4,5-trichlorophenoxy acetic acid and 2,4-dichlorophenoxy acetic acid, was used as a deforestation agent during the Vietnam war. It contained TCDD in significant concentrations so that one can today still observe the health consequences in the affected Vietnamese population and in Vietnam veterans. However, dioxins most significantly became a topic of public discussion in 1976 when a chemical factory exploded in the small north Italian town of Seveso and released massive quantities of TCDD into the surrounding area.

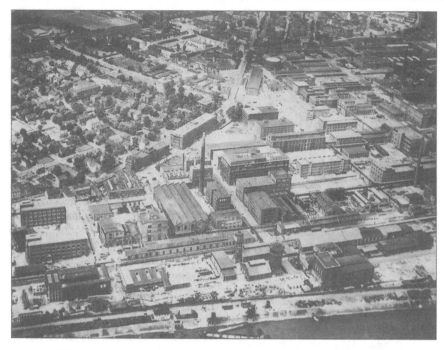

4

Fig. 27
One of the most well-known examples of a German industrial catastrophe in which dioxin was released is the explosion at BASF in 1953. A picture of the plant in 1952 is shown here

The epidemiological studies that have contributed the most to an overall quantitative evaluation of the carcinogenic effect of TCDD deal with the exposure of industrial workers. Of these four studies, one originates in the USA, one is from the Netherlands, and two were conducted in Germany. Among the latter studies is the one on the Boehringer cohort (employees of Boehringer Ingelheim), which was compiled at the Krebsforschungszentrum and at the Medical Center of Chemical Workers Health in Hamburg.

The Boehringer Cohort

A group of 1,189 male employees who worked for Boehringer Ingelheim at the factory in Hamburg-Moorfleet from 1952 to 1984 currently provides the most exact database for evaluating the cancer risk following exposure to dioxin and for the necessary dose/effect analyses. The company produced various herbicides and insecticides that included (2,4,5-trichlorophenoxy)acetic acid and lindane. In this context, substantial exposure not only to TCDD, but also to higher chlorinated dioxins (hexa-, hepta-, octa-) and furans (hexa- and hepta-) occurred. This cohort was marked by the presence of an especially large number of dioxin and furan measurements conducted on the blood or fat tissue of the participants. In contrast, earlier studies usually limit their characterization of the exposure to membership in certain production processes, the duration of such memberships or the appearance of chloracne.

The possibility of using concentrations in biological materials such as blood or fat tissue as surrogate variables is based on great advances made during the past several decades in analytical chemistry and in the detectability of dioxins. However, even today this procedure is still very complicated and expensive. A single measurement costs approximately DM 2,000.

The first important step in determining the exposure in that part of the cohort for which at least one measurement was available entailed examining the kinetic behavior of the individual congeners. There was good agreement with first order kinetics; this means an exponential decay with time. Furthermore, the half-life, i.e. the time period until half the substance has been eliminated,

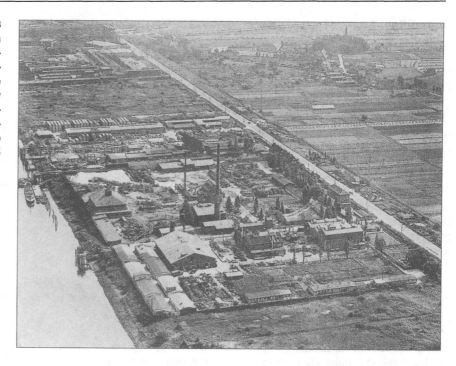

Fig. 28
Employees of the Boehringer Ingelheim factory at Hamburg-Moorfleet were exposed to dioxins and furans at their workplace until 1984. Measurements of these substance classes in the blood and fatty tissue provided scientists with the necessary data to assess the carcinogenic effect of dioxin. The factory is shown here in 1955

could be estimated. This value, for example, was 6.9 years for TCDD. Based on backward extrapolations that used the measured values and estimated workplace-specific assimilation rates, it was possible to evaluate models for the exposure to individual congeners that depended on the work history of individual employees. This model could subsequently be applied to all the members of the cohort so that for every person and at every time an estimate of the concentration or the cumulative (accumulated) exposure was available. Overall, this cohort study made possible the determination of the quantitative relationship between exposure and mortality due to cancer under the consideration of important accompanying exposures as the starting point of a risk evaluation for the individual dioxins and furans.

Overall, 413 people died during the observation time period; of these, 124 deaths were due to cancer. This is significantly more than would be expected based on the general mortality rate for the population at large. Stated more precisely, the cancer mortality rate is 41 percent higher. In contrast to many other carcinogenic substances, this concentration of cancer deaths is distributed to many cancer locations; this observation could be made in all available studies that have been conducted on a worldwide basis. Our evaluations confirm the state of knowledge that has existed to this day, namely that 2,3,7,8-TCDD should be classified as carcinogenic to human beings.

The estimated magnitude of the risk of developing cancer among the Boeh-

ringer employees must be viewed in relation to the magnitude of the exposure that existed at their workplace. Values exceeding 1,000 ng TCDD per kg of blood fat were still measured in several workers a long time after they had completed their employment. This means that an actual concentration at the time that they actively participated in their job can be calculated to be still higher, specifically by a factor of approximately 10 to 100. If one compares this to the concentrations in the general population, there is no reason to be extremely worried or even to panic. However, we would like to emphasize the importance of continuing with the very successful measures to reduce the exposure of the environment to dioxins and furans that have been undertaken during the past several years.

Dose-Effect Analyses and Risk Evaluation

On the basis of the data obtained in the Boehringer cohort and by applying adequate statistical methods, it is possible to estimate a dose-effect function. Using this model, it is then also feasible to make estimates in the low dose range. To this purpose it is first necessary to determine whether or not the risk of developing cancer increases with an increasing dose. This was clearly the case; individuals in the group receiving the greatest exposure were subject to a risk that was approximately twice as large.

However, the validity of a function that describes the relationship between dose and cancer risk must always be carefully interpreted. According to our results, the risk increases sublinearly with the dose. This means that the increase of the dose/effect function is stronger in the low dose range. But the statistical difference to a linear function is only slightly developed so that additional interpretations of the functional form are not possible.

To estimate the risk associated with dioxin in the general population under the prevailing conditions of exposure and also compared to other hazardous substances in the environment, the so-called unit risk concept may be used. For the german population, values for TCDD concentration in the ambient air are given at 8.7 femtograms (fg) per cubic meter in industrial areas or 1.3 fg per cubic meter in the countryside. Applying the unit risk, it follows that the average additional risk over a lifetime lies in the rage of ten to a power of minus six. Therefore, the portion of environmentally caused cancer deaths due to TCDD in the form of an air pollutant, even when compared to other such pollutants, is estimated at being very small indeed.

Priv.-Doz. Dr. Heiko Becher
Dr. Karen Steindorf
Division of Epidemiology

Participating staff
Sabine Holzmeier

In collaboration with

Dr. Dieter Flesch-Janys
Prof Dr. Alfred Manz
Dipl. Stat. Petra Gurn
Medical Center for
Chemical Workers Health,
Hamburg

Dr. Manolis Kogevinas
Dr. Paolo Bofetta
Dr. Rodolfo Saracci
International Agency for
Research on Cancer,
Lyon, France

Selected publications

Flesch-Janys, D., Becher, H.: Risk assessment for dioxins: Using epidemiological data from cancer mortality cohort studies in exposed workers. Informatik, Biometrie und Epidemiologie in Medizin und Biologie 25, 283-291 (1994)

Steindorf, K., Becher, H.: Absolute risk estimates and related parameters in quantitative risk assessment. Informatik, Biometrie und Epidemiologie in Medizin und Biologie 25, 225–232 (1994)

Becher, H., Steindorf, K., Wahrendorf, J.: Epidemiologische Methoden der Risikoabschätzung für krebserzeugende Umweltstoffe mit Anwendungsbeispielen. Hrsg.: Umweltbundesamt Berlin. Erich Schmidt Verlag, Berlin (1995)

Becher, H., Flesch-Janys, D., Kauppinen, T., Kogevinas, M., Steindorf, K., Manz, A., Wahrendorf, J.: Cancer mortality in German male workers exposed to phenoxy herbicides and dioxins. Cancer Causes and Control 7, 312–321 (1996)

Flesch-Janys, D., Becher, H., Gurn, P., Jung, D., Konietzko, J., Manz, A., Päpke, O.: Elimination of polychlorinated dibenzo-p-dioxins and dibenzo-furans (PCDD/F) in occupationally exposed persons. J Toxicol Environ Health 47, 363–378 (1996)

Kogevinas, M., Becher, H., Benn, T., Bertazzi, P.-A., Bofetta, P., Bueno-de-Mesquita, B., Coggon, D., Colin, D., Flesch-Janys, D., Fingerhut, M., Green, L., Kauppinen, T., Littorin, M., Lynge, E., Matthews, J., Neuberger, M., Pearce, N., Saracci, R.: Cancer mortality in workers exposed to phenoxy herbicides and dioxins. An international cohort study. Am J Epid 145, 1061–1075 (1997).

4.3 Familial Breast Cancer: A Risk Assessment

by Jenny Chang-Claude
and Heiko Becher

There is now unequivocal evidence that genetic factors are involved in the etiology of breast cancer. Approximately 5 percent of all breast cancers result from a hereditary susceptibility to the disease. In these cases, the mutation of a predisposing gene is deemed responsible for the early manifestation of this disease in several female members of a family. In 1990, using genetic linkage analysis of families with multiple cases of breast cancer or breast and ovarian cancer, a gene (BRCA1, breast cancer gene 1) was located on chromosome 17. The BRCA1 gene was isolated in 1994 and several of the mutations responsible for causing the disease were identified. One year later,

another dominant breast cancer susceptibility gene, BRCA2, was located and then isolated on chromosome 13.

Despite the fact that familial breast cancer is a relatively rare disease, these findings have attracted a great deal of attention in scientific journals as well as in the daily press. This has led to increased concern and hope among attending physicians as well as in families with a familial aggregation of early and late onset breast cancers. This has regenerated an urgent need for individualized counseling. Women from families in which one or more relatives are or have been affected with breast cancer now wish to learn about their own risk and the risk of their daughters. Some of

Fig. 29
A family-based study of breast and ovarian cancer conducted by the Center since 1991 intends to determine the probability of these diseases with respect to certain genes. Among other activities, the participating women complete a questionnaire

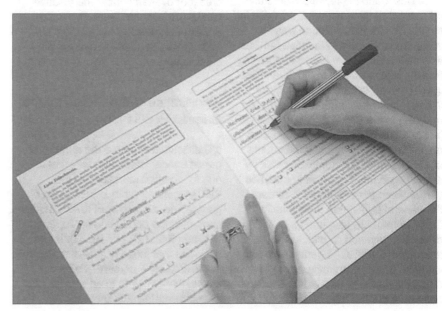

the contributions that we have made in the context of an ongoing project will be presented.

There have been enormous advances in our knowledge with regard to the genetic basis of breast cancer in the last few years. A risk assessment conducted in a manner that was still common only five years ago must today be viewed as being for the most part outdated.

Breast Cancer Genes

The BRCA1 (breast cancer gene 1) gene is located on the long arm of chromosome 17. This gene is not only involved in the development of breast cancer, but also plays a role in ovarian cancer. Linkage analysis in families with several members affected by early onset breast cancer was used to localize this gene. However, linkage between the DNA markers and the disease was found in only approximately 45 percent of all the families included in the study. The BRCA1 gene was involved most frequently in those families with multiple cases of breast cancer before the age of 45 and in those families in which ovarian cancer also occurred. Women who have inherited a germ-line mutation in the BRCA1 gene are subject to an extremely high risk for developing breast cancer during the course of their lifetime. The cumulative risk by age 70 is about 85 percent in mutation carriers compared to about 7 percent in the general population. Additionally, these women are also at high risk for developing ovarian cancer. In the meantime, the BRCA1 gene has been isolated. It is an extremely large gene that stretches over nearly 100,000 base pairs of genomic DNA. Many mutations

that are predicted to have functional relevance have been identified in this gene.

A second breast cancer gene, the BRCA2 gene, is located on the long arm of chromosome 13. Extending over more than 70,000 base pairs and composing of 25 coding exons, it is even larger than the BRCA1 gene that was first discovered. Mutations in this gene also confer a very high risk of developing breast cancer. Furthermore, men who are carriers of BRCA2 mutations are also at increased risk of developing breast cancer: it amounts to approximately 6 percent by age 70 compared to a roughly 0.1 percent risk in the general population. The risk for ovarian cancer is elevated over the general population, but lower than for BRCA1. This gene also shows a broad mutation spectrum.

It is estimated that in 70 to 80 percent of all families with four or more cases of breast or ovarian cancer the disease can be attributed to these two genes. Additional breast cancer susceptibility genes must be involved and remain to be discovered.

Significance of the Genes for the German Population

It is difficult to estimate the number of breast cancer cases annually that are due to inherited mutations of the BRCA1 gene or other breast cancer genes. The number of BRCA1 mutation carriers in the population could range between 5 and 20 per 10,000. If one assumes that these numbers represent approximately 5 percent of all the cases, this amounts to an annual total of approximately 2,200 hereditary

breast cancer cases among an estimated 43,000 new cases of breast cancer that occur each year in Germany. Thus, the majority (95 percent) of breast cancer is sporadic; the aetiology of these cases is still not clarified.

Risk Assessment

During genetic counseling, women can be provided with estimates of their risk of developing breast cancer by a certain age. At present, the accuracy of such a risk estimation depends on the information that is available from the family history and the results of molecular genetic analysis as well as additional assumptions (e.g., with respect to the mode of inheritance) that must be made.

According to the current state of knowledge, it is appropriate to consider two different cases separately.

Case 1:

The woman seeking counseling has one to two relatives affected with premenopausal breast cancer. The relationships among the family members and the ages at diagnosis are available. The mode of inheritance is not obvious and a molecular genetic analysis cannot be necessarily recommended since the possible benefit when compared to the required effort and expense is minimal.

Case 2:

In three generations of this family, several cases of breast or ovarian cancer have occurred in members who are first or second degree relatives of one another. Therefore, the likelihood is higher that an autosomal dominant breast cancer gene is being inherited in this family. A molecular genetic analysis can be recommended.

The vast majority of individuals seeking counseling today will be compatible with the first case.

Risk Assessment for Case 1:

A counselee at a genetic counseling unit can be a woman (here number 1), who would like to be informed about her own risk of disease, because her mother and grandmother have both developed breast cancer.

The risk calculation is based on a large American epidemiological study, the so-called "Cancer and Steroid Hormone Study (CASH)", whose results were published in 1990. Based on these data, detailed tables were constructed that predict the cumulative risk of breast cancer according to a specific family history of breast cancer. For example, a woman in the USA whose mother and grandmother were affected with breast cancer at ages 42, 45, respectively, has a cumulative lifetime risk of developing breast cancer of 38 percent. This estimate uses methods of survival time analysis for women with a certain family history of the disease. In contrast to Germany, the rate of developing breast cancer in the USA is approximately 20 percent higher. This means that a correction of the tables is required before they can be applied to our population. We have developed the necessary mathematical/statistical methods that form the basis for adapting this information and have published appropriately revised tables. Using these tables, one can determine the

risk for developing breast cancer depending on the age at onset of affected relatives. For the given example, the risk for a woman in Germany is 35 percent.

However, these tables do not consider all the possible combinations of affected first-degree and second-degree relatives. Furthermore, the number of unaffected relatives is not accounted for. The risk can, however, be calculated using a further method which accounts for the probability of being a gene carrier based on the actual family history and family structure. By considering both the number and the age of unaffected relatives, the risks determined with this method are significantly different from those risks estimated with the tables. This method can handle much more complex pedigrees, given that the appropriate computer software is available.

Risk Assessment for Case 2:

For high risk families in which breast cancer and/or ovarian cancer appear as a dominant disease in successive generations and a genetic basis for the disease is sufficiently likely, molecular genetic analysis can provide a better estimate of the risk for developing breast cancer and ovarian cancer. Identifying the mutation that predisposes for the disease in the family enables one to distinguish between those family members who carry the mutation and those who do not. In families with a confirmed mutation in the BRCA1 or BRCA2 gene, female mutation carriers will have a risk of developing breast cancer by age 70 that is approximately 80 percent. The risk for ovarian cancer is also elevated. Inherited mutations in the

BRCA1 or the BRCA2 gene have been confirmed in breast cancer patients from many families including those in our own study as well as families that have been examined at other clinics. In such families, women who do not carry the mutation still have the same risk for developing breast cancer as women in the general population of approximately 7 percent.

Generally, predictive genetic testing is offered only to those aged 18 years or more when they are able to give informed consent. An additional necessary prerequisite involves identifying and confirming the nature of the mutation in an affected member of the family. The logistical and ethical considerations are described in the next section.

Molecular Genetic Analysis ("Gene Testing")

The large size of the two genes and the heterogeneous mutation spectrum render the mutation analysis very cost- and time-intensive. The analysis of mutations in the BRCA1 or BRCA2 gene is currently not routinely available. For the time being, mutation analysis can only be offered to large families with multiple cases of breast or ovarian cancer. These should primarily be premenopausal breast cancer patients because of existing data indicating a lower probability of inherited mutations for cancer at an older age. For example, it is estimated that 70 to 80 percent of the families with four or more cases of breast and ovarian cancer before the age of 60 are due to the BRCA1 gene. In breast cancer only families with at least 4 cases diagnosed before the age of 60 or with 3 cases under 50 years, only about 30 percent is attributed to

BRCA1. The gene is estimated to explain less than 20 percent of families with only 2 cases diagnosed under the age of 50 years. Such estimated a priori probabilities for the BRCA1 gene can be used to determine who should be offered BRCA1 gene testing. However, such probability estimates should only be used as a rough guideline since the probability of finding a mutation will also depend on the degree of relationship among those affected with the disease and the overall size of the family. Families with several affected individuals over several generations are rare nowadays since families generally have a smaller number of children.

Inclusion of Environmental Risk Factors for Breast Cancer

In addition to the genetic disposition, there are many exogenous factors that increase the risk of developing breast cancer. These include a young age at onset of menopause, a later age (after the age of 35) at first pregnancy, late onset of menopause (after the age of 55) and a history of benign breast disease. However, the data of the previously mentioned epidemiological studies indicates that risk estimation based on a certain family history for breast cancer cannot be significantly improved by including additional risk factors. Based on the data of a large, prospective, mammography screening study, a model was developed to assess the risk of developing breast cancer in American women who are examined annually in which the four major risk factors were considered: age at menopause, number of previous breast biopsies, age at first pregnancy and the number of first-degree relatives with

breast cancer. However, this model is not used for risk assessment in the context of genetic counseling, because of existing uncertainties in the estimates used. In our study, we have investigated whether some of these risk factors are associated with an earlier age at diagnosis in carriers of a breast cancer gene. We found indications for such an effect modification. However, since the findings are based on a limited number of cases, they cannot yet be used in genetic counseling.

Conclusions

In Germany, approximately one in fourteen women develops breast cancer over a lifetime. Approximately 10 to 15 percent of those affected women have a mother or a sister who is also affected with breast or ovarian cancer. Especially in such a situation, the female relatives will want to know whether they are at increased risk for breast or ovarian cancer. These concerns also apply to their daughters and to future family planning.

It should be pointed out that only a few breast cancer patients (approximately 5 percent) carry a mutation in a dominantly inheritable breast cancer gene. Most of the breast cancer cases in the general population are sporadic. We are still in the process of identifying the genetic and non-genetic components in the etiology of breast cancer. Genetic testing can improve risk assessment for the unaffected female members in selected families in which a genetic predisposition for breast cancer is highly likely. Information about the difficulties associated with risk assessment should be provided to physicians and patients

to avoid rash and simplistic interpretations of gene testing.

The preceding discussions concerning risk assessment for different family and individual situations should have made clear that the estimate of risk for a given person by using information from the molecular genetic analyses of a large number of family members is a complex task whereby most recent informations should be incorporated. Furthermore, it is the responsibility of the genetic counsellor to explain and discuss the risk assessment in the context of genetic counseling. Before genetic testing, both the counselee and the family members must be informed of the risks, benefits and limitations of the methods used and the type and meaning of results that can be obtained. Discussions should be carried out to assist the counselee in understanding what the estimated risk means for her at her particular age.

One must communicate the fact that the risk may remain even after a negative test result. This comprehensive information should include the indication of the possibility of obtaining unwanted results that may prove distressful to other family members. Implicit in all discussions of the options for genetic testing is the right of the individual not to be tested or not to be informed of the test result. Nonetheless, it may be necessary to also obtain test results from such individuals in order to answer the questions of the woman who is seeking advice.

Despite improvements in early detection, breast cancer remains a disease for which no preventive measures exist. The psychologic stress caused by the threat of breast cancer and the understandable fear of a deforming prophylactic or curative removal of the breast or also the ovary require intensive consultation, guidance, and medical care. Molecular genetic services are becoming increasingly available to women from families with a significant history of breast cancer as adjunct to cancer risk counseling. They can also avail themselves of the services offered at ten centers for "familial breast cancer" supported by the Deutsche Krebshilfe covering the genetic counseling, clinical, and psychological management of persons at high risk. Additionally, we will be involved to coordinate a comprehensive interpretation and evaluation of the rapidly increasing body of available knowledge about the susceptibility genes with respect to its application in informing, advising and guiding affected individuals and their families.

We have been recruiting families with at least three cases of breast or ovarian cancer since 1991 for a family study of hereditary breast and ovarian cancer. This project has received support from the Deutsche Krebshilfe since 1993 and was initially designed with the objective of localizing breast and ovarian cancer susceptibility genes and to identify families with a high probability of linkage to these genes. A large number of our families are being analyzed for mutations in the BRCA1 and BRCA2 genes. We inform both the index patients and their attending physicians of the genetic counseling services which are available to the patients and interested family members in the vicinity of their place of residence. Most of the families do not harbor causal mutations in these genes and will be included in further analyses to localize still unknown breast cancer susceptibility genes.

Dr. Jenny Chang-Claude
Priv.-Doz. Dr. Heiko Becher
Division of Epidemiology

Selected publications

Chang-Claude, J., Eby, N., Becher, H.: Die Bedeutung genetischer Faktoren für die Entstehung von Brustkrebs. Zentralblatt für Gynäkologie 116, 660–669 (1994)

Chang-Claude, J., Becher, H., Hamann, U., Schroeder-Kurth, T.: Risikoabschätzung für das familiäre Auftreten von Brustkrebs. Zentralblatt für Gynäkologie 117, 423–434 (1995)

Becher, H., Chang-Claude, J.: Estimating population specific disease risks for a given family history with an application to breast cancer. Genetic Epidemiology 13, 229–242 (1996)

Chang-Claude, J., Becher H., Eby, N., Bastert, G., Wahrendorf, J., Hamann, U.: Modifying effect of reproductive risk factors on the age at onset of breast cancer for German BRCA1 mutation carriers. J Cancer Res Clin Onc 123, 272–279 (1997)

4.4 Chemoprevention of Cancer: Mechanisms and Strategies for Cancer Control

by Clarissa Gerhäuser
and Norbert Frank

In 1995, about 210 000 people in Germany died of cancer. Statistical analyses reveal that every third German will get cancer during his lifetime, every fourth will die of it. Currently, the mean 5-year survival time after cancer therapy is about 50%. Taking this into account and comparing cancer death rates of the past years it becomes apparent that present strategies of cancer therapy by medication, surgery or radiation are insufficient to lower the number of cancer death in the long term.

Cancer is caused by multiple and divers factors. Smoking is considered as one of the major risk factors. As a fact, about 30% of all cancer death are related to smoking, and every seventh smoker will die of lung cancer. In addition, overweight and wrong eating habits contribute to the cancer risk with up to 30%. Further, recent analyses indicate that a significant rate of cancer cases are based on chronic inflammation and infection. As indicated by these data, a high percentage of cancer incidence is actually preventable, and the most logical and effective means to prevent cancer should be seen in the avoidance of these cancer risk factors – so called primary cancer prevention. However, as an example, anti-smoking campaigns and dietary recommendations have not been widely accepted by the general public. It also should be kept in mind that reduction of cancer risk factors does not necessarily prevent cancer. Beside a more general risk to develop cancer due to bad eating habits, smoking or excessive UV radiation, specific risk factors include familiar or genetic predisposition (e.g., some types of breast, colon, or lung cancer). Naturally, tumors that are not caused by exogenous factors

are hardly preventable by primary prevention. These cases, i.e., second primary tumors, recurrences, and tumors developing from preneoplasia, cause an elevated cancer risk for a specific part of the population. Since primary prevention will not be successful in modifying the risk of these endogenously-caused cancer types, another possibility of prevention is seen in secondary prevention targeted at and interfering with cellular and molecular tumor development.

A potential means of primary as well as secondary prevention is seen in cancer chemoprevention, describing the use of chemicals or dietary components to delay, inhibit or reverse the development of cancer, i.e., the prevention of carcinogenesis prior to diagnosis of a tumor.

This strategy of cancer control is by no means new. In 1934, J.R. Davidson demonstrated that skin tumors of rats were preventable by feeding a vitamin E rich diet. Observation and statistical analysis of eating habits of the general public and epidemiological studies have further indicated that increased uptake of fruits and vegetables are positively linked to a reduced cancer risk.

During the past 30 years numerous natural or synthetic compounds have been tested for their potential to prevent cancer in various animal models. Especially the vitamins A (and related compounds), C, D, and E and plant-derived compounds like phenolic antioxidants, coumarins, aromatic isothiocyanates, thiocarbamates, indoles, flavonoids, and tannins were found to be effective.

Additionally, cancer therapeutic agents, for example the anti-estrogen

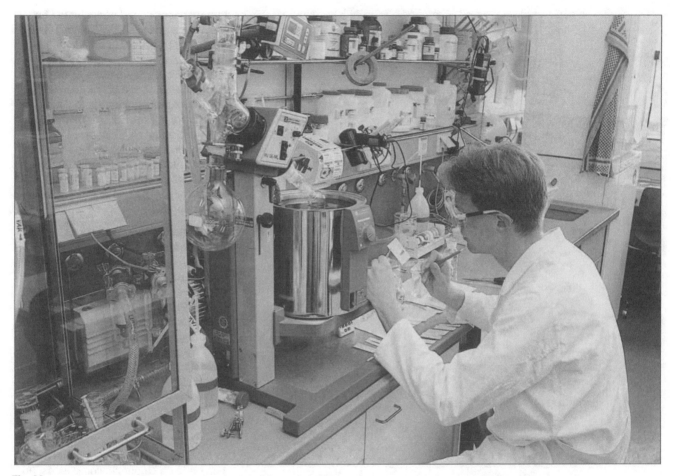

Fig. 30
It is an objective of the working group for "chemoprevention" to optimize the activity of certain natural substances. Scientists identify important structural characteristics of these substances by reproducing them. The product is being tested for purity in this case

tamoxifen used in the treatment of breast cancer, were tested clinically for their efficacy to delay or prevent carcinogenesis with patients belonging to high-risk groups. Tamoxifen binds to the estrogen receptor and, thus, inhibits the transmission of mitogenic signals stimulating cell division and cell proliferation. It could be demonstrated that tamoxifen-treated breast cancer patients had about a 40% reduced risk to develop second primary tumors in the healthy breast. The potential of tamoxifen to prevent breast cancer in healthy individuals belonging to high risk groups (i.e., from families with high breast cancer incidence) is currently tested in three large clinical trials in the USA, Great Britain, and Italy. However, the future use of tamoxifen as a chemopreventive agent might be limited by the fact that tamoxifen was found to elevate the risk to develop endometrial cancer by a factor of three, even though this type of cancer is generally less widespread than breast cancer. Another example of a

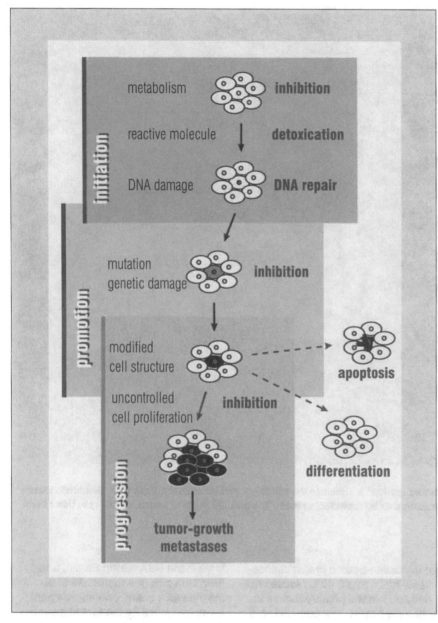

Fig. 31
The diagram shows the different stages of carcinogenesis which are called the initiation, promotion, and progression phases. Furthermore, possible approaches for various natural substances, nutritional components, and synthetic compounds to slow down, inhibit or reverse carcinogenesis are presented

therapeutically used agent tested for preventive activity is finasteride, effective in the treatment of benign prostate hyperplasia. This compound was found to inhibit 5α-reductase, an enzyme catalyzing the conversion of the sex hormone testosterone to dihydrotestosterone. Since dihydrotestosterone was found to be involved in the development of prostate hypertrophy and prostate cancer, the potential of finasteride to prevent prostate cancer is currently being tested in a chemoprevention trial.

As mentioned above, safety aspects are important in selecting natural or synthetic compounds as chemopreventive agents. Since the success of cancer prevention often involves long-term application of preventive agents, these compounds have to fulfill strict criteria regarding side effects and toxicity which exceed those required for therapeutic agents, especially if they are intended to be applied to the healthy general population. On the other hand, for high risk groups, i.e., families with high cancer incidence, individuals with a genetic cancer predisposition (breast or colon cancer) or high workplace exposure to carcinogenic compounds, an elevated risk of side effects might be acceptable if linked to a potential benefit.

The development of cancer is a slow, multistage process that might take up to 20 years, and it would be wrong to consider a person as healthy until a tumor has been diagnosed. Carcinogenesis can be regarded as an accumulation of genetic or biochemical cell damage which offers a variety of targets for chemopreventive agents during the initiation, promotion or progression stage (scheme) .

80

Activation of Drug Metabolism

Modulation of enzymes involved in metabolic activation and excretion of carcinogens is one of the best investigated mechanisms of chemopreventive agents. Phase 1 enzymes activate xenobiotics by addition of functional groups which render these compounds more water-soluble. Then, Phase 2 enzymes conjugate the activated compounds to endogenous ligands like glutathione, glucuronic, acetic or sulfuric acid, thus, enhancing their excretion in form of these conjugates. Since Phase 1 enzymes might contribute to the activation of carcinogens while Phase 2 enzymes are involved in their detoxication, inhibition of Phase 1 enzymes concomitantly with induction of Phase 2 enzymes is considered a logical strategy in chemoprevention, which is especially beneficial in early stages of carcinogenesis. Compounds able to activate Phase 2 drug-detoxifying enzymes include agents like sulforaphane, an isothiocyanate isolated from broccoli, sulfur-containing components of Allium species like onion and garlic, dithiolethiones like oltipraz, which is currently tested for its efficacy in preventing liver cancer in a large scale prevention trial in China, flavonoids, or indoles and glucosinolates from cruciferous vegetables like broccoli, cauliflower, Brussels sprouts, or cabbage.

Antioxidants and anti-mutagens

Insufficient oxygen consumption in mitochondria during fat metabolism (lipid peroxidation) might result in the production of reactive oxygen species (ROS). Generally, in a healthy organism formation of ROS is controlled by endogenous mechanisms including enzymes, like catalase or superoxide dismutase, and glutathione, a cellular antioxidant. Manifestation of oxidative stress (immune diseases, chronic inflammation, infection) disturb the intracellular homeostasis of pro-oxidants and antioxidants. Overproduction of ROS results in DNA damage, for example the formation of oxidized DNA bases. This might lead to mistakes during DNA replication (mutations) causing genetic alterations of the cell. Compounds like vitamins C and E, chlorohyllin, a compound related to the green color of leaves, coumarins, curcumin, a component of curry, ellagic acid found in high concentrations in various kinds of fruits and nuts, and polyphenolic agents including epigallocatechin-gallate from green tea were identified as potent inhibitors of cellular oxidation and lipid peroxidation processes. The components of green tea were shown to possess chemopreventive activity in a variety of animal models. In Japan, it could further be demonstrated that drinking of at least 10 cups of green tea per day delayed cancer onset in females by almost 9 years. Yet, in two long-term large scale chemoprevention trials, the antioxidant β-carotene, a major carotenoid found in orange or red-colored vegetables like carrots failed to prevent lung cancer in heavy smokers; in both trials, lung cancer incidence was elevated in smokers receiving β-carotene.

Curcumin, ellagic acid, green tea polyphenoles, and isocyanates derived from watercress were further shown to reduce cellular damage caused by reaction of carcinogens like aflatoxins or components of cigarette smoke with DNA or proteins (adducts) resulting in mistakes during DNA duplication. N-acetylcysteine, a cough remedy dissolving mucous secretions, seems to act by a similar mechanism and is currently tested in the 'European Study on Chemoprevention' (EUROSCAN) for prevention of head and neck cancer.

Inhibition of arachidonic acid metabolism

Epidemiological studies indicate that regular use of aspirin (acetylsalicylic acid) is linked to a reduced cancer risk. Acetylsalicylic acid irreversibly inhibits enzymes playing a substantial role in the biosynthesis of prostaglandins from arachidonic acid, i.e., cyclooxygenase 1 and 2 (COX-1 and -2). Prostaglandins are hormone-like endogenous mediators of inflammatory processes. Since prostaglandin levels are often elevated in tumor tissue in comparison to normal tissue and COX-2 activity is inducible during the development of tumor cells, non-steroidal anti-inflammatory drugs (NSAIDs) including aspirin, piroxicam, indomethacin or sulindac, and plant-derived inhibitors of the arachidonic acid cascade are regarded as promising chemopreventive agents. Examples of natural COX inhibitors include curcumin, green tea polyphenols, sulfur-containing components of onions and garlic, and resveratrol, which is contained in high concentrations in grapes and red wine and was identified recently as a potential new chemopreventive agent. Interestingly, in addition to the inhibition of the arachidonic acid cascade, NSAIDs seem to activate programmed cell death (apoptosis) of damaged cells. Since long-term use of NSAIDs might cause severe side-effects like intestinal ulceration and gastrointestinal bleeding, further studies have to evaluate the potential of NSAIDs to be used as chemopreventatives for high risk individuals. Prof. Hans Osswald from the Deutsches Krebsforschungszentrum and Dr. Günther Winde (Department of General Surgery, Westfälische Wilhelms-University, Münster) are currently investigating the influence of sulindac on the regression of adenomatous polyps in a small trial with 38 familial polyposis (FAP) patients. To avoid common gastrointestinal side effects, sulindac is applied as a low dose regimen in form of rectal suppositories as opposed to the conventional oral route. After a four year treatment, complete reversion of adenomatous polyps was observed in 78% and partial reversion in 13% of patients.

Inhibition of Polyamine Synthesis

Ornithine decarboxylase (ODC) catalyses the decarboxylation of ornithine to putrescin, which is further converted to higher polyamines essential for duplication of DNA. Since this pathway is the only source of putrescine in mammalian cells, ODC is regarded as a key enzyme in polyamine biosynthesis. Although ODC and the resulting polyamines are essential for cellular proliferation, induction of ODC is involved in tumor promotion and cell transformation. Cultured tumor cells often contain high levels of ODC. Based on these characteristics, ODC is considered an attractive target in both chemotherapy and chemoprevention. ODC activity is irreversibly inhibited by difluormethylornithine (DFMO), a synthetic analog of ornithine. This compound is currently being tested at the National Cancer Institute (USA) in a small clinical trial with about 100 participants for its potential to prevent breast, cervical, prostate, bladder, colon, and skin cancer. In addition to the direct inhibition of ODC enzyme activity by DFMO, compounds like vitamin A and its derivatives (retinoids), curcumin, epigallocatechin-gallate, rotenoids, and silymarin, a mixture of three flavonoids isolated from the milk thistle Silybum marianum, were found to inhibit the induction of ODC by tumor-promoters without reducing intrinsic ODC activity. Extracts from rosemary or ginger have similar activities on tumor promoter-mediated induction of ODC. However, the active principle of these extracts is not identified yet. Chemopreventive activity of these compounds and extracts has been demonstrated in animal models.

Signal Transduction

Further insight into the molecular mechanisms of signal transduction and characterization of essential receptors and enzymes has revealed a variety of new targets for chemoprevention. These include various kinases and phosphatases, which by transient phosphorylation (transfer of phosphate groups) or dephosphorylation of target proteins deliver extracellular mitogenic signals to the nucleus. Genetic damage and mutations can cause continuous activation of these proteins resulting in uncontrolled proliferation and cell growth. As an example, mutations in the Ras oncoprotein were found to induce cell transformation. Ras mutations were detected in 15% of all diagnosed tumors, the incidence being especially high in patients with pancreatic cancer (up to 90%). Ras protein is activated by transfer of a lipophilic farnesyl group. This post-translational modification facilitates the association of Ras with the cell membrane which is essential for Ras-mediated activation of target proteins in the signal transduction pathway. Interestingly, monoterpenes like limonene and perillyl alcohol, which are contained in high concentrations in citrus fruit oils, were found to inhibit enzymes essential for synthesis and transfer of this farnesyl group and subsequently prevented the activation of Ras. In animal models, these compounds inhibited chemically induced breast, lung, stomach, and liver cancer. First clinical prevention trials with limonene and perillyl alcohol are currently under way in the UK and USA, respectively.

Induction of Cell Differentiation

Cancer can be regarded as an imbalance of cell proliferation and cell differentiation, i.e., cell maturation and development to a defined cell type. Consequently, induction of cell differentiation to a normal, not cancerous phenotype is regarded as an important mechanism of cancer chemoprevention. The potential of retinoids (vitamin A and derivatives) to induce cell differentiation is well established. These compounds were found to potently reduce the growth of head and neck cancers, which are mainly caused by high alcohol consumption and heavy smoking. Vitamin D and derivatives as well as genistein found in high concentration in soy products were also identified as potent inducers of differentiation. Genistein additionally seems to inhibit angiogenesis, i.e., the formation of blood vessels important for tumor growth.

Cancer is a disease caused by a complex network of multiple factors. Based on established targets and mechanisms in the multistage process of carcinogenesis, the group 'Cancer Chemoprevention' at the Krebsforschungszentrum is developing in vitro test systems suitable for the detection of novel cancer chemopreventive agents. Investigation of molecular mechanisms of preventive activity of these compounds as well as new insights into the causes of cancer and carcinogenic processes will provide additional targets for potential chemopreventive agents.

The practical use of chemopreventive strategies is still in its infancy. In addition to more general health recommendations like the consumption of a diet rich in fruit and vegetables, cancer chemoprevention is thought to reduce a defined cancer risk by selected chemopreventive agents. At the moment, definite proof of chemopreventive efficacy in man is limited to expensive long-term, large scale chemoprevention trials recruiting thousands of participants and monitoring reduction in cancer incidence by the tested agent. Successful development and application of chemopreventive agents will partly depend on a reduction of these costs and the duration of observation by application of validated biomarkers as surrogate endpoints. Suitable biomarkers might include genetic cell damage or cellular and histological alterations during development of cancer. Ideally, modification of these biomarkers should correlate with the reduction of cancer incidence and provide early evidence of the chemopreventive potential of a test agent. Recent progress in chemoprevention should stimulate intensive investigations in this promising area of current cancer research.

The planned investigations are made possible by generous financial support by the „Verein zur Förderung der Krebsforschung in Deutschland e.V.".

Dr. Clarissa Gerhäuser
Dr. Norbert Frank
Division of Toxicology and Cancer Risk Factors

Participating staff

Christian Herhaus
Jutta Knauft

In cooperation with

Dr. Hans Rudolf Scherf
Division of Toxicology and
Cancer Risk Factors,
Deutsches Krebsforschungszentrum

Prof. Dr. Hans Becker
Pharmacognosy and
Analytical Phytochemistry,
University of Saarland, Saarbrücken

Prof. Dr. Susanne Grabley
Hans-Knöll-Institute of Research on
Natural Substances,
Jena

Dr. Manfred Jung
Institute of Pharmaceutical Chemistry,
Westphalian Wilhelms-University,
Münster

Prof. Ha Van Mao
Center for Cancer Research,
Central Hospital Tran Hung Dao,
Hanoi, Vietnam

Prof. Onyechi O. Obidoa
Department of Biochemistry,
University of Nigeria,
Nsukka, Nigeria

Selected publications

Gerhäuser, C., Mar, W., Lee, S.K., Suh, N., Luo, Y., Kosmeder, J.W., Luyengi, L., Fong, H.H., Kinghorn, A.D., Moriarty, R.M., Mehta, R.G., Constantinou, A., Moon, R.C., Pezzuto, J.M.: Rotenoids mediate potent cancer chemopreventive activity through transcriptional regulation of ornithine decarboxylase. Nature Med. 1, 260–266 (1995)

Gerhäuser, C., You, M., Liu, J., Moriarty, R.M., Hawthorne, M., Mehta, R.G., Moon, R.C., Pezzuto, J.M.: Cancer chemopreventive potential of sulforamate, a novel analog of sulforaphane that induces phase 2 drug-metabolizing enzymes. Cancer Res. 57, 272–278 (1997)

Udeani, G.O., Gerhäuser, C., Thomas, C.F., Moon, R.C., Kosmeder, J.W., Kinghorn, A.D., Moriarty, R.M., Pezzuto, J.M.: Cancer chemopreventive activity mediated by deguelin, a naturally occurring rotenoid. Cancer Res. 57, 3424–3428 (1997)

Gerhäuser, C., Lee, S.K., Kosmeder, J.W., Moriarty, R.M., Hamel, E., Metha, R.G., Moon, R.C., Pezzuto, J.M.: Regulation of ornithine decarboxylase induction by deguelin, a natural product cancer chemopreventive agent. Cancer Res. 57, 3429–3435 (1997)

Bartsch, H., Frank, N., Bertram, B.: Prävention. In: Hämatologie/Onkologie, Kapitel 12. Hrsg.: Ostendorf, P.C., Seeber, S., Verlag Urban und Schwarzenberg, München, 123–132 (1997)

4.5 Advances in Secondary Cancer Prevention: Regression of Precancerous Lesions by a Nonsteroidal Anti-inflammatory Drug (NSAID)

by Hans Osswald

I. Long-term Sulindac Therapy in Patients with Familial Adenomatous Polyposis (FAP) as a Form of Cancer Prevention

Familial adenomatous polyposis (FAP) is an autosomal, dominantly inherited disease characterized not only by the increasing development of predominantly colorectal polyps but also other benign and malignant neoplasias in different organs because of the extracolic manifestation of the underlying disease. Colectomy with ileorectal anastomosis (IRA) represents standard therapy in several polyposis centers, because it is a procedure with low mortality and morbidity rates and good functional outcome. A newer standard method is the ileoanal pouch anastomosis. After removing the large intestine, the polyps remaining in the rectum and the duodenum regress for several years. Because of the dissemination of the polyps that will later once again develop, the possibilities of future surgical intervention are limited.

Therefore, many studies have been conducted to evaluate appropriate drugs that may influence polyp formation. Certain nonsteroidal anti-inflammatory drugs (NSAIDs), especially sulindac, have proven themselves to be effective. The unwanted side effects of NSAID treatment in the usual dose, especially bleeding and mucosal damage of the gastrointestinal tract as well as reduced sodium and water excretion through the kidneys due to the inhibition of prostaglandin synthesis, contribute to possible risks during the required long-term treatment. The withdrawal of NSAID results in a reoccurring of adenomatous polyps within about 6 to 9 weeks.

In our study, which was conducted in collaboration with Oberarzt Prof. Dr. Günther Winde of the Clinic and Polyclinic for General Surgery at the University of Münster, we sought out possibilities for avoiding the unwanted effects ("side effects") that are to be expected when administering sulindac in the usual dose of 300-400 mg daily per patient. In comparison to taking the drug orally, rectal administration of sulindac should result in a delayed uptake and a lower concentration of the drug in the gastric mucosa. Within the context of a dose finding study, we primarily intend to ascertain the minimally effective dose of sulindac that proves adenoma-reversion and prevents a new formation of adenomas.

Beginning with an induction therapy of 2 x 150 mg sulindac daily per patient for a period of 12 weeks, the daily dose per patient was subsequently reduced to 2 x 100 mg, 2 x 75 mg, 2 x 50 mg and 2 x 25 mg of sulindac. The results obtained indicated that a maintenance dose of 2 x 25 mg of sulindac was sufficient for all but 3 patients who required 2 x 75 mg of sulindac daily.

The non-randomized, controlled phase 1 pilot study includes 10 FAP patients who had undergone a colectomy (removal of the colon - large intestine) in the control group that did not receive treatment. Within the group receiving sulindac therapy, the beginning number of 15 FAP patients who had undergone a colectomy has in the meantime increased to a total of 36 individuals participating in the study. The presence of FAP is confirmed in all the study participants by means of heredity and gene analysis as well as histological analysis. The usual, chance assignment to study groups, the randomization

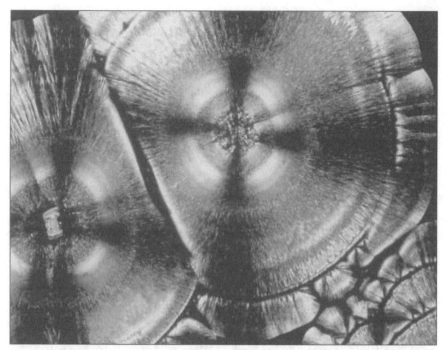

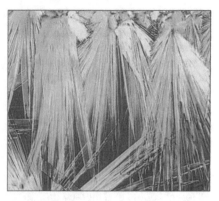

Figs. 32, 33, 34
Vitamins E and C as well as provitamin A (β-carotene) are suitable for cancer prevention. Cancer precursors in the oral mucous membrane regress when this antioxidant combination is taken continuously in a certain dose, and alcohol and tobacco consumption are avoided

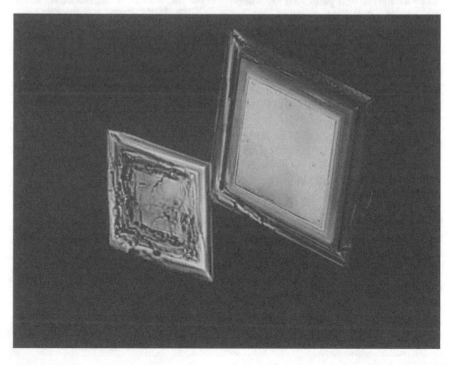

of FAP patients into control or therapy groups, was not performed because of the differing distribution of the adenomatous polyps in the stomach, duodenum, and rectum on the one hand and the different benign tumors in individual patients, on the other hand. It made more sense to include those patients in the control group who had declined to participate in long-term drug therapy. Thereby, the problem of assigning members of the same family to different control and therapy groups could also be avoided.

The possibility of attaining a regression of adenomas by means of a low-dose, maintenance sulindac therapy, using one sixth the usual sulindac dose, is confirmed for the current observation time period of 62 months. Meanwhile, the possibility of immediately beginning a low-dose, long-term sulindac therapy in FAP patients who have undergone a colectomy has been considered, because the required time until complete regression of the adenomas indicates no significant differences from the originally used induction therapy at the usual dose of 2 x 150 mg sulindac per day.

The antidysplastic effectiveness of the low sulindac dose is probably due to the limited formation of sulindac acyl-glucuronide within the organism. In vitro, the highest possible dose of sulindac that can be tolerated by human beings (in vivo) does not even induce any inhibition of cell growth.

The abnormal activation of the ras oncogene plays a role in the development of adenomas. After nine months of low-dose sulindac maintenance therapy, the abnormal activation is completely reversed. The overexpression of the bcl2 gene prevents the occurrence of programmed cell death in various types of cells. Sulindac maintenance therapy inhibits the overexpression of bcl2. The level of mutated p53 protein is also reduced during low-dose sulindac maintenance therapy. Thereby, normal apoptosis, the ability (and natural task) of individual cells to die some day, is reestablished. This provides a possible explanation for the mechanism of action; but also indicates the necessity of long-term therapy. Furthermore, this tumor prevention study also confirms the possibility of intervening in genetically caused, inheritable diseases at a level that follows the regulation of cell growth, namely translation.

The low-dose, maintenance therapy with the NSAID sulindac effects a regression and prevents the new formation of adenomas in a group of patients with FAP who have undergone a colectomy for almost five years. So far, there have been no unwanted effects and neither a short-term interruption nor a termination of the treatment has been required. A long-term therapy with sulindac is necessary in order to prevent the new formation of adenomas that will reoccur if treatment is terminated. The regression of adenomas under sulindac long-term therapy appears to be due to the reestablishment of apoptosis. The polyposis of the exit opening of the biliary and pancreatic ducts in the duodenum (papilla Vateri) that exists in some of the FAP patients requires additional biochemical and pharmacological investigation so that a complete regression of adenomas can also be achieved at this localization.

Prof. Dr. Hans Osswald
Division of Toxicology and Cancer Risk Factors

In collaboration with

Prof. Dr. Günther Winde
Clinic and Polyclinic for General Surgery, University of Münster

Selected publications

Winde, G., Gumbinger, H. G., Osswald, H., Kemper, F., Bünte, H.: The NSAID sulindac reverses rectal adenomas in colectomized patients with familial adenomatous polyposis: clinical results of a dose-finding study on rectal sulindac administration. Int. J. Colorectal Dis. 8, 13–17 (1993)

Winde, G., Schmid, K. W., Schlegel, W., Fischer, R., Osswald, H., Bünte, H.: Complete reversion and prevention of rectal adenomas in colectomized patients with familial adenomatous polyposis by rectal low-dose sulindac maintenance treatment. Dis. Colon Rectum 38, 813–830 (1995)

Winde, G., Schmid, K. W., Brandt, B., Müller, R., Osswald, H.: Clinical and genomic influence of sulindac on rectal mucosa in familial adenomatous polyposis (FAP) Dis. Colon Rectum 39, A8 (1996)

Winde, G., Schmid, K. W., Brandt, B., Müller, R., Osswald, H.: Clinical and genomic influence of sulindac on rectal mucosa in familial adenomatous polyposis (FAP) Dis. Colon Rectum 40, 1156–1169 (1997)

II. Preventive Treatment of Oral Dysplasias as a New Method of Cancer Prevention

The long-term survival in the treatment of oral cancer with a combination of surgery, chemotherapy and/or radiotherapy is limited by the possibility of a renewed formation of tumors in the oral mucosa, so-called local recurrences, and the formation of metastases in the neighboring lymph nodes. In comparison to other forms of cancer such as those affecting the lung, the breast or the colon, distant metastases develop relatively late. In advanced stages of oral cancer, the recurrence rate amounts to approximately 70 % within three years after the onset of treatment. The high rate of reoccuring carcinomas within the oral mucosa seems to be caused by dysplasias existing simultaneously or occuring delayed. First reports concerning the appearance of re-developing carcinomas go back to Theodor Billroth (1879). The proposed field theory (1945) of Rupert A. Willis assumes that the carcinoma develops from several tumor precursors that are found in a field of varying size. Not only the mucous membrane of a single organ, but the entire region of the upper aerodigestive tract that has been exposed to chronic damage can be affected by the multicentric development of cancer. In the case history of the majority of patients, tobacco and alcohol consumption play a role as factors that cause chronic damage.

Since the multimodal concepts for the treatment of advanced oral cancer that have been used until now have made no decisive progress, it appears that the prevention of dysplasias in the oral mucosa may be a promising advantage. However, a prerequisite for this is that the necessary long-term therapy has no unwanted effects and is not likely to induce resistance in the target tissue to the substances used. Based on experience, the effectiveness of a cancer-preventing substance (this means a substance that prevents the formation of a carcinoma or causes the regression of a dysplasia) can be recognized within three months. In the case of effective cancer-preventing substances, a number of study participants ranging between 10 and 15 proves sufficient to decide whether or not to end or continue the study. In contrast to earlier, comprehensive, long-term studies , the use of biomarkers (in this case of dysplasias for later cancer development) has proven itself to be a feasible procedure for rational cancer prevention. However, most of the chemopreventive (antidysplastic) substances that prevent cancer must be administered for the long-term in order to guarantee a permanent dysplasia regression (this means preventing the development of a form of cancer).

In a study consisting of two groups of 24 patients each that we conducted in collaboration with Prof. Dr. Dr. Joachim Zöller from the Clinic and Polyclinic for Oral and Maxillofacial Surgery of the University of Heidelberg, we used a combination of antioxidants that consisted of β-carotene (provitamin A), β-tocopherol (vitamin E), and ascorbic acid (vitamin C). This combination offers many advantages because of its very good tolerability. Its intended use is not to prevent vitamin deficiencies by means of minimal doses, but instead is administered in a supernutritionally, pharmacologically effective dose for cancer prevention.

The first group of patients suffered from leukoplakia (white spots caused by proliferation of the epithelium), a form of dysplastic lesions. After withdrawal of alcohol and tobacco, these spots did not regress within the three month period that followed. The second group consisted of patients whose primary carcinoma of the oral cavity had been treated with cisplatin and 5-fluoruracil as well as subsequent surgical removal of the carcinoma. Of these patients, however, only four had stopped consuming alcohol and tobacco. In order to assess the possible influence of the cancer-preventing treatment with the selected antioxidant combination, the following examinations were performed during the subsequent three months at a distance of approximately two centimeters from the former tumor resection line: histological evaluation of the oral mucous membrane in a hematoxylin-eosin stained section, DNA flow cytometry, staining of the nucleolus organizer region, determination of the micronuclei (the micronuclei originate from chromosome regions that split irregularly during anaphase.) and the cytokeratin expression as an epithelial differentiation marker.

In both groups of patients, the antioxidant combination induces a decrease in the elevated initial values of the cell proportion that is found in S-phase within the dysplastic area. In a similar manner, the number and size of the nucleolus and the nucleolus organizer region clearly decreases in both patient groups; the increased micronuclei also indicate a striking decrease. Furthermore, in both groups, the antioxidant combination achieves a statistically sig-

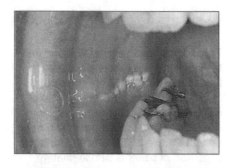

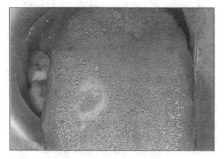

Figs. 35, 36
In 47 of 48 patients, the oral mucosa normalized itself during the regular ingestion of β-carotene and vitamins E and C. Flat, white changes in the mucous membrane which are early dysplasias of oral cancer regress within 12 weeks (fig. 35). These flat, white nodules of the skin and mucous membrane, shown in fig. 36, are described as "sugar cookies" in the vernacular. These also regress when the antioxidants in supranutritional doses are regularly consumed

nificant decrease of the cytokeratin gene expression that was elevated before treatment (especially the suprabasal expression of keratin 10). In a similar manner, the histological examination yields a significant „redifferentiation" of the dysplastic changes in the oral mucosa for both groups of patients. This is probably due to apoptosis of the dysplastic cells. However, these changes in the dysplastic area can only be maintained by continuing the use the combination of antioxidants; stopping their ingestion for more than 7 to 12 weeks leads to a renewed development of dysplasias. The antioxidant combination used during the 58 month course of this study caused no unwanted effects, with the sole exception of discrete skin tanning due to the β-carotene.

Additional cancer-preventing (chemo-preventive) studies are planned in the clinical area.

The following requires further investigation:

– the required duration of the long-term treatment with the antioxidant combination;

– measuring the tissue concentration of the used antioxidants in dysplastic and normal mucosa;

– the mechanism by which the „redifferentiation" of dysplastic changes caused by the antioxidants occurs.

Apoptosis, programmed cell death, could represent the most effective mechanism and would also provide a logical explanation for the reoccurence of dysplasia(s) after the withdrawal of antioxidant drugs; the effectiveness of

other cancer-preventing natural substances combined with ascorbic acid and α-tocopherol.

Thanks are owed to Merck AG, Darmstadt, for supporting this research.

Prof. Dr. Hans Osswald
Division of Toxicology and Cancer Risk Factors

In collaboration with

Prof. Dr. Dr. Joachim Zöller
Clinic and Polyclinic for Oral, Maxillofacial, and Plastic Surgery of the University of Heidelberg

Selected publications

Zöller, J., Flentje, M., Born, I.A., Osswald, H.: Influence of cisplatin and 5-fluorouracil in the oral mucosa. Oral Oncology. Eur. J. Cancer 30B, 200–203 (1994)

Zöller, J., Flentje, M., Maier, H., Born, I.A., Osswald, H.: Influence of beta-Carotin, vitamin C and E on oral dysplasia. Anal. Cell Pathol. 6, 420 (1994)

Zöller, J., Maier, H., Flentje, M., Born, I. A., Osswald, H.: Der Einfluß einer Cisplatin-5-Fluorouracil-Kombinationschemotherapie auf die maligne Transformation des Epithels der Mundschleimhaut. HNO 42, 257–263 (1994)

Zöller, J., Flentje, M., Born, I.A., Osswald, H.: Die Redifferenzierung oraler Präkanzerosen durch die Antioxidantienkombination β-Carotin, α-Tocopherol und Ascorbinsäure – eine Möglichkeit der Chemoprävention? Z. Onkol. 28, 29–41 (1996)

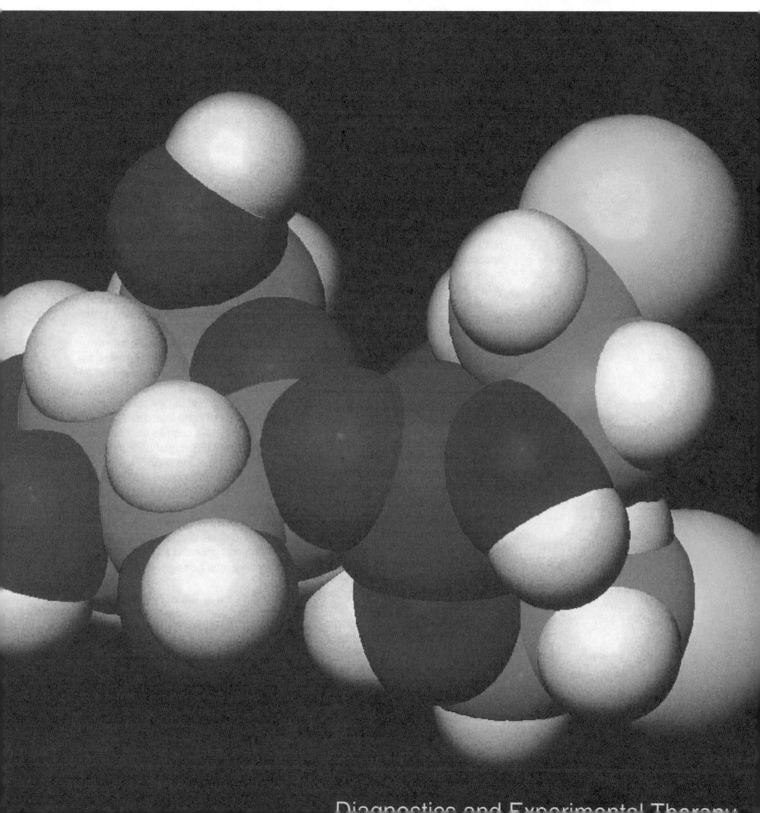

Diagnostics and Experimental Therapy

5

Diagnostics and Experimental Therapy

This Research Program has set itself the task of providing the prerequisites for developing new therapeutic and diagnostic procedures, an aim which it pursues by bringing together clinical- and fundamental-research groups.

The Division of Cell Growth and Division is pursuing investigations of the centromer/kinetochor complex, the point of contact between the distribution apparatus and the chromosome. For many tumor cells, an imbalance occurs in the distribution of genetic material between the daughter cells. This gives rise to aneupleoidy, a loss or gain of chromosomes. Such distribution errors cause additional damage to the cells and are a typical feature of malignant tumor cells. Their analysis with molecular-biological, biochemical, and morphological methods can lead to improved therapy.

Studies in the Division Perinatal Toxicology concentrate on sensitizing and protective factors for chemotherapy. The division's work also contributes to the development of new substances and their application. Together with the construction of pharmacokinetic and pharmacodynamic models, topics of study include carcinogenesis by heavy metals and efforts to reduce the side effects of radiotherapy and anticancer drugs. A new activity of this division is the culture of blood precursor cells which carry the surface molecule CD34. They are taken from the patient and cultured and amplified outside the body so that they can be reinjected when the patient is undergoing chemotherapy.

The Division of Experimental Therapy, founded in 1994, has as its central topic the genetic basis of disease processes and therapy. With the elucidation of the molecular basis of the defect that leads to loss of thymus function in the nude mouse, the isolation of the „nude" gene, the first genetic feature of the differentiation of lymph tissue was identified. An analysis of the function of the nude gene promises to give insight into the processes by which lymph cells mature and acquire a functioning T-cell repertoire. Finally, such efforts should improve our understanding of the role of the immune system in the process of cancer and in its therapy. These investigations of the development of the immune system are closely related to the questions addressed by the clinical cooperation units. With respect to designing genetic therapy procedures, the division is concerned with functional approaches to gene analysis. The primary aim here is to understand as a whole the function of large interconnected gene complexes such as the gene locations for the immunoglobulins. A prerequisite for tackling such questions is the availability of methods for the selective cloning of DNA fragments in the megabase range. Through the selective fragmentation of genomic DNA it is intended to clone such fragments of predetermined structure as artificial yeast chromosomes („designer YAC").

The Division of Tumor Progression and Immune Defense tackles questions related to metastasis and tumor therapy. A particular focus of the work is the functional analysis of various forms of the adhesion molecule CD44, which plays an essential role in the production of blood, in the activation of lymphocytes, and in metastasis via the lymph system. Our investigations concentrate on a cascade of reactions that serve to transmit signals within the cell and are initiated by particular variants of the

CD44 molecule. It should be mentioned in connection with this that the division was able to isolate an enzyme, phospholipase C, which splits phosphatidylcholine and plays an important role in the transmission of growth signals. Investigations will be pursued of those enzymes activated by the attachment of phosphate groups that regulate the signal transmission. Along with the studies of function, the work also concentrates on possible therapeutic applications in bone marrow transplantation and on attempts to develop a tumor specific immune therapy. In this context special attention must be paid to the costimulating properties of CD44 and the directed and tissue specific migration of certain well-defined CD44 variants.

The clinical cooperation unit Molecular Oncology/Pediatry was started at the beginning of 1995. Its projects are concerned with the regulation of physiological cell death (apoptosis) in hematological-oncological diseases. Apoptosis is essential for maintaining normal tissue homeostasis. Disruption leads to uncontrolled cell replication and resistance to conventional therapy or to premature death of the cells. The possibility of identifying genetic defects in apoptosis molecules or apoptosis programs can yield new approaches for understanding and treating tumor diseases. Selective molecular intervention, for example, the sensitzing of tumor cells to apoptosis signals or the initiation of apoptosis by gene transfer and antibody constructs, open up new prospects in tumor therapy, and future research will test the potential of such approaches.

For a large number of leukemias, malignant lymphomas, and also solid tumors, specific genomic modifications have been identified as the cause of the malignant growth; thus, these offer a possible point of attack for somatic gene therapy. One of the projects of the clinical cooperation unit Molecular Hematology/Oncology is concerned with correcting the abnormal regulation of gene expression in chronic myelogenous leukemia using antisense nucleic acids and ribozymes. In order to employ antisense RNA and ribozymes, appropriate vectors are needed to transport inhibitory genes into normal blood stem cells and leukemia cells. The cooperation unit is thereby concentrating on the adeno-associated virus vector system (AAV-2). The target cells for the gene transfer are the stem cells of the blood producing system. Thus, these cells are being taken from patients with malignant hemoblastoses and solid tumors. The cells are then cultured so as to allow immunological and molecular characterization.

A further project involves investigating the blood stem cells of HIV infected patients in order to lay the foundations for a future genetic therapy using, for example, RNA inhibitors.

The activities of the cooperation unit Dermatooncology were launched in May 1997. This unit is a joint endeavor of the Mannheim City Hospital and the Deutsches Krebsforschungszentrum. It offers skincancer sufferers the opportunity to seek information and to receive treatment at an advanced stage of the disease, as well as providing follow-up aftercare. The research activities focus on malignant melanoma. The scientists are attempting to elucidate the mechanism by which particularly the daughter tumors of this cancer become resistant to anticancer drugs. Other important topics will include the identification of new tumor specfic surface molecules of melanoma cells and also the rapid translation of research results into experimental therapy and clinical pilot studies.

Coordinator of the Research Program:
N. N.

Divisions and their heads:

Histodiagnostics and Pathomorphological Documentation:
Prof. Dr. Dymitr Komitowski

Perinatal Toxicology:
Prof. Dr. Jens Zeller

Cell Growth and Division:
Prof. Dr. Neidhard Paweletz

Applied Immunology:
N. N.

Tumor Progression and Immune Defense:
Prof. Dr. Margot Zöller

Experimental Therapy:
N. N.

Clinical Cooperation Unit Molecular Oncology/Pediatry:
Prof. Dr. Klaus-Michael Debatin

Clinical Cooperation Unit Molecular Hematology/Oncology:
Prof. Dr. Rainer Haas

Clinical Cooperation Unit Dermato-Oncology:
Prof. Dr. Dirk Schadendorf

5

5.1 Diagnosis of Breast Cancer – Current Radiological Procedures

by Gerhard van Kaick
and Dietrich von Fournier

The examination methods for breast cancer have attained notable clinical significance and have also become an important issue in health policy matters. There are several reasons for this:

– During the past 25 years, the frequency of breast cancer has steadily increased in industrial nations. Every eighth woman in the USA will during her lifetime become ill with breast cancer.

– A dominant causal factor for the development of breast cancer is unknown. Therefore, cancer prevention (primary prevention) has hardly been possible.

– There have been significant advances in the treatment of breast cancer. In early stages of tumor growth, the breast can be preserved with very good therapeutic results (15 year survival rate of 80 percent).

Therefore, it is the objective of diagnostic procedures to detect the tumor at an early stage; this means less than 1 cm in diameter, if possible.

Approximately 70 percent of women who are afflicted with breast cancer themselves seek out medical care, because they have detected a lump in their breast. It is rarer for them to also note retractions of the breast or bloody secretions from the nipple. Therefore, regular (monthly) self-examination by women remains an important foundation for the early detection of breast cancer. The annual palpation examination conducted by a physician is part of the statutory early detection program.

Not every palpated lump corresponds to a malignant tumor. Among women under 50 years old, only 5 percent of the lumps are caused by breast cancer; among women older than 50, almost 25

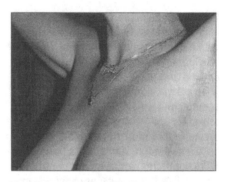

Fig. 37
The aim of diagnostics is to detect tumors as early as possible so that the breast can be preserved. During the 15 years following treatment, no metastases or secondary tumors developed in this patient. The image was taken three years after completion of radiotherapy

percent are due to breast cancer. Pain or retractions of the nipple require further diagnostic clarification, but are more rarely the result of cancer.

Tumors often cause a very substantial formation of connective tissue in the surrounding area. This gives them a hard consistency. Usually, a tumor exhibits irregular and radial growth, but a small number of tumors are round and have a relatively smooth boundary.

For the recognition and evaluation of tumors, mammography is the most frequently used and also the most important procedure. This method is very reliable when the technical quality is good and the examiner is very knowledgeable in its use. However, it is repeatedly criticized in public for two reasons:

– Patients occasionally complain about pain during breast compression.

Figs. 38, 39
The two possibilities of mammography: Dense regions within the surrounding fatty and glandular tissue as well as microcalcifications belong to the most important mammographic signs of breast cancer. Using direct magnification mammography (left image), this dense focus can definitely be identified as breast cancer. By applying a four-fold magnification to unclear microcalcifications (right image), this woman can avoid an unnecessary operation. This is a benign type of calcium deposit

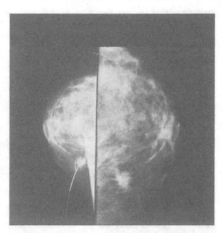

Fig. 38

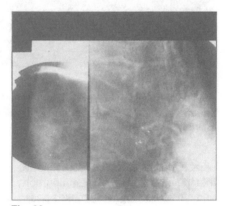

Fig. 39

– Reservations exist concerning the effects of radiation in younger women under 50 years old.

The proper positioning of the breast with compression proves decisive for the quality of the x-ray image and also for the timely recognition of a small tumor. Today, compression of the breast lasts for less than two seconds and is experienced as being tolerable by most women if they are properly informed beforehand. Complaints associated with breast compression can be significantly reduced when mammography is performed approximately one week following menstruation.

Exposure to radiation has been significantly reduced in new mammography equipment to below 2.5 cGy for images taken in two planes. Using mammography in a patient with suspected breast cancer is not disputed. However, what has been discussed is whether regular early detection examinations applied to the population as a whole increase the risk of getting breast cancer due to the radiation exposure. According to the results obtained in larger Swedish stud-

ies, the mortality for breast cancer has certainly decreased under conditions of regular early detection examinations. Therefore, it appears that the benefit of early detection far outweighs any possible risks associated with the radiation dose.

The most important characteristics of breast cancer as seen in a mammogram are:

– regions of increased density within the surrounding fat and glandular tissue,

– grouped microcalcifications typical of cancer,

– filling defects or irregularities upon introduction of a contrast medium into the milk duct (galactography), and

– appearance of a new region of density when compared to earlier images.

In women after menopause, fatty tissue in the breast usually dominates so that the tumor node contrasts strongly against the more radiopaque fatty tissue. In women between 40 and 50 years of age, the diagnosis is complicated, because the comparatively dense glandular tissue in the background provides a less favorable contrast for the tumor. Therefore, the diagnostic results for women before menopause are of poorer quality than for women over 50 years old. However, even for this age group mammography usually enables a tumor to be detected months to years before it actually becomes palpable.

So-called microcalcifications arise from calcium deposits in necrotic tumor cells of the milk ducts. They are so small that one must often use a magnifying glass in order to recognize them. The experienced radiologist can distinguish between the benign type and the malignant type of calcifications. However, microcalcifications typical of cancer are seen only in approximately 50 percent of breast cancers. They can be observed in tumors that are limited to the lumen of a milk duct. Therefore, they are a true, early sign of cancer that can only be detected by mammography.

Today, standard procedures employed in examining the breast in symptomatic women also include ultrasound (mammosonography) in addition to palpation and x-rays. The ultrasound procedure examines the breast with high frequency applicators (5 to 10 MHz). The echo structure of a normal breast varies depending on the age of the patient. Mammosonography requires a great deal of experience. The results obtained very much depend on the examiner since no overall image of the breast is taken as in the case of mammography. Only small sectional images of certain regions are produced by the examiner. A significant diagnostic advantage of sonography is seen in being able to distinguish with certainty suspicious solid foci from harmless cysts. Cystic changes occur very frequently in the context of mastopathy; they are encountered in more than 60 percent of women who have attained the age of sexual maturity. They are usually difficult to interpret in a mammogram.

It is more difficult to detect and classify solid foci of the breast when using sonography. Differentiating between benign and malignant tumors is possible, but the available criteria can only be applied with a certainty of approximately 80 percent. The classic sign of a malignant tumor is the ultrasound shadow which is caused by the high proportion of connective tissues contained in most tumors. Furthermore, one notes an indistinct boundary that is due to the radial growth of the tumor. Reduced elasticity is an important sign. Using sonography to detect microcalcifications proves hardly possible even today. Fibroadenomas, benign tumors that are often already observed in women under 25, typically have a smooth boundary and do not exhibit a dorsal ultrasound shadow. However, individual tumors, such as a medullary or mucinous carcinoma, can look just like a fibroadenoma in the

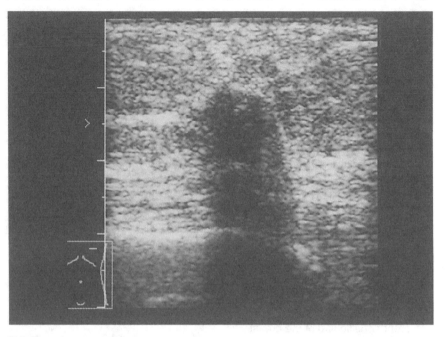

Fig. 40
Ultrasound image of breast cancer. The high proportion of connective tissue in most tumors "swallows" the ultrasound and leaves behind a typically broad "ultrasound shadow" (black indentation)

ultrasound image. From this it follows that the combination of mammography and mammosonography makes possible the detection and classification of changes with a relatively high level of certainty. However, in doubtful cases, further clarification by means of biopsy is urgently needed.

Mammography and mammosonography are the two examination methods used for the focused removal of tissue samples. A needle must be placed in such a manner that it is located in the suspected tumor region. An advantage of mammosonography is the possibility of continuously observing and following the needle as it enters the appropriate tissue. Suspicious microcalcifications

cannot be depicted with sonography. In such a case, the placement of the needle occurs with mammography. Depending on the technique used (needle or punch biopsy), a tissue sample is obtained by suction or cutting; the sample then undergoes either cytological or histological processing. If the suspicious focus must be removed, it is necessary to mark the area insofar as it is not palpable. This is accomplished by introducing sterile, marking wires with a hook so that they cannot change their location and the focus can be located with certainty during the operation or the tissue biopsy. In order to be certain that the desired focus has been removed in the excised tissue sample, radiography is performed on the dissected tissue. This means that an x-ray is taken of the removed tissue. These images should again contain the suspicious focus.

The diagnostic procedures are not very stressful and are conducted under local anesthesia within 3 to 10 minutes on an outpatient basis. Because of this, the tendency usually exists to conduct a punch biopsy for histological clarification should suspicious findings be discovered in the mammogram or with ultrasound. Depending on the clinic and the experience of the physician in question, a carcinoma is discovered for every 3 to 5 conducted biopsies. The remaining cases are benign tumors that, however, did require additional clarification.

Newer examination techniques for the female breast are color Doppler sonography and dynamic magnetic resonance imaging (MRI). Color Doppler sonography shows blood flow in the ultrasound image. Smaller blood vessels can be depicted, but not the capillaries. During the past several years, it has been discovered that malignant tumors have more substantial vascularization than benign changes do. This can be confirmed for 80 to 90 percent of malignant tumors. However, the approximately 15 percent of breast carcinomas that remain exhibit very little vascularization. This procedure provides additional information in a non-invasive manner that does not suffice to completely distinguish between benign and malignant changes with certainty.

The increased vascularization exhibited by a tumor is also the basis for magnetic resonance imaging (MRI) examinations of the female breast. This procedure requires injecting a special contrast medium (e.g., gadolinium-DPTA).

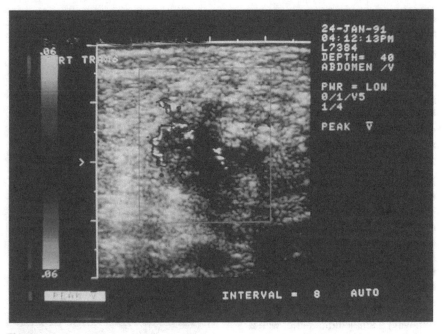

Fig. 41
Color Doppler sonography assists in the distinction between benign and malignant changes. It measures and presents the velocity of the blood flow in a color-coded form. Malignant tumors usually exhibit especially strong vascularization and present significantly more color signals than benign tumors do

During the first minute after injection, the signal intensity in carcinomas increases by at least 90 percent and attains its peak during the second minute. Thereafter, a flat decline follows. Recording this dynamic process is only possible, because many images are taken one following the other at short time intervals. This is very complicated since every image requires that both breasts be examined in 15 sectional planes. Evaluating such a large number of images (several hundred) is only possible by using a computer program. Such a procedure developed at the Deutsches Krebsforschungszentrum then indicates the pathological dynamics exhibited by the contrast medium

through a colorful overlay so that the physician can more easily recognize the tumorous region. The background for this type of MRI diagnostics is seen in the fact that the tumor induces the growth of small blood vessels through special substances (e.g., vascular endothelial growth factor). Only when the microscopically small tumor has constructed a vascular net can it develop further.

During this examination, the patient lies on her stomach. The breasts hang in two receptacles that are contained within a special support into which antennas have been installed. These send and receive the signals. Comparatively speaking, the procedure is time consuming and expensive.

MRI of the breast is currently the most sensitive procedure for detecting breast cancer although 5 to 10 percent of the tumors escape detection. Diagnostic limitations are especially noted when depicting the so-called in situ carcinoma in which the tumor vasculature has not yet been sufficiently developed.

An indication for a breast MRI is currently given for: Patients with breasts that are difficult to evaluate both with mammography and sonography and patients with silicon breast implants. Detecting grouped microcalcifications in an x-ray is not an indication for this procedure.

Therapy that preserves the breast by removing a small tumor either with a sufficient margin of safety or by excising a single breast quadrant, requires supplemental radiotherapy of the remaining breast tissue. This irradiation causes reactions in the tissue so that an evaluation using mammography and also MRI proves more difficult during the 18 month period that follows. An edema (a diffuse deposit of fluid in the tissue) and a thickening of the skin are most readily noticed; this gradually regresses during the second half of the second year. Only after approximately two years is the mammogram again sufficiently reliable. The scar that develops at the site of the operation is not easily distinguishable from a recurrence of the tumor since it too exhibits a radial arrangement. During both of these years following radiotherapy, examinations with ultrasound are an important supplemental diagnostic procedure.

In the presence of breast implants, the diagnosis must consider that tumors

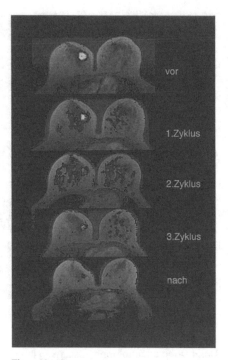 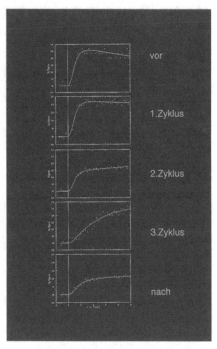

Figs. 42, 43
Functional mammography using MRI. The images from a patient with breast cancer (yellow) were taken before and after the completion of individual cycles of chemotherapy. After the first cycle of chemotherapy, the signal time curve from the tumor region in question (Fig. 43) shows a flattening of the curve's slope which can be seen as a positive reaction to therapy

can also develop behind the implant. Because of their location, they cannot be depicted by mammography and also partially not by sonography. Tears in the implant must also be recognized. In these matters, MRI of the breast provides relevant information.

Future Developments

Improvements in the named diagnostic procedures are being intensively pursued on a worldwide basis. Interesting developments in mammography in-

clude the possibility of direct magnification mammography. The procedure permits identifying even the smallest microcalcifications. However, additional technical improvements in the equipment are still necessary and clinical experiences must be expanded upon.

Digital mammography is a goal that has been pursued for a long time. This means that the analog signal of the film exposure must be converted into a digital data format. With digital mammography, image creation, image presentation, data transmission, and data storage can be separated from one another. Furthermore, the acquired data can be processed by computer to optimize the image. Finally, a technique that can automatically detect pathological changes by means of computer-supported image analysis is being actively pursued. Also an evaluation of findings by an expert using teleradiology will become technically simpler. Such an application is especially interesting for screening procedures.

Among other problems, difficulties have so far arisen related to the requirement that the data matrix should be 4,000 x 4,000 pixels in size so that microcalcifications can also be detected with certainty. This necessitates a significant amount of data that can today, however, be more successfully managed using modern computer technology. One can assume that during the next few years digital mammography will be used more frequently in clinics. The combination of magnification mammography and digital mammography can mean an additional, important step in improving breast diagnostics in the future.

Progress also continues to be made in the field of sonography. Newer equipment permits examining the breast with frequencies between 10 and 14 MHz. This results in greater spatial resolution, but with a more significantly limited depth of penetration. Ultrasound contrast media will continue to improve examinations that employ the color Doppler technique and will contribute to the differentiation of focus-like changes.

For MRI of the breast, the initial offering of specialized breast scanners by certain companies could become significant. The main tasks for the next several years will mainly be a standardization

of the examination technology itself and obtaining additional knowledge about tumor physiology both with respect to vascularization and contrast media kinetics.

The introduction of regular mammography as an early detection test for women after the age of 40 or 50 is an objective that has been striven towards for a long time in Germany. Several neighboring European countries (Sweden, Netherlands, England) have partially realized this goal. Tumors should be detected and treated at an early stage in order to reduce the mortality due to breast cancer. The earlier diagnosis that results in this process could incorrectly give the impression of a longer survival rate ("lead time bias"). However, the reduction of breast cancer mortality, confirmed in several studies, proves the effectiveness of early detection methods that also employ strict quality control; breast cancer mortality in women over 50 years old could be reduced by approximately 25 percent and in women between age 40 and 49 by up to 15 percent.

It is presently still being disputed whether or not mammography should already be employed as an early detection technique in women between the ages of 40 and 49 (apart from formal studies). In this context, one must consider that the frequency of cancer in this age group is lower and that the probability of discovering a tumor will also be lower. A study conducted over a 10 year period and published in 1995 yielded no statistically significant difference between the age group of women between 40 and 49 and the group between 50 and 64 with respect to tumor size, lymph node status, and tumor stage. Using mammography for

the early detection of cancer on a nationwide basis only makes sense when the quality of the equipment and the examiner can be guaranteed. Quality control and review by a second expert is demanded by almost all proponents of a screening program.

Applying the modern technique of mammography results in an integral radiation dose between 1 to 4 mSv. Based on calculations, several critics proposed that a breast dose of 0.1 mSv could theoretically result in an additional four breast carcinomas among one million women undergoing mammography after a latency period of 10 years. This means that the individual risk for breast cancer would increase from 9 percent to 9.001 percent. If one transfers this risk to the general risks that one is subjected to in life, it would be comparable to the likelihood of dying in an automobile accident while driving one's car for a distance of 18 km. In screening studies, however, women who regularly received a mammogram never exhibited an increased breast cancer rate when compared to the women in the control group who did not submit to mammography.

Medical diagnostics has assumed a new role in being increasingly better able to detect a predisposition to cancer. The discovery of the breast cancer genes, BRCA1 and BRCA2, was a significant step in understanding the heredity of factors that can cause breast carcinoma. According to the statistics currently available, the cumulative risk for carriers of the BRCA1 genetic defect to develop breast cancer until the age of 70 is 82 percent compared to 9 percent for the general population. In this context, it is typical for these patients to more frequently develop breast cancer at an earlier age (60 percent before the age of 50). Furthermore, the affected patients also frequently develop ovarian cancer (44 percent). This genetic predisposition, the result of a germ line mutation, is inherited in an autosomal dominant manner. The proportion of genetically caused breast cancers is currently estimated at approximately 3 to 5 percent. Females with breast cancer that occurs before the age of 35 are found to have a genetic predisposition in 25 to 40 percent of the cases.

If such a predisposition is known, the patient should be offered both oncological as well as genetic counseling. Since the appearance of tumors must already be expected at an early age, early detection examinations are indicated for such a patient after the age of 25. In this context, it is recommended that until age 40 both ultrasound and MRI be used in addition to breast palpation. Thereafter, regular mammograms as part of a clinical examination should be conducted. This opens a new field for medical diagnostics, one that not only affects the area of breast carcinomas.

Prof. Dr. Gerhard van Kaick
Department of Oncological Diagnostics and Therapy

Prof. Dr. Dietrich von Fournier
Department of Gynecological and Obstetrical Radiology, Radiological University Clinic Heidelberg

Selected publications

Kubli, F., Fournier, D. von, Bauer, M., Junkermann, H., Kaufmann, M. (Eds.): Breast Diseases: Breast-Conserving Therapy, Non-Invasive Lesions, Mastopathy, Springer Verlag (1989)

Fournier, D. von, Anton, H.-W., Junkermann, H., Bastert, G., Kaick, G. van: Brustkrebs-screening, Radiologe 33, 227–235 (1993)

Teubner, J., Bohrer, M., Kaick, G. van, Georgi, M.: Echomorphologie des Mammakarzinoms. Radiologe 33, 277–286 (1993)

Huber, S., Delorme, S., Knopp, M.V., Junkermann, H., Zuna, I., Fournier, D. von, Kaick, G. van: Breast tumors: computer-assisted quantitative assessment with Color-Doppler. US Radiology 192, 797–801 (1994)

Knopp, M.V., Brix, G., Junkermann, H.J., Sinn, H.J.: MR mammography with pharmakokinetic mapping for monitoring of breast cancer treatment during neoadjuvant therapy. MRI Clinics of North America 2, 633–658 (1994)

5.2 Virtual Operation Planning in Liver Surgery

by Gerald Glombitza,
Christian Herfarth, Wolfram Lamadé
and Hans-Peter Meinzer

Hepatic resection is the only treatment for patients with colorectal cancer metastatic to the liver that has resulted in long term survival and may be potentially curative. Without treatment 5 year survival is less than 2%. Liver resection in selected patients has led to an increase of 5 year survival rates to 20-40%. None of the chemotherapeutic regimens could demonstrate similar results. Therefore, surgery remains gold-standard in treatment of limited hepatic disease in colorectal cancer patients. Selection of patients out of the continuum of metastatic tumor progression is the crucial step. Generalization to more than two organs excludes the patient

from hepatic resection. Furthermore three cornerstones have to be considered in liver surgery: the liver tumor has to be resected completely within sound liver parenchyma, liver function is dependent on sufficient functionally active liver volume, and (sub-)segments of the liver which might get devascularized by liver resection have to be removed as well. Thus, the surgical strategy is dependent on the 3D localization of the liver tumor in relation to the three liver vascular trees. One of the limiting factors is postoperative liver function which is dependent on remaining liver tissue. A prediction of absolute or relative rest liver volume has been very dif-

Fig. 44
This CT image depicts the spine and the ribs as light structures. The tumor is seen as a dark mass in the left side of the image. Within the liver, the blood vessels can be recognized as light regions full of a contrast medium. Such two-dimensional cross sections do not provide the necessary three-dimensional orientation that is so very important in the planning of an operation

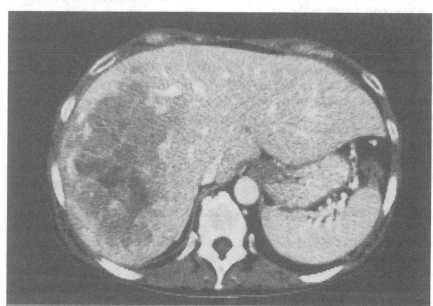

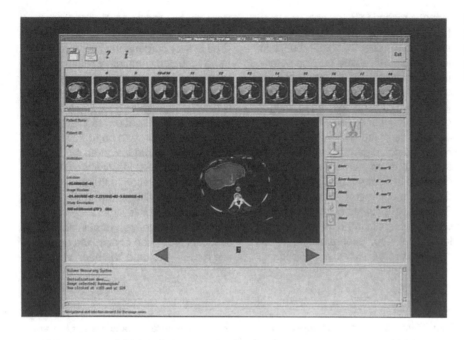

Fig. 45
By using a special image processing program, the depicted organs can be precisely differentiated from their surroundings

ficult and has widely been substituted by simple imagination and rough estimation. A computer based calculation was up to now not practical due to missing extraction systems for the plain liver and its tumor. Especially in patients with multiple liver lesions operation planning is getting difficult as resection plains may cut in a complicated way through the vascular trees leading to devascularized (sub-)segments which have to be removed as well. To circumvent these problems the following operative strategies have been pursued.

Liver Segment Oriented Surgery

In toto extirpation of all liver segments which are affected by the tumor. Disadvantage: patients might erroneously be categorized as irresectable due to great loss of liver parenchyma.

Metastasectomy

Peeling out the tumor together with some security margin without anatomic orientation

Disadvantage: Necrosis of devascularized subsegments may lead to septic state.

Anatomy Oriented Liver Subsegment Surgery

It does not exist yet due to missing preoperative operation planning and intraoperative navigation systems. There are no existing computer based analysing systems which recognize, extract, and separate the vascular trees within the liver. Prediction of postoperative liver function is still not practicable due to missing liver volume measurements. All preoperative liver function tests

must surrender as long as there is no prediction of remaining liver volume.

The knowledge of the exact three dimensional relation of the tumor and the vascular trees within the liver decides on the preoperative selection of patients for hepatic resection. Despite low perioperative mortality (0-2%) there is still a high complication rate of up to 35%. Therefore objective selection criteria should be mandatory.

Problem

Operability of a liver tumor is dependent on its three dimensional relation to the intrahepatic vascular trees. According to Bismuth and Couinaud, the substructure of the vascular trees defines the eight segments of the liver which are theoretically functioning autonomously. The situation is complicated by the great anatomic variability of the liver vascular trees.

The liver tumor has to be resected completely within sound liver parenchyma using a typical security margin of 1 cm. Sufficient functional active liver volume has to be preserved. Potentially devascularized (sub-)segments of the liver must be recognized and removed as well.

The aim of this study is to establish a computer based, quantitative, three dimensional operation planning system in liver surgery. An individualized operation strategy will be facilitated which takes into account the great anatomic variability of liver architecture in the individual patient. A quantitative operation planning including subsegments would be possible. Patients with multiple liver metastases would have a benefit as the resected liver volume would be minimized and the risk of devascularized parenchyma with partial liver necrosis would be reduced.

Prerequisite of doing so the system has to

– recognize and separate parenchyma, vessels and tumor.

– calculate the absolute and relative volumes.

– recognize, reconstruct, and symbolically describe the three dimensional vessel trees.

– calculate a potential resection proposal, which may be modified by the user interactively.

To reach this goal, surgery, radiology and informatics are co-operating.

The ongoing developments might optimize patient selection in the future as operation planning will become quantifiable and objective. Complication rates

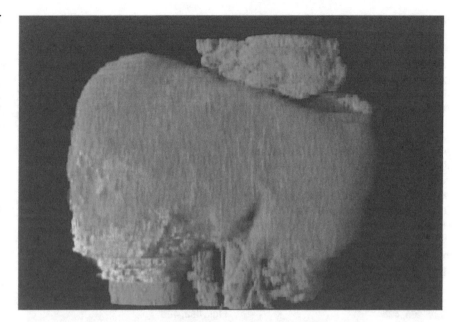

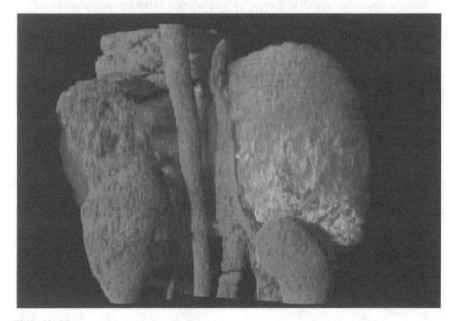

Figs. 46, 47
The liver (brown) and the tumor (gray) that is to be removed are shown in a three-dimensional form. In Fig. 47, red indicates neighboring organs, e.g., the kidneys, the aorta, and the inferior vena cava

might decrease due to an improved patient selection and by a highly individualized operation planning and resection. Besides of the advantages for the patient there might be a reduction of the expenditure for intensive care and hospital stay.

CT scans taken from routine diagnostics are the input for image processing. According to the actual problem two different methods of contrast medium applications may be used; bolus tracking: contrast medium injection through a high pressure pump is triggered by a computer so that the contrast medium reaches the liver just in time as the CT scan starts sampling the data from the

liver. Reasonably good results for 3D reconstruction can be obtained. Angio-CT: an arterial catheter is introduced into the iliac artery from a skin puncture in the groin. The inflow of the contrast media into the liver is highly selective, thereby increasing image contrast.

Slice thickness and concomitant image resolution has been increased dramatically since introduction of spiral CT imaging.

Image Transfer

The image data generated by the CT scanner has to be transferred to the

workstations installed in the Krebsforschungszentrum because they offer the capacity and performance which is necessary. The teleradiology system CHILI®, developed by the Division of Medical and Biological Informatics at the Krebsforschungszentrum, supports this data transfer. Picture formats can easily be transformed on this platform.

Image Processing and Standard Visualisation

After the completion of the image transfer three-dimensional image data with millions of voxels (volume picture elements) are available to the computer. For further image processing it is necessary to segment the data, i.e., to assign the pixels to different anatomical structures. Fundamental informations for resection planning are the structure of liver parenchyma, liver tumor and the vessel trees.

Image data vary greatly from patient to patient. Liver metastases may present from hypo-, to hyperintens compared to sound liver parenchyma. The identification of diseased areas of parenchyma cannot be performed completely automatically. So at the moment a semi-automatic analysis is performed, where the liver and the diseased parenchyma are marked manually.

This means a two-dimensional image processing program is used for marking the interesting regions slice by slice. Basic image processing algorithms like region growing and edge detection are used. This program was designed with particular interest in an ergonomic graphical user interface in order to minimize the time used for processing the

Figs. 48a, 48b
The tumor is massively shown in gray; in contrast, only the transparent integument of the liver is depicted

Figs. 49a, 49b
The location of the tumor relative to the blood vessels is shown here. This location is a main factor in deciding whether or not the tumor can be surgically removed

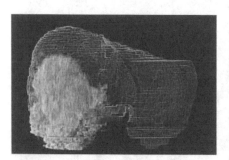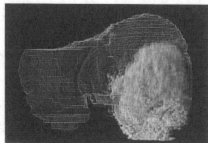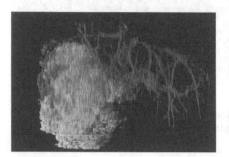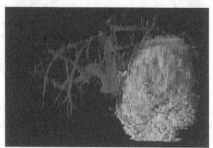

whole three-dimensional data set, a basic requirement for the integration into clinical routine.

After this manual segmentation the remaining image processing steps are performed automatically. Dependent on the imaging mode, especially the bolus length and bolus time, the portal vessel tree or both the portal and the hepatic vessel tree are segmented by means of entropy thresholding methods. Now all necessary informations for evaluation of the relative position of diseased areas and liver vessel trees are available. The quantitative assessment of these informations is performed automatically.

Actual Level of Operation Planning

For operation planning two aspects are important. The first aspect is the generation of a quantitative report about the data, i.e., relative and absolute volume measurements of the liver and the tumor. These values are calculated during the manual segmentation process and are used during the following automatic data analysis process.

Another quantitative statement concerns the resection index. This combined volumetric measure tries to predict the loss of functionality caused by the planned resection. The diseased areas of the parenchyma do not add to total liver function. So the loss of functionality is mainly caused by the resection of sound parenchyma, which has to be removed because of the relative position of the tumor and vessel trees and the resulting operation strategy. So an important result of the preoperative analysis is estimation of the resection index.

Therefore, it is necessary to simulate the planned resection virtually in order to estimate the volume of sound, resected and remaining liver parenchyma. So the modeling of different operational strategies is a working package for the near future.

The other aspect of three-dimensional data analysis is visualization. Different visualization methods show the spatial relation between the tumor, the liver surface, and the vessel trees. For this purpose standardised visualizations are calculated which present the complex spatial information in an intuitive way.

These visualizations are calculated by means of the „Heidelberg Raytracing

Model". The three-dimensional data set is viewed „virtually" by the computer. Artificial light sources illuminate the body and the included organs consisting of image data.

In additional to the liver and the tumor, the whole vessel system is visualized. The portal system (the venous inflow of the liver) gathers the blood from the alimentary tract. The hepatic veins represent the venous outflow of the liver into the inferior vena cava. In the visualization process, every organ is assigned a certain color in order to structure the complex spatial information. Although a randomly chosen observer position and viewing direction is possible in our visu-

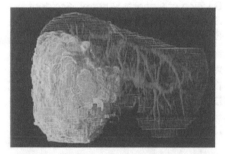
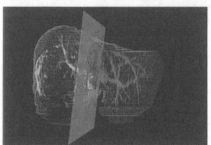

Figs. 50a, 50b
The tumor must be removed with a safety zone of one centimeter into healthy tissue. This is depicted as a green covering in Fig. 50a. The vascular regions within the safety zone are yellow in Fig. 50b

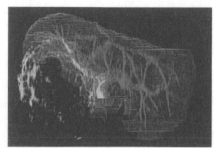
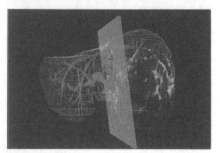

Figs. 51a, 51b
The computer has calculated the recommended sectional plane (blue) for the operation

alizations, only rotations around the liver are shown. By standardizing the visualizations, they become common to the surgeon and comparable between different patients.

All quantitative and qualitative statements are available at the latest the day after the image acquisition. So the computer-aided image data analysis may be integrated into the operation planning procedure. The methods developed for this project are, in principle, also applicable for operation planning concerning other organs.

This work is being supported by the Tumorzentrum Heidelberg/Mannheim.

Dr. Gerald Glombitza
Priv.-Doz. Dr. Hans-Peter Meinzer
Division of Medical and
Biological Informatics

Prof. Dr. Christian Herfarth
Dr. Wolfram Lamadé
Division of General Surgery, Accident Surgery and Outpatient Clinic,
Surgical University Clinic Heidelberg

Cooperating scientists

Dipl.-Inform. Med.
Athanasios M. Demiris
Marc-Roger Göpfert
Division of Medical and
Biological Informatics,
Deutsches Krebsforschungszentrum

Prof. Dr. Gerd Otto
Priv.-Doz. Dr. Thomas Lehnert
Division of General Surgery, Accident Surgery and Outpatient Clinic,
Surgical University Clinic Heidelberg

Prof. Dr. Günter Kauffmann
Priv.-Doz. Dr. Götz Richter
Dr. Matthias Brado
Division of Radiodiagnostics,
Radiological University Clinic,
University of Heidelberg

Selected publications

Hohenberger, P., Schlag, P., Schwarz, V., Herfarth, Ch.: Tumor recurrence and options for further treatment after resection of liver metastases in patients with colorectal cancer. J. Surg. Oncol. 44 (4), 245–251 (1990)

Lehnert, Th., Otto, G., Herfarth, Ch.: Therapeutic modalities and prognostic factors for primary and secondary liver tumors. World J. Surg. 19, 252–263 (1995)

Herfarth, Ch., Heuschen, U.A., Lamadé, W., Lehnert, Th., Otto, G.: Rezidiv-Resektionen an der Leber bei primären und sekundären Lebermalignomen. Chirurg 66, 949–958 (1995)

Engelmann, U., Schröter, A., Baur, U., Schroeder, A., Werner, O., Wolsiffer, K., Baur, H.J., Göransson, B., Borälv, E., Meinzer, H.-P.: Teleradiology System MEDICUS, Proc. International Symposium CAR'96 Paris, 537–542 (1996)

Wolsiffer, K., Mayer, A., Niebsch, R., Meinzer, H.-P.: Die Integration des Heidelberger Raytracers in OpenGL zur integrierten Segmentierung und Visualisierung dreidimensionaler medizinischer Volumendaten. In: Bildverarbeitung in der Medizin. Proceedings des Aachener Workshops 1996. Hrsg.: Lehmann, Th. et al., 143–148, RWTH Aachen (1996)

5.3 A New Approach to the Improvement of Tumor Therapy: The Use of Glucose-Coupled Substances

by Barbara Bertram
and Manfred Wießler

If cancer were caused by bacterial agents, tumor chemotherapy would be much easier and more effective than it has been until now. The therapy of bacterial diseases primarily targets the pathogens: penicillins prevent the proper formation of the bacterial cell wall, tetracyclines inhibit bacterial protein synthesis; sulfonamides interfere with the synthesis of nucleic acids, and so forth. In this process, it is the pathogens and not the healthy cells that die or are at least inhibited in their growth. However, cancer is not a disease that can be traced to bacteria, but instead is based on a disturbance of the growth control processes in body cells. Thereby, the cell attains immortality and divides more or less continuously. At the root of this disturbance lies a mutation which is a change in the genetic material. As long as the mutation is not repaired or the cell does not die, the altered genetic material is passed on to daughter cells at each cell division. The change in the hereditary material occurs at the molecular level. For example, the DNA is altered to such a degree by the formation of so-called adducts (products that are the result of DNA reacting with carcinogenic, chemical substances) that it is incorrectly read during the chromosome duplication process. The result of such a mutation can express itself in an incorrect activation of growth factors or in an improper exclusion of growth-inhibiting substances. In both instances, this causes a deterioration in the control mechanisms governing cell growth. The course of events from the first mutation to the formation of a tumor is a protracted process indeed. It can often take many years.

Two decisive questions arise at this point:

How can cancer formation be prevented?

If the formation of cancer cannot be prevented or can only be imperfectly attained, how can this disease be treated?

The answer to the first question reads: prevention reduces the formation of tumors. This entails a wide-ranging avoidance of exposure to safety hazards (primary prevention), but also the consumption of antineoplastic substances (secondary prevention). During the past several years, the idea of prevention has received a significant boost after people have come to realize that it is clearly more intelligent to avoid potential safety hazards (e.g., not to smoke) or to ban them from the environment (e.g., prohibit using asbestos for insulation) than to wait long enough for cancer to finally occur.

The answer to the second question, how cancers should be treated, is very complex and can only be discussed cursorily here. The three classical methods of cancer treatment are surgery, radiotherapy, and chemotherapy. During the past few years, the new techniques of immunotherapy and the still experimental gene therapy have been introduced. These new types of therapy are still of limited usefulness, because of a lack of specificity, inadequate stability of the transferred material, and its limited life in the organism. New therapeutic methods are still very much in demand.

The path that we have chosen to follow in treating malignant tumors focuses on improving the conventional (available) drugs used in cancer treatment. In this context, one must know that the medications used until now, with few exceptions (e.g., hormone-coupled therapeutic agents), are not tumor-specific. They do not only attack the cancer cell, but also the healthy cell, especially when it is rapidly dividing. Such cells, for example, can be found in the hair, the walls of the intestines and in the nails. This is the reason for the well-known and pronounced side effects associated with such treatment that can express themselves in damage to the bone marrow, dizziness, nausea, and hair loss. Furthermore, a resistance to therapy develops after a period of treatment that varies in length. It is usually directed against several antineoplastic agents and is, therefore, called „multidrug resistance."

The primary focus of our research involves the modification of already established cell poisons (cytostatic agents). It is the objective of our studies to impart to these employed substances a more pronounced capability to recognize tumor cells. Thereby, the described side effects should be mitigated. The central theme entails coupling the active principle to a sugar component. Presently, we are pursuing two concepts of sugar-mediated „drug targeting." The term, „drug targeting", includes acting upon a specific type of tissue in a focused manner by using a particular medication or transporting a drug to the desired site of action.

The first concept is based on the different energy demands of tumor cells and normal cells. Because of their increased growth, tumor cells require more „fuel" than normal, healthy cells do. Glucose is this cellular fuel; it is passed into the cell by means of special transport proteins. However, the glucose transport proteins do not only process free glucose, but also sub-

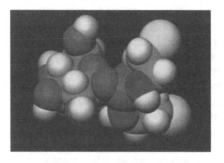

Fig. 52
The molecular model depicts the bond between glucose and ifosfamide mustard. Each sphere symbolizes an atom; each color represents an element

stances that are coupled to glucose. These so-called glucosides, for example, are ubiquitous in the plant kingdom. They are used by the plants as storage forms for different substances. It is possible that tumor cells may take up a larger quantity of a glucose-coupled cytostatic agent than normal cells do. The workability of this concept has been demonstrated by a sugar-coupled substance, (β-D-glucosyl-ifosfamide mustard (Glc-IPM), that was developed in our department and is currently undergoing clinical trials.

Ifosfamide mustard (IPM) forms in the metabolism during the breakdown of ifosfamide (Holoxan®, IFO-cell®) which belongs to the three most commonly used cancer drugs. Ifosfamide is used to treat leukemias, neuroblastoma, Ewing's sarcoma and carcinomas of the ovaries, the testicles and the female breast. Its mechanism of action involves alkylating the DNA; it belongs to the group of alkylating agents. Alkylating the DNA (binding it to drugs or other chemical substances) causes it to become fragile and breaks in the DNA strands occur or it is „read" incorrectly during the cell duplication process and changes in the hereditary material result. These occurrences can ultimately lead to the destruction of the cell. IPM is extremely poisonous and unstable; it

cannot by itself be administered as a drug. By binding it to glucose it becomes stabilized as a „prodrug" which is the precursor of a drug. This precursor, itself, does not possess any or only minimal activity and it is only converted into the active form of the drug at the site of action. In animal experiments, (β-D-glucosyl-IPM exhibits an antitumor effect comparable to that of ifosfamide, but its poisonous effects are significantly less.

The second concept focuses on being able to specifically recognize complex sugar structures. On their surface, all cells possess sugar-binding proteins which are called lectins. The lectin pattern of degenerated cells differs from that of healthy cells. By using complex sugar structures (oligosaccharides) that preferentially bind to tumor-associated lectins, it is conceivable to imagine that tumor cells can be targeted in a focused manner. If the oligosaccharide is coupled to a cytostatic agent, an active principle can result that is specifically directed against the tumor. The uptake mechanism into the cell is assumed to involve lectin-modulated endocytosis.

Before such oligosaccharide-bound therapeutic agents can be produced, the lectins of the tumor cell in question must be isolated and its sugar-binding behavior must be characterized. Affinity chromatography methods can assist in this process. Branched oligosaccharides are used as the affinity material to bind the tumor cells. Because of a special effect (cluster effect), these sugars are able to bind lectins so tightly that they are not immediately rinsed off when the affinity column is washed. The affinity of a lectin for a specific oligosaccharide not only depends on the type, but number of terminal sugars; the binding pattern is also decisive for the strength of the interaction. By varying the binding pattern of the terminal groups, it should prove possible to probe the ligand specificity of a lectin in a focused manner.

The first concept (coupling to sugar, specifically to glucose and other monosaccharides) resulted in the development of several new substances in our department. The initial syntheses and screening procedures were carried out by Michael Dickes in his dissertation from 1985 to 1988. As of 1990, the ASTA Medica company primarily participated in research of the substance (β-D-glc-IPM, already mentioned above and which subsequently proved to be very promising. Since July of 1996, this substance is being examined in phase I and phase II studies for its suitability as a tumor medication in clinical use. According to the German Arzneimittelgesetz [of 1976, last changed by the 5th amending statute of 1994], for a newly developed substance to come this far it must first have attained good results in a so-called preclinical phase, a phase before actual clinical use in human beings. Therein it must prove itself to be nontoxic to a large degree and useful for the intended area of application. Furthermore, data concerning its metabolism and its distribution in the body

(phamacokinetics) and its method of reaction in living organisms (pharmacodynamics) must be collected.

The preclinical studies involving our substance yielded many results when compared to the ifosfamide that was not coupled to sugar. The most important results will be mentioned here: Toxicity for rats is lessened by a factor of 4.5 when compared to ifosfamide. The leukocyte count in the bone marrow of mice decreases by only 10 to 30 percent, whereas it temporarily decreases by up to 90 percent following administration of ifosfamide. The therapeutic effectiveness on transplantation tumors of the mouse is comparable to that of ifosfamide and superior to that of cyclophosphamide. In solid tumors, therapy with glc-IPM results in more long-term survivors than does ifosfamide. The previously discussed resistance phenomena, that very frequently appear following treatment with cytostatic drugs, were not observed after treatment with glc-IPM. Quite to the contrary, our substance even proved effective in cells that are resistant to the related substance, cyclophosphamide.

In order to examine the distribution of the active principle in the organs, it makes sense to employ a radioactively marked substance whose path throughout the body can more readily be followed by specialized measurement procedures than an unmarked substance can. In our department, in which studies employing radioactively marked substances can be conducted, we synthesized the appropriate substances. For investigations focusing on the mechanism of the reaction, we also produced the β-L, the α-L and the α-D forms. Such variants are called structural isomers.

Total body autoradiography is a procedure used to determine the distribution of substances in the body. Surprising results were obtained when we conducted this procedure with our substance: Following injection in rats, the β-D form accumulates in the brain while

An overview of the phases in clinical trials

	Test Substance
preclinical studies (in the test tube and in animal experiments)	screening
	pharmacokinetics (distribution and elimination of the substance in the body)
	pharmacodynamics (effect of the substance in the body)
clinical studies	phase I (tolerance, metabolism, (in humans) mechanism of action, maximal tolerable dose)
	phase II (effectiveness, relative harmlessness)
	phase III (proof of effectiveness and harmlessness). Approval (initially for 5 years as an ethical drug)
	phase IV (proof of effectiveness in a new application/indication)

the β-L form does not. Additionally, substance accumulation in a so-called transplantation tumor was only observed after injection with the β-D, but not with the β-L form. It is very likely the case that the already named glucose transporters, which facilitate the transport of D-glucose, but not of the mirror image molecule L-glucose across the membrane, are responsible for this behavior. If this membrane transport hypothesis of D-glucosides by means of specialized glucose transporters can be confirmed, a fundamentally new means would be available for introducing active principles into the brain in the form of their glucose conjugates. This method could result in an improved therapy of brain tumors and other diseases of the central nervous system (e.g., Alzheimer's disease). Possible approaches for preventing such illnesses could eventually also be developed.

Submitting the preclinical data described above along with proof of the substance's satisfactory stability both in its undissolved and dissolved forms to the Federal Institute for Drugs and

Fig. 53
This model depicts the bond between glucose and ifosfamide mustard in a different manner

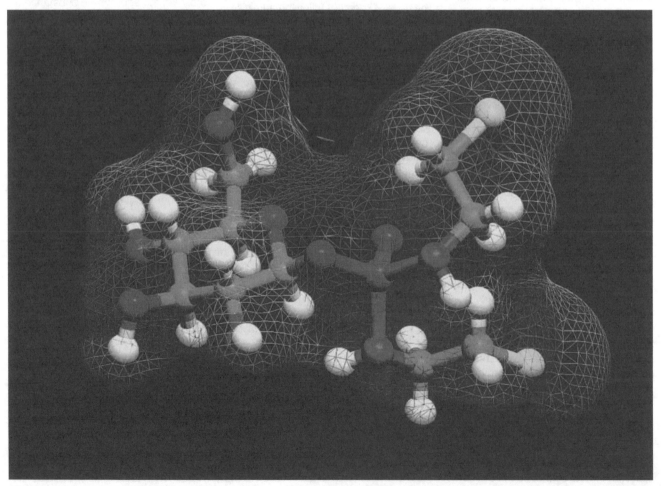

Medical Products, satisfied the preconditions for being able to begin the clinical studies. In July of 1996, phase I and phase II studies commenced. In general, initial applications of an active substance are tested on healthy individuals. However, since cancer drugs usually possess carcinogenic potential themselves, initial testing is conducted on cancer patients (Declaration of Helsinki, Good Clinical Practice 1992, GCP). If it is demonstrated that a more effective tumor therapy can be conducted with glc-IPM than with the related compounds, ifosfamide and cyclophosphamide, while simultaneously remaining at a lower toxicity level, the principle of glucose coupling will be expanded to include other drugs. In addition to its clinical relevance, glc-IPM also plays a very unimportant role in basic research. With the assistance of this substance it becomes possible to study the significance and the mechanism of action of the above-mentioned transport proteins, the glucose transporters.

If glc-IPM successfully passes through all the hurdles of the required studies through phase III and IV, it could, by a conservative estimate, be available on the market as a new drug in the year 2003. Until then a total of 18 years will have passed from the first idea for a new antineoplastic agent until its market introduction. This represents half of a researcher's career.

Dr. Barbara Bertram
Prof. Dr. Manfred Wießler
Division of Molecular Toxicology

Participating scientists

Dr. Jörg Stüben, pharmacist
Marianne Schaper, pharmacist
Dipl.-Chem. Stefan Menzler
Division of Molecular Toxicology,
Deutsches Krebsforschungszentrum

Prof. Dr. Manfred Volm
Priv.-Doz. Dr. Uwe Haberkorn
Division of Oncological Diagnostics
and Therapy,
Deutsches Krebsforschungszentrum

Dr. Claus-Wilhelm von der Lieth
Dr. William Hull
Central Spectroscopy,
Deutsches Krebsforschungszentrum

Dr. Rüdiger Port
Division of Perinatal Toxicology,
Deutsches Krebsforschungszentrum

Prof. Dr. Jürgen Engel
Dr. Bernd Kutscher
Dr. Uli Niemeyer
Dr. Joerg Pohl
ASTA Medica, Frankfurt

Prof. Dr. Hermann Koepsell
Anatomical Institute of the Bavarian
Julius Maximilian University, Würzburg

Selected publications

Pohl, J., Bertram, B., Hilgard, P., Nowrousian, M.R., Stüben, J., Wießler, M.: D 19575 – a sugar-linked isophosphoramide mustard derivative exploiting transmembrane glucose transport. Cancer Chemother. Pharmacol. 34, 364-370 (1995)

Stüben, J., Bertram, B., Wießler, M.: Antitumor activity and distribution of β-D-lactosylisophosphoramide mustard: a potential cytostatic agent exploiting lectin mediated transport. Int. J. Oncol. 7, 225–231 (1995)

Stüben, J., Port, R., Bertram, B., Bollow, U., Hull, W.E., Schaper, M., Pohl, J., Wießler, M.: Pharmacokinetics and whole body distribution of the new chemotherapeutic agent β-D-glucosylifosfamidemustard (D 19575) and its effects on the incorporation of [^{3}H-methyl]-thymidine in various tissues of the rat. Cancer Chemother. Pharmacol. 38, 355–365 (1996)

5.4 Molecular Therapy in the Treatment of Hematological and Oncological Diseases

by Ralf Kronenwett and Rainer Haas

The three pillars in the treatment of malignancies are surgical tumor removal, radiotherapy, and chemotherapy. Thanks to intensive research efforts these treatment methods have been undergoing continuous development. Because of this, the cure rate for cancers has significantly improved during the past several years. In this context, one observes that operating techniques in surgery have become increasingly more sophisticated; the dose distribution in radiotherapy can be optimally adapted to the location and form of the tumor by using computer simulation so that healthy tissue can be protected, and in chemotherapy blood stem cell transplantation permits the dose of drugs used to combat cancer to be increased to many times that used in earlier treatment methods. Although the successes of these classical therapies are indisputable, they remain unspecific in their nature and are associated with damage to healthy body cells. Therefore, it is our goal to develop new forms of treatment that eliminate the causes of malignant tumor cell growth in a focused manner.

Changes in the genotype as a target for gene therapy

For many malignancies specific changes in the genetic make-up, the genome, that are responsible for tumor development can be characterized. In humans the genome of every cell consists of tens of thousands of genes that are arranged as deoxyribonucleic (DNA) chains on 23 chromosome pairs. The germ cells in the testicles and the ovaries are an exception in that they possess only single and not paired chromosomes. The DNA itself is composed of four different building blocks (nucleotides). The unique order of these building blocks specifically encodes the information for a gene. In order to make the information stored in this manner available to the cell, a gene must first be rewritten (transcription) in the form of messenger ribonucleic acid (mRNA) which serves as a template for the synthesis of proteins (translation). The proteins are mainly structural building blocks, enzymes and hormones for the cells. If a gene defect arises in a cell, this can lead to a disturbance of growth regulation that is accompanied by uninhibited cell reproduction and the subsequent development of a tumor disease. These cancer-causing genes are called oncogenes and can be found in their intact form (as proto-oncogenes) in healthy cells. Their nucleotide composition or chromosomal location is changed by means of still unknown factors so that a cancer cell either forms directly from a normal cell or by way of several intermediate steps.

An example of the pathological activation of a proto-oncogene can be seen in chronic myeloid leukemia (CML). In this disease an exchange (translocation) of fragments between two chromosomes occurs in a hemopoietic stem cell. The so-called abl proto-oncogene on chromosome 9 combines with another gene on chromosome 22 to form the bcr-abl oncogene. Because of its new surroundings, the abl gene has a pathogenic effect and causes the uncontrolled reproduction of these blood cells. Since this form of leukemia has only been curable through bone marrow transplantation (a type of treatment that only proves feasible for a selected few patients and is always associated with a high risk), new forms of therapy are urgently needed.

Another disease in which an incorrectly regulated gene participates is the centroblastic, centrocytic form of Non-Hodgkin's lymphoma (cb-cc NHL), an affliction of the lymphatic system. In this case, a chromosomal translocation causes an activation of the bcl-2 proto-oncogene located on chromosome 18. Activating the bcl-2 proto-oncogene prevents the cell from dying (programmed cell death; apoptosis) and, thereby, changes the natural process of growth regulation. Also this disease is only rarely curable by means of conventional chemotherapy. Since specific changes in the genome are known for both these diseases, CML as well as cb-cc NHL, these abnormal genes can serve as targets for a therapeutic approach. Another group of diseases that could be treated with molecular therapy are several viral infections. An infection with the human immunodeficiency virus (HIV) leads to the immunodeficiency disease AIDS (acquired immunodeficiency syndrome). After infection, the HIV genes can be incorporated into the

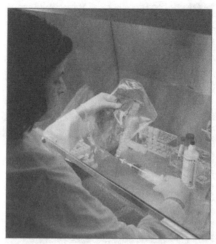

Fig. 54
The hemopoietic stem cells from leukemia patients are worked with under sterile conditions

chromosomes of the affected cells where they remain for many years. The infection with HIV serves as an example of an acquired change in the genome of a healthy cell. Viral genes are

also possible targets for molecular therapy.

Inhibition of improperly regulated genes using the antisense principle

In each instance two of the four nucleotides that form the DNA and RNA chains can form a complementary pair (hybridization) and in this manner can construct a double-stranded molecule consisting of opposite nucleotide chains. The messenger RNA (mRNA) which serves as a template for protein synthesis is called „sense" RNA (German: Sinn); the complementary sequence is designated „antisense" RNA (German: Gegensinn). A possible means of correcting an error in the genome of a tumor cell is the use of antisense nucleic acids (DNA/RNA). If these are introduced into a cell, the complementary mRNA cannot be transcribed to the corresponding protein; this results in the inactivation of the gene.

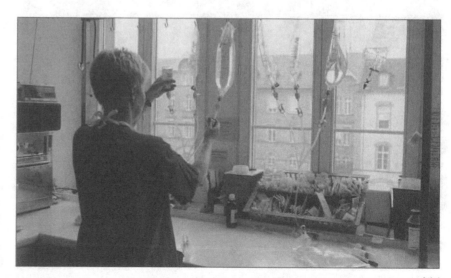

Fig. 55
In the Clinical Cooperative Unit for Molecular Hematology/Oncology, infusions with chemotherapeutic agents are being prepared

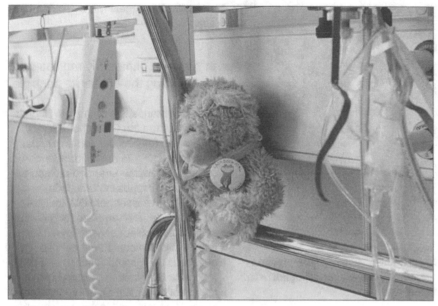

Fig. 56
The teddy bear is a constant companion of the younger patients

Fig. 57
During the transplantation of blood stem cells, patients require much rest

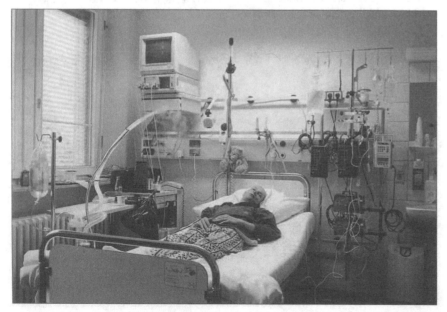

We are working to develop antisense molecules that are directed against the bcl-2 proto-oncogene in centroblastic, centrocytic Non-Hodgkin's lymphoma and against the bcr-abl oncogene in chronic myeloid leukemia. By means of investigations conducted in a cell-free system with purified sense and antisense RNA molecules, we were able to determine sequences that selectively bind to bcr-abl RNA. These sequences were synthesized as antisense DNA molecules having a length of up to 30 nucleotides and were tested in cell cultures. In our experiments, such constructs used in a test tube were able to partially inhibit the degeneration of malignant leukemia cells. A next step will include clinical studies and will entail the introduction of antisense DNA molecules into leukemia patients.

Introduction of antisense genes into cells by using viral vectors

So far we have used synthetic antisense DNA molecules (antisense oligonucleotides) in cell culture experiments that are directly introduced into the nutrient solution of tumor cells. Additionally, we are also attempting to develop genes that, after their introduction into leukemia cells, continuously produce antisense RNA against the bcr-abl oncogene. In this manner, the therapeutic molecules are available in the tumor cell until it dies; this should result in improved inhibition of cell reproduction.

A prerequisite for employing such a therapeutic technique is the development of „gene ferries" (vectors) in order to introduce the therapeutic genes into the sick cells. For the introduction of foreign hereditary material into cells (also called transduction), viruses have primarily been used during the past several years. In this process, one uses a principle that is already available in nature, because viruses are naturally capable of introducing their foreign genes into the cells of organisms that they infect. In our division, we have focused our attention on the adeno-associated virus type 2 (AAV-2) since this virus can also infect resting cells such as the hemopoietic stem cell. In order to be able to verify the incorporation of foreign genes into hemopoietic cells, we use so-called reporter genes that are integrated into the genome of AAV-2 during the production of the viral vector. After the target cell has been infected by the virus, the foreign gene is transported into the cell and is activated. If transduction proves successful, products of the reporter genes can be detected by a staining reaction or by means of fluorescence analysis in the cell when using a microscope. Using the described vector system, we were able to introduce reporter genes into leukemia cell lines. However, only a relatively small number of the cells were successfully hit. A successful gene transfer requires a large quantity of viral vectors. Therefore, we are working on improving vector production and the transduction conditions so that the number of transfected stem cells can be increased. Afterwards, the reporter genes are replaced with therapeutic genes that are then introduced into the tumor cells to inhibit malignant growth.

Therapeutic genes such as the antisense genes cannot be introduced only into tumor cells, but also into healthy cells. For example, one can take advantage of this fact in HIV infections. If one introduces an HIV-inhibiting, antisense construct into hemopoietic stem cells, these cells and the T-helper cells (the main target of HIV) that develop from them are resistant to infection. This could prevent the further spread of the virus throughout the body of an AIDS patient. A successful gene therapy for HIV infections is, however, only possible when the hemopoietic stem cells, that are supposed to be given a virus-inhibiting gene, have not already been infected with HIV. Therefore, we have employed the procedure of ultrasensitive fluorescence in situ hybridization (FISH) to detect HIV DNA in the chromosomes. The method was established by using HIV-infected cell lines in which more than 60 percent of the integrated viral genomes could be detected. Furthermore, we could identify the chromosomes in which HIV is integrated in the examined cell lines. In the future, we would like to use this method to determine whether hemopoietic stem cells from patients are infected with HIV or contain genetic material from HIV and are thus infected with this virus.

Clinical application of molecular therapy

The use of this molecular therapy is supported by the Clinical Cooperation Unit Molecular Hematology/Oncology of the Deutsches Krebsforschungszentrum. This unit was founded in March 1995 with the objective of improving the diagnostics and therapy of malignant diseases through a rapid transfer of results from basic research into clinical applications. The opening of the associated hospital ward in the building of the Medical Clinic at the University of Heidelberg in November 1996 gives the Center control of a ward with a total of eight beds. This facility enables the attending physicians and the basic research scientists to work together. An initial therapeutic application entails administering the synthetic antisense DNA which we developed to patients with CML and cb-cc NHL much in the same way as antibiotic therapy or chemotherapy can be given. Although the antisense oligonucleotides are taken up by most of the body's cells, their specific effect can, in the case of chronic myeloid leukemia, only be realized in tumor cells that carry the bcr-abl oncogene. Therefore, no side effects are expected in healthy body cells. This is a decisive advantage when compared to chemotherapy in which all rapidly reproducing cells are attacked; this causes the unpleasant side effects of chemotherapy.

Another possible application of antisense nucleic acids is the treatment of hemopoietic stem cells outside of the patient's body. For this purpose, stem cells are removed from the blood of tumor patients following chemotherapy and the administration of hemopoietic growth factors. After high dose chemotherapy and radiotherapy which destroys the bone marrow, the patient is again given the hemopoietic stem cells that had been previously removed. This allows hemopoiesis to become reestablished. The procedure is called autologous blood stem cell transplantation. It was conducted worldwide for the very first time 12 years ago in the Medical Clinic and Polyclinic V of the University of Heidelberg. During the past several years, it has undergone further development especially for the treatment of non-Hodgkin's lymphomas of low malignancy. In order to prevent tumor cells from being reintroduced into patients, stem cell preparations are either selectively concentrated or are cleaned with monoclonal antibodies ("purging"). Possibly leukemia cells can also be eliminated by treating stem cells with antisense DNA outside of the patient's body.

To what extent molecular therapy can result in a cure of chronic myeloid leukemia or non-Hodgkin's lymphomas of low malignancy or can enhance the successes attained by autologous blood stem cell transplantation will be shown in clinical studies. Such research will be conducted in a collaboration between the University Clinic, Heidelberg, and the Krebsforschungszentrum in the near future.

The project is supported by the Tumor Center Heidelberg/Mannheim.

Dr. Ralf Kronenwett
Prof. Dr. Rainer Haas
Clinical Cooperation Unit Molecular Hematology/Oncology

Participating scientists

Dr. Martin Deichmann
Dr. Elisabeth Ogniben
Dr. Maria-Teresa Voso

In collaboration with

Priv.-Doz. Dr. Jürgen Kleinschmidt
Division of Tumor Virology,
Deutsches Krebsforschungszentrum

Priv.-Doz. Dr. Georg Sczakiel
Division of Genome Modifications and Carcinogenesis,
Deutsches Krebsforschungszentrum

Prof. Dr. Jens Zeller
Division of Perinatal Toxicology,
Deutsches Krebsforschungszentrum

Dr. Stefan Fruehauf
Dr. Stefan Hohaus
Dr. Marion Moos
Dr. Simona Murea
Department of Internal Medicine V
(Specialty: Hematology, Oncology, Rheumatology),
University Medical Clinic
and Polyclinic V,
Heidelberg

Dr. Andreas Hochhaus
III. Medical Clinic,
Clinic of the City of Mannheim

Selected publications

Haas, R., Brittinger, G., Meusers, P., Murea, S., Goldschmidt, H., Wannenmacher, M., Hunstein, W.: Myeloablative therapy with blood stem cell transplantation is effective in mantle cell lymphoma. Leukemia 10, 1975–1979 (1996)

Haas, R. Murea, S.: "State of the Art": Hochdosistherapie mit Stammzellsupport. In: Onkologie Service aktuell, Springer Verlag, Berlin, Heidelberg, 4, 4–11 (1996)

Kronenwett, R., Haas, R., Sczakiel, G.: Kinetic selectivity of complementary nucleic acids: bcr-abl-directed antisense RNA and ribozymes. J. Mol. Biol. 259, 632–644 (1996)

Deichmann, M., Bentz, M., Haas, R.: Ultrasensitive FISH is a usefull tool in studying chronic HIV-infection. J. Virol. Meth. 65, 19–25 (1997)

Voso, M.T., Hohaus, S., Moos, M., Haas, R.: Lack of t(14;18) PCR-positive cells in highly purified CD34 positive cells and their CD19 subsets in patients with follicular lymphoma. Blood 89, 3763–3768 (1997)

5.5 CD 95: Recipient of the Death Message

by Klaus-Michael Debatin and Peter H. Krammer

The most frequent form of cell death in an organism is apoptosis. In certain defense cells of the immune system, the T lymphocytes, apoptosis occurs after the CD95 (APO-1/FAS) receptor has been activated by the CD95 ligand to which it is connected. By means of the CD95 system, T lymphocytes can themselves commit suicide as well as kill other T lymphocytes and target cells. Eliminating apoptosis-sensitive T lymphocytes is of decisive significance for the equilibrium of the immune system, self-tolerance, immune suppression (suppression or weakening of the immune response), and turning off an immunological response. Outside of the lymphatic system, the CD95 system also plays an important role in tissue homeostasis. Reduced apoptosis can lead to the development of tumors. On the other hand, increased apoptosis can result in a weakening of the immune system such as in the case of HIV infection or, in the case of other diseases, tissue destruction. Cancer drugs that are successfully used in tumor therapy activate the CD95 system. Disturbances in CD95-mediated apoptosis are probably one of the reasons for developing drug resistance and the ineffectiveness of antitumor therapies. Understanding the molecular mechanisms of apoptosis would permit the development of rational clinical therapies for diseases in which apoptosis is incorrectly regulated.

In our immune system, the activation and production of antibody-producing B lymphocytes and T lymphocytes that execute cellular immune reactions occur constantly. Nevertheless, the number of lymphocytes as well as the quantity of other tissues remains relatively constant in a healthy adult organism. Therefore, regulatory processes must exist that determine the constancy of the lymphocyte pool and the overall cellular mass.

T lymphocytes in the peripheral immune system that effect defensive reactions react with antigens (e.g., parts of viruses or bacteria) by means of specific receptors. These antigens are presented in the form of peptides, small protein molecules, by antigen-presenting cells. After antigen contact has been made, the T lymphocytes reproduce. The army of lymphocytes is now in the position to successfully combat the enemy, the antigen, and to either neutralize or eliminate it. After the battle has been won, most of the antigen-specific lymphocytes are no longer needed. They are eliminated by means of focused cell death; the immune response is thereby turned off or suppressed. Even self-reactive T lymphocytes are killed by apoptosis.

Under the light microscope, the death struggle of cells that die by means of apoptosis presents a dramatic and spectacular image. They begin to conduct wild movements, a process that is described by the term "boiling" (German "kochen"). Afterwards, they experience the stage of zeiosis in which the cells cast off small vesicles. Finally, the center of the cell nucleus becomes lumpy. During apoptosis that occurs within tissue, dead cells are devoured by neighboring cells or by phagocytes without any accompanying inflammation.

The hereditary material of the dying cells, the DNA, has previously been split into small fragments by DNA-digesting enzymes.

On the surface of most of our body cells there are thousands of

CD95(APO-1/Fas) molecules, the apoptosis-causing "death receptor". This could be an indication of the fact that the receptor plays a role in the apoptosis program of many types of cells. The most well-known example is the role that CD95 plays in the immune system. Molecules that bind to a receptor are called ligands. CD95 also has a natural ligand, the CD95 (APO-1/Fas) ligand. In cells that carry CD95 on their surface, apoptosis can be triggered by means of anti-CD95 antibodies (e.g., anti-APO-1 or Anti-Fas) as well as by the "death ligand", CD95L. Both the binding of anti-CD95 antibodies and CD95L cause a cross-linking of the CD95 receptors on the cell surface, a process that triggers the death signal in the interior of the cell. In order to better understand this process, one must take a closer look at the structure of CD95.

CD95 is constructed of three parts: an intracellular part that protrudes into the interior of the cell, a transmembrane part that reaches through the cell membrane, the cellular envelope, and an extracellular part that protrudes out of the cell. The extracellular part shows a great deal to the members of another receptor family, the tumor necrosis receptor family. The extracellular part of CD95 establishes contact to the external environment of the cell; anti-CD95 antibodies and CD95L bind to it. In contrast, the intracellular part of CD95 is important for the initiation of signals required for apoptosis. Of special significance for this is a segment of the intracellular part of CD95 that is called the "death domain".

Major elements of the signal path of CD95 have been clarified. According to this we assume that the initial steps of CD95-mediated apoptosis proceed in the following manner: CD95L binds to CD95, whereby three ligands and three receptor molecules unite to form a complex. In doing so, the intracellular death domains of the three CD95 receptors approach one another in such a manner that they bring together additional molecules, called CAP ("cytotoxicity dependent apoptosis associated proteins"), which are already present in the cell interior, to form a complex with CD95. This process is called DISC ("death-inducing signaling complex"). The formation of the DISC initiates apoptosis. If the DISC is not formed, apoptosis is not triggered and the cells are apoptosis-resistant. However, the processes that directly follow the formation of the DISC are still mainly unknown. Their clarification will permit experimental access to several signal switches that determine whether cells are sensitive or resistant to CD95-mediated apoptosis. It is easy to predict that knowledge of this process will have both experimental and clinical significance. A signal defect that is caused by a disturbance in the formation of the DISC is found in genetically defective mice (lprcg mice) that have a CD95 receptor with altered hereditary material in the death domain. This defect, a reduced density in CD95 receptors (in lpr mice) or the expression of a dysfunctional CD95L (in gld mice: CD95L is mutated and can no longer bind to CD95), interferes with CD95-mediated apoptosis.

All three cases, lpr, lpr^{cg} and gld mice, showed a similar symptomology: first, a significant enlargement of the spleen and lymph nodes, which can be traced to a pathological collection of defective T lymphocytes, and second, autoimmunity with autoantibodies that is similar to the human disease, lupus erythematodes. This affliction is similar to an autoimmune disease that involves the entire body. Almost the same signs of disease were found in children with genetic defects in the CD95 system. In children and animals with a CD95 gene defect, the symptoms could be explained by the fact that CD95-mediated apoptosis was reduced in both the T lymphocytes and the B lymphocytes. Therefore, the lymphocyte death rate that is physiologically important for the preservation of the equilibrium in the immune system is pathologically low. The collection of malfunctioning T and B lymphocytes causes the lymphoid organs to become enlarged and results in the formation of antibodies directed against the organism itself.

The findings described above led one to the assumption that the CD95 system was especially important for the proper functioning of the immune system and that a disturbance in its processes is not noticed as readily in other areas of the organism. This assumption has been confirmed. One of the main questions with respect to the CD95 system focused on whether T lymphocytes could kill themselves, their neighbor T cells or other cells such as B lymphocytes with the assistance of the CD95 system. Our working group and other scientists were able to demonstrate that T lymphocytes produce the death receptor, CD95, and also the death ligand, CD95L, after they have been activated by antigen through the T cell receptor. Both CD95 and CD95L could be found on the cell membrane and in soluble form.

Therefore, a T cell possesses both the "death receptor", CD95, and the "murder weapon", CD95L, and can thereby destroy itself by inducing apoptosis. This form of T cell death, called "autocrine suicide", exists in addition to other forms of death that are mediated by the CD95 system. For example, T cells with CD95L on their cell membrane can commit "fratricide" and kill neighboring T cells, that are CD95+. Furthermore, CD95L can be secreted and can kill neighboring cells. Through similar mechanisms, non-T cells can also be sacrificed by T lymphocytes. In any case, T lymphocytes can kill other cells as well as commit suicide.

CD95 appears in B and T lymphocytes after activation on the cell surface. However, the sensitivity for CD95-mediated apoptosis requires a longer lasting stimulation of the T cells. Immature T cells that develop as thymocytes in the thymus also secrete CD95, but they are mainly resistant to CD95-mediated apoptosis.

This spectrum of sensitivity and resistance to apoptosis in CD95-secreting cells is again seen in T cell leukemias. Tumor cells from patients with adult T cell leukemia, in which the leukemia cells externally correspond to activated T cells, are very sensitive to CD95-induced apoptosis. In the case of this very rare form of leukemia, we were able to show several years ago that intact apoptosis programs exist in tumor cells and can in fact be triggered.

In contrast to adult T cell leukemia, many leukemias exhibit a T cell phenotype. The leukemia cells correspond to immature differentiation stages of T lymphocytes (thymocytes) and are resistant to CD95-mediated apoptosis.

The molecular determination of sensitivity and resistance to CD95-mediated apoptosis in cancer cells still remains unclear for the most part. In principle, disturbances of the CD95 system can be caused by mutations or functional defects of the CD95 ligand, the CD95 receptor and the molecules of the signal path. However, initial experiments show that mutations in the CD95 receptor, occur in genetically determined diseases that are present with lymphoproliferation and autoimmunity, but not in T cell leukemias. It appears much more likely that CD95 resistance in T cell leukemias is the consequence of an internal anti-apoptosis program in which the CD95 signal path is blocked.

Apparently, the activation of the CD95 program (e.g., by triggering a "suicide" or the killing of neighboring cells in tissue) or the direct activation of the CD95 signal path cannot only be triggered by physiological occurrences, but also by means of cancer drugs (cytostatic agents). It does appear to be the case that the sensitivity to chemotherapy (and radiotherapy) of various lymphatic and non-lymphatic tumors depends upon the existence of an intact signal path. Drugs that are usually used in the treatment of leukemias and tumors that are sensitive to chemotherapy promote the expression of the CD95 ligand in cells or increase the expression of the receptor. The interaction between the CD95 ligand and receptor is caused by drugs such as doxorubicin, methotrexate, and cytarabine in concentrations that are usually employed in chemotherapy. Blocking the CD95 signal path results in resistance to cytostatic agents in cell culture.

It was surprising to discover that the effect of cytostatic agents, specifically the killing of tumor cells, requires an intact CD95 system and an intact CD95 signal path. This has far-reaching conse-quences. Figures 58 and 59 illustrate a dramatic difference in the ability to kill CD95-sensitive and CD95-resistant leukemia cells when using a drug such as doxorubicin wich is frequently employed in leukemia therapy. In one case, all cells are rapidly killed. Other cells in which the CD95 signal path has been blocked are not affected at all by the drug. These findings have great significance for the therapeutic use of known drugs and the development of new cytostatic or cytotoxic principles of action in cancer therapy.

In addition to triggering "autocrine suicide" or „fratricide" in activated T cells in the context of regulating the immune response, this mechanism possibly plays a significant role in various diseases. For example, studies conducted by many working groups show that in HIV infections it is especially the CD4+ helper cells that die at an increased rate. In HIV infection, one assumes that this dying of the T lymphocytes is not directly related to the viral infection of the cells, but is instead caused by indirect mechanisms in which viral gene products participate. In fact, viral gene products such as Tat and gp120 can, under certain experimental conditions, trigger CD95-mediated apoptosis in activated T cells. T lymphocytes from patients with an HIV infection have a massively increased expression of the CD95 receptor and a clearly elevated constitutive expression of the CD95 ligand. Therefore, we assume that in HIV infection an activation and/or an increased activity of the CD95 system leads to an increased elimination of T cells. This type of accelerated apoptosis, which is possibly caused by activation of the CD95 system, is also found in other diseases of lymphohemato-

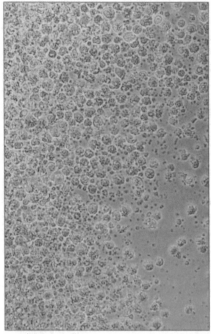
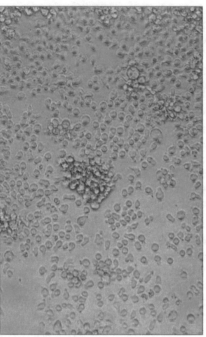

Figs. 58, 59
The cancer drug, doxorubicin, can trigger programmed cell death or apoptosis in leu-kemia cells (Fig. 58): The cells disintegrate into small vesicles. The cells shown in Fig. 59 survive doxorubicin treatment, because they have a defect in the apoptosis pathway: Programmed cell death is not triggered

poietic cells such as aplastic anemia. Therapeutic strategies wich are able to stop apoptosis in HIV infections and other diseases may possibly advance the treatment of a variety of diseases that are accompanied by accelerated cell death.

Clarifying the function of the CD95 system could lead to a better understanding of diseases that are marked by "too much" or "too little" apoptosis. Increased tumor mass is also explainable as the sum of unregulated growth and reduced cell death due to a lower rate of apoptosis. In such a case, intracellular anti-apoptosis programs could

negatively influence the sensitivity to apoptosis and play a role in tumor formation as well as the development of tumor resistance as, for example, occurs in the course of chemotherapy.

Prof. Dr. Klaus-Michael Debatin
Clinical Cooperation Unit Molecular Oncology/Pediatrics

Prof. Dr. Peter H. Krammer
Division of Immunological Genetics

Selected publications

Trauth, B.C., Klas, C., Peters, A.M. et al.: Monoclonal antibody-mediated tumor regression by induction of apoptosis. Science 245, 301–305 (1989)

Krammer, P.H., Dhein, J., Walczak, H. et al.: The role of APO-1-mediated apoptosis in the immune system. Immunological Reviews 142, 175–191 (1994)

Dhein, J., Walczak, H., Baumler, C. et al.: Autocrine T-cell suicide mediated by APO-1/FAS/CD95. Nature 373, 438–441 (1995)

Friesen, C., Herr, I., Krammer, P.H., Debatin, K.-M.: Involvement of the CD95 (APO-1/Fas) receptor/ligand system in drug-induced apoptosis in leukemia cells. Nature Medicine 2 (5), 574–577 (1996)

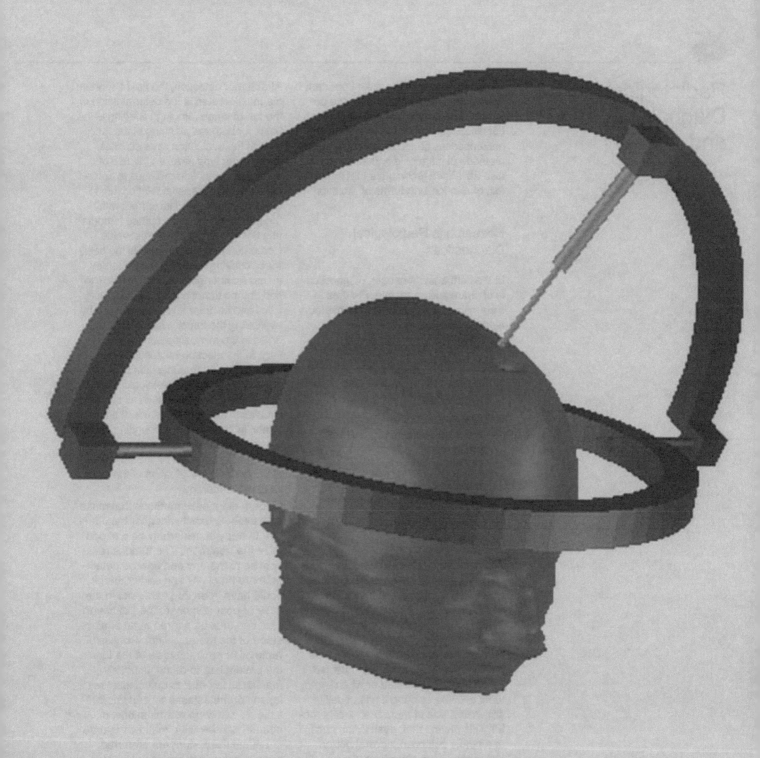

Radiological Diagnostics and Therapy

Radiology is one of the most important specializations in medicine for the detection, treatment, and follow-up of cancer diseases. Today, radiology not only encompasses conventional radiological methods of diagnosis and therapy, but also advanced techniques that make use of non-ionizing forms of radiation.

Research in Radiological Diagnostics

In the fight against cancer, diagnostics is of strategic importance. Failures in diagnosis can hardly be compensated by therapy.

Tumor diagnostics basically has the following tasks:

1. Detection of the tumor in the earliest possible stage;

2. Determination of its size, localization, relationship to organs, and spread ("staging");

3. Characterization of the tumor tissue through morphological, physiological, and biochemical parameters;

4. Control of the course of therapy, and

5. Diagnostic postoperative care.

The decisive first step in treating the individual cancer disease is the earliest possible detection of the tumor. Diagnostic procedures should put little strain on the patient so that they can be used as soon as suspicion arises. In general, the tumor develops without symptoms for several years before it is detected. At the time it is detected or when symptoms become evident, it has usually grown to a size of more than 1 centimeter. This means that, even in the case of an early detection, several million tumor cells have already grown.

After tumor detection, the next important diagnostical step is the determination of the tumor stage (staging). Staging is the basis for both the planning of the therapy and the evaluation of its success. Each tumor type requires the use of specific examination methods to determine its size, its spatial relationship to other structures, and its spread within the organism. Here, computed tomography has proven to be of great value. Computed tomography also is the basis for calculating advanced radiotherapy plans. Another goal of diagnostics is to find out the tumor's individual characteristics and its "internals". This is done by evaluating the tumor's histological properties in the microscope and, if necessary, in the electron microscope (grading). Recent approaches aim at detecting and quantifying physiological and biochemical parameters such as blood circulation and metabolism within the tumor, in the healthy surrounding tissue, and in metastases. This data provides important information for therapy planning and for the evaluation of the success of the therapy.

Modern diagnostic methods that make it possible to exactly monitor the effect of a therapy considerably help to optimize the treatment. The tumor's response to therapy can now be detected more precisely and earlier than it could have been 20 years ago. In the case of poor response, the treatment plan can thus be altered at an earlier stage of the therapy. After successful removal or apocatastasis of the tumor, the patient has to be continuously monitored in order to detect local relapses or metastases as early as possible. In follow-up examinations, of course, non-invasive methods that do not strain the patient are preferred over invasive techniques.

Various diagnostic methods are available for the detection and evaluation of the cancer disease.

1. Biochemical and immunologic examinations of body fluids (blood, urine, discharges, etc.);
2. Detection of tumor tissue with imaging techniques:
   a) radiodiagnostics
   b) endoscopy
   c) ultrasound diagnostics
   d) computed tomography
   e) magnetic resonance tomography
   f) scintigraphy, including immunoscintigraphy
   g) positron emission tomography;
3. Detection of individual tumor cells (cytodiagnostics) in the sputum, in smear, or in puncture fluid;
4. Pathological detection of tumor cell clusters through sampling of suspicious tissue.

Imaging techniques make it possible to detect tumors and metastases that are larger than 1 to 2 centimeters. Due to physical and biophysical limitations, however, it cannot be expected to enhance the resolution in the near future. Instead, the development in diagnostics is aimed at better specifying the characteristics of the detected foci.

In the recent past, diagnostic research focused on improving the evaluation of the tumor's size, its structure, and its functional performance on the basis of newly developed, advanced radiological methods. Such examinations have now become possible with magnetic resonance tomography and positron emission tomography.

Magnetic resonance tomography (MRT) images a specified portion of the body slice-by-slice; the slice images can then be evaluated by the physician. For the examination, the patient is placed in a strong magnetic field. Certain atomic nuclei, which have an intrinsic angular momentum (spin), behave like small magnets and align with the external magnetic field. They may be excited by radio waves whose frequency corresponds to the nuclei's precession frequency. The excited nuclei emit high-frequency signals that give information on the state of the tissue they are located in. However, these signals have to be decoded with the help of modern data processing methods. The use of even stronger magnetic fields makes it possible to also investigate specific metabolic processes occurring in the tissue (magnetic resonance spectroscopy).

Parallel to and supplementing MRT, the tumor tissue is also examined with positron emission tomography (PET). PET renders slice images of the distribution of radiolabeled organic substances within the body. A radiolabeled molecule, in which one of its atoms is replaced with a radioactive atom of the same kind, has the same biological properties as the corresponding unlabeled molecule. A fact of great importance for the analysis of metabolic processes is that radiolabeling makes it possible to measure quantitatively.

Positron emission tomography and magnetic resonance tomography make it possible to non-invasively measure important metabolic parameters (perfusion, the metabolisms of glucose, phosphorus, and proteins, catabolism) of cancer drugs in the tumor. By comparing the treatment data with the data collected prior to and at the beginning of the treatment, the physician can draw conclusions about the success of the therapy or optimize the treatment protocol.

Therefore, both techniques are used in the search for tumors, in tumor staging, for monitoring the course of therapy and, most importantly, for the characterization of tumor tissue in the living organism.

Radiological Therapy Research

The term "cancer" does not mean one specific disease but is a comprehensive term for a multitude of different tumor types. Thus, it cannot be expected that all malignant tumors can be influenced or cured with one and the same therapy. One basic difficulty for some therapeutic techniques comes from the fact that the tumor cell has developed from a normal cell. Consequently, much lesser differences to normal cells can be exploited for therapy than, for example, in the case of bacteria.

There are various approaches to cancer therapy: surgical removal of the tumor tissue, radiotherapy, hyperthermia, hormone therapy, chemotherapy, gene therapy, and immunotherapy. Surgery and radiotherapy are local tumor treatments. They cannot be used, however, if the tumor has infiltrated vital organs, as a consequence of which radical removal or destruction of the tumor is no longer possible without damaging the healthy tissue. Preliminary results show that radiotherapy of various tumors can be effectively supplemented by local hyperthermia.

Chemotherapy is used for several types of solid tumors after they have metastasized. Chemotherapy has shown important results in the treatment of malignant diseases of the hematopoietic tissue (leukemia). Positive effects on primarily malignant tumors of the lymph nodes can be achieved through radiotherapy and/or chemotherapy, depending on the tumor's stage. In general, hormone therapy is limited to tumors whose cells carry hormone receptors.

In the field of radiotherapy, the activities of the Deutsches Krebsforschungszentrum aim at the complete elimination of the tumor while optimately sparing the neighboring healthy tissue. This objective can be realized by improving radiotherapy planning, in particular, by using computerized tomography and magnetic resonance tomography, as well as electronic data processing.

A particularly powerful radiotherapeutic technique being developed at the Deutsches Krebsforschungszentrum is photon conformation therapy. In conformation therapy, the tumor is irradiated from various directions, and an adjustable multi-leaf collimator adjusts the shape of the irradiating beam to that of the tumor for each direction of irradiation. Thus, the dose is concentrated and homogeneously distributed within the tumor, while the neighboring tissues are protected.

Another technique used for precision radiotherapy, stereotactic convergent beam irradiation, has been developed for the treatment of small tumors in the brain or in the region of the head and neck. The patient's head is immobilized, and the tumor is irradiated from various directions with highly collimated photon beams. Again, the dose is concentrated within the tumor and the neighboring healthy tissue is spared. This technique is used for single-high-dose irradiations of tumors, metastases and vessel deformations in the brain.

Presently, a combined therapy of irradiation and hyperthermia is being tested for the treatment of tumors of the esophagus, the bile duct, the cervix, and the rectum. Controlled local hyperthermia can be produced with special antenna systems.

For many years, pulsed high-energy ultrasound has been used to destroy nephroliths. Experimental studies have shown that a modified form of this technique, in combination with radiation, heat, and chemical substances, is suitable for the local treatment of tumors. Clinical trials are planned to follow these preliminary experiments.

Another promising concept which is being further developed and applied at the Deutsches Krebsforschungszentrum is photodynamic therapy. A photosensilizer is introduced into the tumor via the circulating blood, and the tumor is irradiated with suitable laser light. The resulting chemical processes destroy the tumor from within. Researchers of the Deutsches Krebsforschungszentrum have succeeded in developing photosensitive substances with considerably higher accumulation rates in the tumor than has been achieved with previous substances. This method may improve the treatment of superficial tumors.

Clinical studies on all of the mentioned techniques are being carried out in close cooperation with the clinics of the Tumor Center Heidelberg/Mannheim and the Department of Stereotactic Neurosurgery of the University of Cologne.

Als an alternative to radiotherapy, researchers at the Deutsches Krebsforschungszentrum are investigating other minimally invasive treatment methods for localized cancers. An important

focus of these activities is the development of stereotactic laser neurosurgery in cooperation with the Institute for Applied Physics of Heidelberg University. This technique uses a probe to target any site within the brain to a very high precision. With the help of this probe, the beam of a special laser traverses the tumor. The interaction of the laser beam with the tissue results in a "cold" resection of the tumor, i.e., no thermal damage to the surrounding healthy tissue is done – a side effect which is often observed with traditional lasers. The absence of thermal damage is due to the extremely short period of interaction between laser beam and tissue. Using such a probe, it is possible to remove a tumor very precisely from the inside. An irrigation and suction apparatus integrated in the probe is used to remove the tissue fragments from the resulting cavity and to stabilize the pressure inside the cavity. This new treatment method will make it possible to remove, in particular, deep-seated brain tumors while sparing the surrounding healthy tissue as much as possible.

The aim of newly established clinical cooperation unit "Radiotherapy" is to develop new radio-oncological treatment methods. One line of research will investigate the possibilities of optimizing the therapeutical effects of radiation on a biological basis. An important task of the cooperation unit will be to carry out clinical trials of the phases I/II and II, in which the new treatment methods are tested for their safety and reliability. If the results are promising, the next step will be to perform randomized trial studies of phase III in close cooperation – both in terms of staff and premises – with the University Radiological Hospital in Heidelberg.

Coordinator of the Research Program:
Prof. Dr. Gerhard van Kaick

Divisions and their heads:

Oncological Diagnostics and Therapy:
Prof. Dr. Gerhard van Kaick

Biophysics and Medical Radiation
Physics:
Prof. Dr. Walter W. Lorenz (until 1997)
Priv.-Doz. Dr. Gunnar Brix

Radiochemistry and
Radiopharmacology:
Dr. Wolfgang Maier-Borst (until 1997)
Dr. Hannsjörg Sinn

Medical Physics:
Prof. Dr. Wolfgang Schlegel

Clinical Cooperation Unit Radiotherapeutic Oncology:
Priv.-Doz. Dr. Dr. Jürgen Debus

6.1 Therapy of Brain Tumors with Laser Neurosurgery

by Wolfgang Schlegel
and Jürgen Dams

The Problem of Treating Brain Tumors

Although computed tomography (CT), magnetic resonance imaging (MRI) and positron emission tomography (PET) have during the past several years significantly contributed to improving the diagnosis of brain tumors, the therapeutic possibilities that are currently available - surgery and radiotherapy - are still very limited, especially for brain tumors exhibiting infiltrating growth.

In the traditional, neurosurgical operating technique (opening of the cranium and the following dissection of the tumor), injury to healthy tissue and subsequent functional losses or limitations are inevitable.

The main advantage of radiotherapy, which employs ionizing radiation, is its ability to avoid the trauma associated with the operation itself. However, very frequently radiosensitive areas are located very close to the tumor. This limits the magnitude of the usable radiation dose in such cases and makes the long-term healing of the tumor through irradiation impossible. Also, the early stages of tumors that exhibit infiltrating growth (e.g., glioblastoma) cannot be treated with sufficiently high radiation doses. Furthermore, radiation necrosis may occur as an undesired side effect, especially in the radiotherapy of larger tumors. Toxic substances that can prove to be a significant burden to the patient are released in the necrotic tissues.

Therefore, it continues to be necessary to search for more efficient and less harmful therapeutic procedures for brain tumors.

The New Method: Surgery with Short-Pulsed Lasers

To broaden the spectrum of treatment possibilities for brain tumors, laser beams were already introduced many years ago in neurosurgery. Laser beams can be conducted to the site of the operation through glass fibers. If they make contact with tissue, they release a large quantity of light energy which results in the tissue being destroyed. These properties mean that laser beams are an ideal tool for minimal invasive surgery which is a more protective and effective method of operating. However, a serious disadvantage of laser surgery as practiced until now has been that only lasers that produce heat when making contact with tissues have been available. Because of the production of heat and the associated side effects in the brain, such thermically effective lasers are unsuitable for neurosurgery.

This situation has significantly changed with the introduction of the short-pulsed laser technique which has been known for approximately the past ten years. Short-pulsed laser equipment enables one to engage in a „cold" removal of tissue without imparting any thermic damage to the surrounding areas. However, such equipment has usually been too complicated, too large, too maintenance-intensive, and, most importantly, too weak in its power output to effectively remove larger tissue volumes such as a tumor. They have previously only been used medically in ophthalmology, for example, to treat ametropia by removing corneal tissue.

The Project Team „Stereotactic Short-Pulsed Laser Neurosurgery": A Coming Together of Scientists from Physics and Medicine

The project team has existed for approximately four years and is supported by the European Union. It consists of scientists from the Institute for Applied Physics at the University of Heidelberg under the direction of Professor Josef Bille, the Division of Medical Physics at the Deutsches Krebsforschungszentrum (directed by Professor Wolfgang Schlegel), and the Neurosurgical Clinic at the University of Cologne (directed by Professor Volker Sturm). These researchers have come together to take up the new method of short-pulsed laser technology and to also make it usable in the treatment of brain tumors. Additional cooperating partners in this project include: the Neurosurgical Clinic at the University of Louvain, the Institute for Control Engineering at the University of Siegen, the Physical Institute at the Swiss Federal Institute of Technology Zurich (ETHZ), and the MRC GmbH company in Heidelberg.

The objective of this cooperative arrangement is to develop a laser surgery procedure that will be based on short-pulsed lasers and will also make possible the less damaging and effective removal of larger tissue volumes. The developed procedure must permit pre-planning and optimization of the operation with computer programs and the entire course of the operation must be able to be exactly monitored and controlled through simultaneous imaging. Such a minimally invasive operating technique will not only be a significant improvement in the treatment of brain

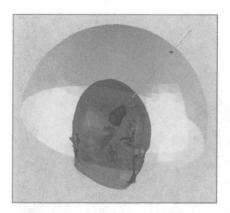

Fig. 60
Using data obtained from CT and magnetic resonance spectroscopy, the location of a tumor (red) can be presented as a three-dimensional computer image before the operation. In this manner, the computer simulation shows where the surgical probe can best be placed within a defined area (gray hemisphere)

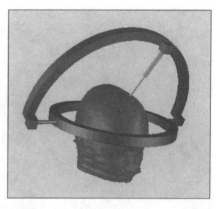

Fig. 61
In order to exactly position the surgical probe, the patient's head is immobilized via attachment to the stereotactic ring. The probe is attached to a rotatable yoke and is brought into proper position based on the calculated data

tumors, but will also prove extremely useful in other difficult to execute and risky surgical procedures (such as slipped disk operations).

Allocation of Duties

At the ETHZ, the working group of Professor Ursula Keller developed compact laser systems that require minimal maintenance („diode-pumped solid state lasers") and that attain previously unheard of power densities. They make possible the cold removal of tissues by means of laser beam impulses with irradiation times in the femtosecond to picosecond range (10^{-15} sec to 10^{-12}). When the 10 W laser that is currently being constructed is completed, it will be possible to remove several cubic

centimeters of tissue in only a few minutes time.

The working group of Professor Josef Bille at the Institute for Applied Physics (University of Heidelberg) is constructing a new type of probe that will facilitate the described technique of minimally invasive surgery in the manner of „keyhole surgery". This probe works in the same way as a periscope in a submarine: At the end of the articulated arm, the laser beam is deflected through a prism at a ninety degree angle. By means of the shifting of different focusing lenses and the rotation of several tubes within a rigid sheath, the tumor can be removed in the form of cylinders. This cylinder geometry, along with the possibility of turning the laser on or off at every point of a cylinder's

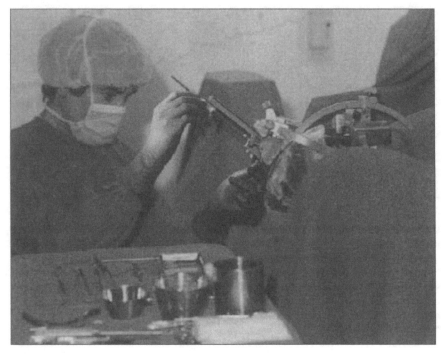

Fig. 62
During the operation, the neurosurgeon guides the probe into the skull through a bore hole approximately six millimeters in diameter

mits an exact localization of any number of points in the brain and, thereby, an exact planning of the therapy. Furthermore, the ring serves as a basis for guiding the probe in the later operation.

To avoid injuring cranial nerves, blood vessels and sensible areas, the planning program developed at the Deutsches Krebsforschungszentrum facilitates the interactive optimization of the access path already before the operation. To this purpose, the exact location of the operating probe is shown in cross-sectional images that run perpendicular to the path of access.

An additional criterion in choosing the access path is the desired objective of attaining an optimal fit of the tissue removal technology to the form of the tumor. A three-dimensional computer graphic showing the anatomy and the operation instruments is planned to provide a complete overview of probe position.

Calculating the dose is the next step, which is also realized in a computer program. It is determined in which direction, for how long and with what power irradiation must proceed in order to completely remove the tumor.

Finally, the computer program calculates the coordinates that are needed to adjust the stereotactic target equipment. During the removal of tumor tissue in the brain with a computer-guided laser probe, work must proceed with extreme precision and utmost care and safety. Constant monitoring of the course of the operation through imaging procedures is, therefore, absolutely necessary. Three different possibilities are presently being examined by the project team:

A confocal laser-scanning microscope was developed at the Institute for Ap-

surface, means that the field of operation can be adjusted for any kind of tumor.

The prototype of the probe has an external diameter of 5.5 millimeters and requires that only a burr hole of this size be made through the cranium; the previously necessary more extensive opening of the cranium common in other operations can be avoided.

Following the removal procedure, the resulting tissue fragments are eliminated from the brain by means of a rinsing and suction mechanism that is integrated into the probe. The rinsing system which contains an automatic pressure control mechanism was developed at

the Institute for Control Engineering, University of Siegen, under the supervision of Professor Werner Düchting.

In the Division of Medical Physics at the Deutsches Krebsforschungszentrum, work is continuing on a computer-aided planning tool to optimally position the probe within the head of a patient and also on methods to calculate the dose needed to remove tumors with laser beams. The first objective of the developed computer programs is to precisely be able to position the probe in the brain. Before the data are entered into the tomograph, a stereotactic ring is fixed to the patient's head just as in the conventional stereotactic operating technique. This stereotactic ring per-

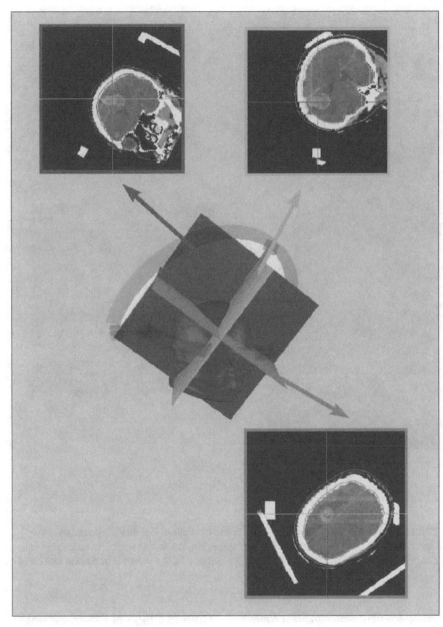

Fig. 63
Using CT, sectional images of the tumor are produced in various planes: vertical (green) and along the surgical probe (red and yellow). The images allow the outline of the tumor to be recognized and, thereby, make planning the course of the operation possible

plied Physics. It is integrated into the operating probe in the form of an endoscope and transmits optical images from the operating field of the probe with highest local resolution and depth of focus to an external computer. The presentation of these images on the computer monitor provides the treating physician with important information about the course of the operation.

An additional means of monitoring the operation is being investigated at the Deutsches Krebsforschungszentrum; this involves a 3D ultrasound probe that is to be inserted into an additional burr hole in the patient's head. The ultrasound images must then be compared with the original images obtained from preoperative CT and MRI data as well as the endoscopic images. This permits an even more detailed evaluation of the removal procedure.

Probably, the most exact, but also the most complicated and expensive option for monitoring the course of the operation is intraoperative magnetic resonance tomography. Conducting the operation in an MR tomograph and showing the operation in MRI images requires that both the stereotactic fixation and target systems as well as the laser probe be manufactured from materials that are suitable for use in the strong and constantly changing magnetic fields of an MR tomograph. Materials that conduct electricity must not be used in order to avoid that image-falsifying electrical currents are induced in the materials. Therefore, only plastic or ceramic materials can be considered for the production of the operating tools. The Deutsches Krebsforschungszentrum, the Institute for Applied Physics, and

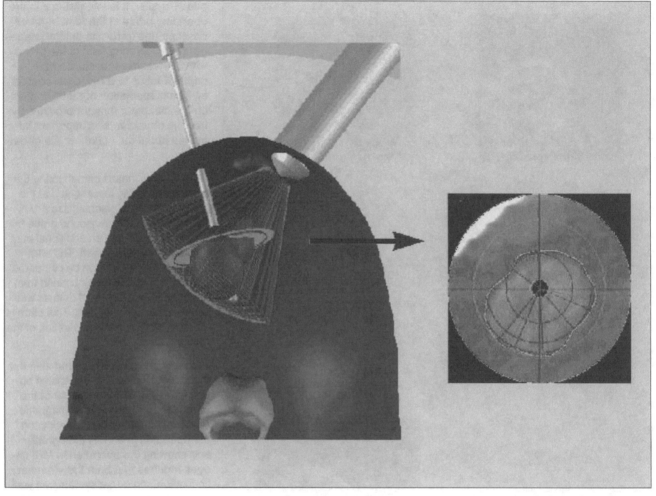

Fig. 64
The use of ultrasound is one of several possibilities for directly following the course of the operation. For this purpose, an ultrasound transducer is introduced into the skull through a second bore hole. During the operation, the tumor region is examined with ultrasound (left). From the ultrasound signal changes in the location of the tumor, which are due to the removal of tissue, can be directly (in real time) displayed (right)

the MRC company in Heidelberg are working together to solve the associated problems (among others, strength, capability to be sterilized, tissue compatibility). MRC, which wants to take over the production of the complete neurosurgical laser system after the successful conclusion of the development project, has its origins in the project team. The firm specializes in the development of MRI-compatible surgical systems.

Current Stage of Development and Next Steps

A 1 W short-pulsed laser system, the stereotactic probe, and the associated computer control programs have been developed to a prototype stage. Following comprehensive experiments on dead brain tissue, the procedure has since the beginning of 1996 been evaluated in animal experiments at the Neurosurgical Clinic of the University of Louvain (Belgium). Experiences collected so far with the prototype system are very encouraging. The procedure's manner of functioning could in principle be confirmed. The precision of tumor removal attained lay within a range of 50 micrometers, and it was possible to demonstrate that healthy tissue bordering on the removal zone was not adversely affected.

The next important steps include the completion of the planning program, the further development of the system, a tenfold increase in laser power output, and also the integration of imaging procedures (ultrasound, MRI) to monitor and control the course of the operation. If, as planned, these tasks can be successfully completed by the end of 1997, Professor Volker Sturm of the Department of Stereotactic Neurosurgery (Cologne) will sometime during 1998 undertake the first clinical use of the probe.

Parallel to tests at participating clinics, MRC will continue to rework the neurolaser system and to proceed with the approval procedure prescribed by the government. It is our objective to be able to offer the very first neurosurgical short-pulsed laser system for clinical use within the next three years.

Image-guided, minimally invasive procedures will continue to play a role of increasing significance in medicine. In an exemplary international cooperative effort between clinics, research institutes in the physical and medical sciences, and the medical technology in-

dustry, a new laser treatment procedure for brain tumors is to be developed. For the first time, short-pulsed lasers (so-called picosecond lasers) are being used. Their output of light energy is sufficiently high enough so that several cubic centimeters of tissue can be removed in a „cold" manner over a few minutes time. The procedure, which makes use of preoperative computer-aided planning and also employs monitoring through real time imaging, is characterized by the highest possible degree of precision and extremely low stress to healthy brain tissue. A successful conclusion of the project that is herein described would be an important step not only in realizing less harmful and more efficient treatment methods for brain tumors, but also in improving other operations that are today still associated with high risks and significant side effects.

Prof. Dr. Wolfgang Schlegel
Dipl.-Phys. Jürgen Dams
Division of Medical Physics

Participating scientists

Dr. Rolf Bendl
Dr. Norbert Suhm

In collaboration with

Prof. Dr. Josef Bille
Institute for Applied Physics of the University of Heidelberg

Dr. Markus Götz
MRC – MRI-Compatible Surgical Systems GmbH, Heidelberg

Prof. Dr. Volker Sturm
Department of Functional Neurosurgery and Stereotactics,
Neurosurgical Clinic of the University of Cologne

Selected publications

Bille, J.F., Schlegel, W., Sturm, V.: Stereotaktische Laser-Neurochirurgie. Physik in unserer Zeit 24, 280–286 (1993)

Dams, J., Bendl, R., Fischer, H.J., Schlegel, W., Sturm, V., Bille, J.: Planung, Simulation und Optimierung der Positionierung einer neuartigen Sonde in der stereotaktischen Laser-Neurochirurgie. In: Medizinische Physik 96. Hrsg.: Leitner, H., Stücklschweiger, G., DGMP, Graz, 187-188 (1996)

6.2 Planning and Monitoring of Gene Therapy with Suicide Genes Using Positron Emission Tomography

by Uwe Haberkorn

A very promising approach in gene therapy involves the introduction of so-called suicide genes into cancerous tumors followed by their subsequent activation. Suicide genes code for enzymes that do not occur in mammals and convert relatively harmless precursor substances into their poisonous (toxic) metabolites. Introducing such genes into tumor cells results in the production of these toxic metabolites. In a manner of speaking, suicide genes, thereby, cause tumor cells to commit suicide. Our working group is predominantly investigating two of these suicide systems: cytosine deaminase (CD) and herpes simplex virus thymidine kinase (HSV-tk). The enzyme cytosine deaminase occurs in fungi and bacteria. It converts the substance 5-fluorocytosine (5-FC), used to treat fungal infections, into the chemotherapeutic agent, 5-fluorouracil (5-FU). Since the enzyme does not occur in mammalian cells, only minimal side effects are to be expected in humans. Approaches employing HSV-tk in gene therapy have already been studied in a variety of tumor models and are currently undergoing initial clinical trials. In contrast to human thymidine kinase which attaches the required phosphate molecules to the "building blocks" during the duplication of the hereditary substance, HSV-tk is less specific. It also converts nucleoside analogues such as acyclovir and ganciclovir to the corresponding monophosphate metabolites. After the metabolites have been incorporated into the deoxyribonucleic acid (DNA) of the tumor cells, the cells die. Transferring the suicide gene can occur by using changed (recombinant) viruses, altered by means of genetic engineering. Since the efficiency of infection and, therefore, the related introduction of the sui-

cide gene is minimal, it is highly likely that several infections will be necessary to attain a therapeutically adequate activity level of the suicide enzyme. It makes sense to detect the enzyme activity in the tumor by means of a noninvasive procedure to decide whether several infections are needed. Since both 5-fluorocytosine and ganciclovir can be marked with the positron emitter 18F, it is possible to use positron emission tomography (PET) to determine the activity of the suicide enzyme. Furthermore, effects on tumor metabolism can be used to provide an early evaluation of the treatment.

Monitoring Gene Therapy by Means of Metabolic Effects

After transferring HSV-tk into rat hepatoma cells, examinations were conducted to evaluate the uptake of various metabolic tracer substances: fluorodeoxyglucose (FDG), 3-o-methylglucose, aminoisobutyric acid (AIB), methionine, and thymidine. When ganciclovir was administered, the uptake of FDG and 3-o-methylglucose increased by up to 195 percent. Experiments which involved control cells and varying proportions of HSV-tk producing cells demonstrated a dependence of these effects on the number of cells that produced HSV-tk. The uptake of the synthetic amino acid AIB decreased to 47 percent. Methionine and thymidine incorporation into the proteins or the DNA fell to 17 and 5.5 percent, respectively.

These data show that PET combined with metabolic tracer substances can be used to monitor approaches that employ gene therapy with suicide genes. Increased uptake of FDG and 3-o-methylglucose in the tissue culture thymidine are consistent with a blocking of amino acid transport as well as protein and DNA synthesis.

The course of treatment with PET proceeds as follows: prior to beginning therapy the metabolism is initially measured with FDG, thymidine or a different tracer. Thereafter, viruses are used as the carrier system to execute the infection. Monitoring measurements with PET are conducted after the toxic precursor substance has been given. However, this procedure has two problems: On the one hand, the length of the time interval between the administration of the precursor substance and PET measurement must be firmly established. This can be solved empirically. On the other hand, the therapist must decide when a therapeutically sufficient activity level of the suicide enzyme has been reached in the tumor. By measuring the uptake of specific substrates for the suicide enzyme this problem, too, can be satisfactorily resolved.

Planning and Monitoring of Gene Therapy Through the Accumulation of Specific Substrates

We have at different times measured the uptake of ganciclovir marked with tritium (^{3}H) in cells that produce HSV-tk as well as in cells that have not been altered by genetic engineering. The former accumulated more 3H-ganciclovir than the control cells did. To simulate this situation in vivo, we experimented with mixtures consisting of control cells and HSV-tk producing cells. Here too, we observed that the accumulation of ganciclovir depends on the proportion of HSV-tk producing cells: the more that cells incorporate the suicide gene, the

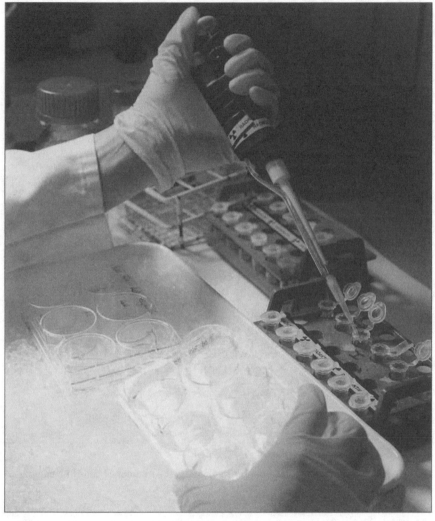

Fig. 65
Radioactively marked thymidine, a building block of the genetic material, is added to tumor cells of the rat liver. At certain time intervals, the uptake is measured. The quantity of incorporated thymidine provides information about whether or not the suicide program of the tumor cells has been successfully activated

can be interpreted as a stress reaction of the tumor cells. A possible mechanism that may explain this is the redistribution of transport proteins from intracellular storage to the cell membrane. Similar results have been observed in conventional chemotherapy. The data for the uptake of AIB, methionine, and greater the enzyme activity. This results in an increased uptake and conversion of ganciclovir and a greater cell death rate which is especially important as an indication of therapeutic success.

Additionally, experiments have been conducted with a second suicide system: cytosine deaminase (CD) from the intestinal bacteria Escherichia coli. The CD gene was transferred to a human glioblastoma cell line in a test tube and the uptake of 5-fluorocytosine was measured. Cells that contained CD produced 5-fluorouracil while the control cells were not able to do this. Furthermore, significant quantities of 5-fluorouracil could be detected in the culture medium. This could explain the "bystander effect" observed in earlier experiments. The term refers to the fact that cells located near those that produce the suicide gene are also affected by the therapeutic effect. Studies focusing on the transport of 3H-5-fluorocytosine indicate that 5-FC diffuses into the cell and that the radioactivity leaves the cell very rapidly. Therefore, the slow uptake and the rapid elimination of 5-fluorocytosine or 5-fluorouracil could prove to be limiting factors for therapeutic success.

When employing multitracer studies to plan and monitor approaches that employ gene therapy with suicide genes one proceeds as follows: first, a so-called baseline measurement is conducted with a radioactively marked, specific substrate for the suicide gene and a metabolic tracer. Following infection, the enzyme activity is estimated by measuring the accumulation of the specific substrate. This information allows one to determine the time at which the precursor substance should be given. Only then can the effectiveness beyond

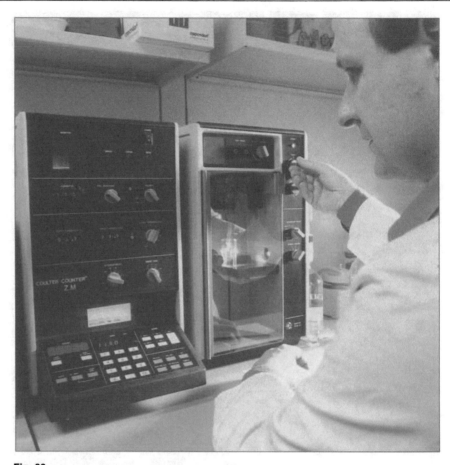

Fig. 66
Dr. Uwe Haberkorn uses the cell counter to measure the number of cells in a sample

the metabolic effects be properly evaluated.

Future Developments

During the next several months, the usefulness of the above-mentioned procedure will be evaluated with various specific substrates for suicide enzymes in the animal model. The working group continues to occupy itself with con-

structing tissue-specific gene transfer systems. The genetically altered, retroviral carrier systems used in this procedure normally infect cells which are undergoing division and are, therefore, suitable for transferring genes into tumor cells. However, other tissues that are undergoing division, such as bone marrow, intestinal epithelium, hair follicles etc., can also be infected. From this observation, it follows that the therapeutic genes must be specifically expressed. On the one hand, this goal can be attained by altering the viral envelope which can result in a specific infection. On the other hand, using tissue-specific, regulatory DNA segments such as promoters and enhancers can also bring about the desired result. Our studies are focused on various promoter/enhancer systems: for thyroid gland tumors on the regulatory elements for thyroglobulin and calcitonin, for some other tumors on the promoter for the carcinoembryonic antigen (CEA), and for liver tumors on the albumin promoter. In comparison to normal cells, most tumor cells exhibit an elevated transport of glucose. This is viewed as one of the characteristic traits of the transformed phenotype. In the meantime, an entire „family" of glucose transporters has been identified. Especially the expression of type 1 (GLUT1) is activated in malignant cells. This change occurs very early in the course of cellular degeneration. Here too, the regulatory elements of gene activation are known and could be employed to attain a tumor-specific expression. By combining methods from molecular biology with measurement techniques from nuclear medicine, it could even prove possible to attain an activation of suicide genes only in the tumor, itself, and to detect this noninvasively.

Priv.-Doz. Dr. Uwe Haberkorn
Division of Oncological Diagnostics and Therapy

Participating scientists

Dr. Franz Oberdorfer
Division of Radiochemistry and Radiopharmacology

In collaboration with

Dr. Khashayarsha Khazaie
Surgical Clinic of the University of Heidelberg

Dr. Anthony Shields
Harper Hospital, Detroit, Michigan, USA

Dr. Yushio Hiasa
Nara Medical School, Kashihara, Nara, Japan

Selected publications

Haberkorn, U., Ziegler, S.I., Oberdorfer, F. et al.: FDG uptake, tumor proliferation and expression of glycolysis associated genes in animal tumor models. Nucl Med Biol 21, 827–834 (1994)

Haberkorn, U., Morr, I., Oberdorfer, F. et al.: Fluorodeoxyglucose uptake in vitro: aspects of method and effects of treatment with gemcitabine. J Nucl Med 35, 1842–1850 (1994)

Haberkorn, U., Oberdorfer, F., Gebert, J. et al.: Monitoring of gene therapy with cytosine deaminase: in vitro studies using ^{3}H-5-fluorocytosine. J Nucl Med 37, 87–94 (1996)

Haberkorn, U., Altmann, A., Morr, I. et al.: Multi tracer studies during gene therapy of hepatoma cells with HSV thymidine kinase and ganciclovir. J Nucl Med 38, 1048–1054 (1997)

Haberkorn, U., Altmann, A., Morr, I. et al.: Gene therapy with Herpes Simplex Virus thymidine kinase in hepatoma cells: uptake of specific substrates. J Nucl Med 38, 287–294 (1997)

6.3 Teleradiology: Improving Communication in Radiological Diagnostics

by Uwe Engelmann
and Malte L. Bahner

According to a definition of the American College of Radiology, teleradiology is the electronic transfer of radiological images from one location to another for the purpose of interpretation or mutual consultation. It is hoped that this will serve to accelerate and improve communication between the different treating physicians, including radiologists. This would be especially important in the treatment of cancers.

Since conventional video conferencing systems and systems for image transmission do not meet the needs of radiologists nor fulfill the strict requirements of the German Data Protection Act, it was the goal of our project to develop a clinically usable teleradiology system. With such a system it should be possible to transmit digital, medical images, such as those produced by computed tomography scans or magnetic resonance imaging, over the telephone lines by using a computer. The Deutsches Krebsforschungszentrum and the Steinbeis Transfer Center for Medical Informatics have developed the teleradiology system called MEDICUS and have evaluated it in a field test after the necessary components were first defined with radiologists and actively practicing clinicians.

It was the objective of the MEDICUS 2 project to develop a teleradiology system which allows for the transfer of radiological images and cooperative work with these images over ISDN lines. The project, the developed software, and the experiences gathered during clinical testing are presented below.

Fig. 67
The partners of the teleradiology association

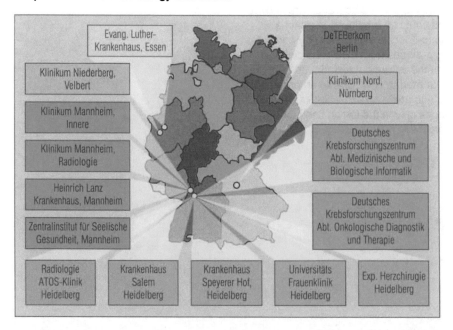

The MEDICUS 2 Project

The project was sponsored by the De-TeBerkom company, a subsidiary of Telekom AG, from August 1994 July 1996. The working group headed by Priv.-Doz. Dr. Hans-Peter Meinzer in the Department of Medical and Biological Informatics jointly conducted this project with the Steinbeis Transfer Center for Medical Informatics in Heidelberg. In this effort, the Deutsches Krebsforschungszentrum was responsible for the scientific supervision of the project; the Transfer Center was responsible for the implementation, installation, and maintenance of the system. A network of 13 radiologists in private practice, small hospitals, university clinics, and at the Deutsches Krebsforschungszentrum was established to test and evaluate the developed system. Most of the partners are located in the general area of Heidelberg/ Mannheim. Additional partners come from Essen and Nuremberg.

After the list of radiological partners had been finalized, a system analysis was conducted to determine the requirements which should be fulfilled by a teleradiology system from the viewpoint of the user. An examination of the commercially available teleconference systems such those used in office communications demonstrated that these do not meet the specific needs of radiologists. Such difficulties begin with the specific image formats used by radiologists which are not used outside the field. Furthermore, radiological images have an image depth of twelve instead of eight bits and can, therefore, not be processed by conventional systems. Typical, radiological image processing functions such as gray

scale adjustment and the analysis of gray scale values in „regions of interest" are missing. Additional disadvantages of commercially available teleconferencing systems are found in their not being integrated into the existing radiological environment. Among other shortcomings, such systems lack the capability to be connected to imaging equipment (e.g., computer tomograph) and to manage patient data. Therefore, specialized teleradiology systems must be developed that meet the requirements of radiologists.

The MEDICUS System

The MEDICUS system integrates images from different sources such as computed tomography (CT), magnetic resonance imaging (MRI), video cameras and ultrasound equipment. The transfer of image data from the imaging equipment is primarily an automatic process. Usually, data transmission originates from an export command in the imaging equipment. The transfer process is based on the communication protocols, DECnet, TCP/IP, and DICOM. Within the scope of this project, eleven different types of MRI and CT scanners from various manufacturers (e.g., Siemens, Philips, Toshiba, GE Medical Systems) were connected to the system. In most of the cases this was a very complicated process since the equipment did not represent the latest technology available and no standard interfaces for data communication (DICOM) were available.

Alphanumeric data (patient name, identification number, date of birth, type of examination, date, study number, and others) contained in the image files are stored in the MEDICUS patient data

base. In this process all personal data is encrypted. The program uses the alphanumeric information to present the examinations and images in a manner that is similar to how medical users (radiological technician or radiologist) have become accustomed to having such information presented to them on CT and MRI consoles. The users are not forced to deal with the operating system, the file system, or the transfer program.

Using a connected video camera, one not only can transmit images of the individual(s) with whom one is communicating, but can also digitize films or other documents such as an ECG curve. Even ultrasound equipment can be easily connected.

The design of the graphical user interface is based on results obtained from cognitive psychology and a style guide for medical applications. With just three clicks of the mouse, complete examinations can be sent to another MEDICUS workstation. It is possible to select only certain parts of an examination and to include a cover letter. The sender of the information also has the possibility to limit the receiver's rights of use with respect to the transmitted data (e.g., the receiver may only look at, print, and export).

During the transmission of personal data over public networks, data protection plays a decisive role. Therefore, a security concept was developed and implemented specifically for MEDICUS. It is based on the Federal Data Protection Act and the IT Security Handbook of the Federal Agency for Security in Information Technology (BSI). Measures take into account the areas of organization, technology, training, and software. With respect to the software, this has

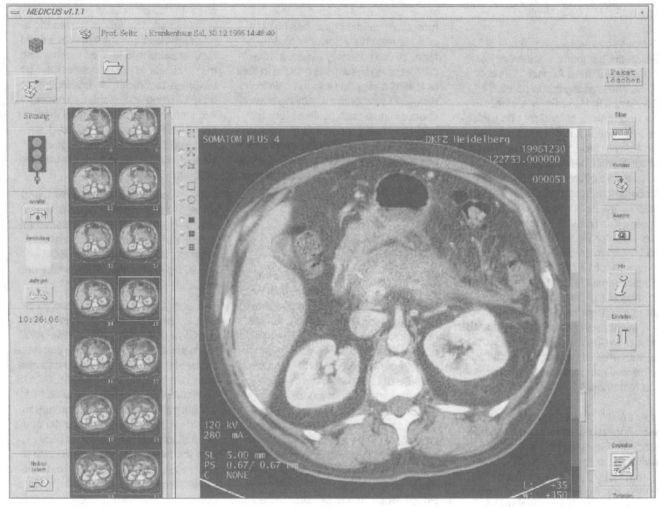

Fig. 68
The screen of the MEDICUS program offers the user the possibility to call up images in original size, enlarged or in the form of an overview with a few mouse clicks. The presentation of interesting regions in graduated gray scales simplifies the evaluation of images

the practical consequences that all local data are encrypted by a symmetric procedure. For the communication process itself, data packets are encrypted by a more complicated, but also safer, public key cryptography system. Furthermore, all data contain

the digital signature of the sender. This ensures the integrity and the authenticity of the data and also the confidentiality of the data transmission process.

After the data are „packed" and encrypted, they are automatically transmitted at a time specified by the user. A computed tomography image consisting of 512 x 512 image points (pixels) and an image depth of twelve bits requires approximately 33 seconds to transmit when both B channels of an ISDN connection (64 KB/sec per channel) are used. This means that the transmission of a typical data record consisting of 30 to 60 CT images takes about 15 to 30 minutes.

The teleconference, itself, begins with a conventional phone call. Thereupon, both conference participants start their MEDICUS program. One of the two partners calls the other by using the program and a red telephone symbol rings on the receiving individual's monitor. The connection is made when the person who is called clicks on the telephone symbol. Thereafter, the available image data on both sides are compared so that only data can still be seen which is available on both sides. Both partners can now select and display images and conduct image processing functions. All actions are processed simultaneously on both sides so that both conference participants always see the same images.

The images can be shown in their original size, can be enlarged, or be presented in fourfold or sixfold divided formats. It is possible to display gray values and to analyze regions of interest (density, size, mean, standard deviation). A magnifying lens feature is available with which selected image sections can be enlarged. The visible gray scale range of the 12 bit images can be changed with the level/window functions. The measuring functions can be used to measure distances, rectangles and circles. In this context, both partners always see exactly the same images and also see the position of the other party's mouse pointer on the imaging screen. Functions to regulate the right of action were intentionally not included. Practical use has shown that the usual conventions of interpersonal communication suffice.

Therefore, control through the computer is not needed.

A possible area of application for teleradiology which is usually mentioned is gaining quicker and better access to an expert's opinion. Since teleradiology is a subdivision of telemedicine, there are still other possible areas of application that can be imagined for this discipline. A regular radiology conference between the physicians of a small or medium size hospital and those at a radiological facility that is responsible for conducting the cross sectional imaging studies that the clinic requires only becomes possible when teleradiology is introduced into the equation. Thereby, time-consuming, daily business trips can be avoided. Less personnel is required when employing teleradiology during nighttime working hours; a single radiologist can provide services to several departments. If a direct network connection does not exist between a radiotherapy planning system and the computer tomograph used in planning such therapy, this connection could be made with teleradiology and an ISDN line that is easily installable. Creating a network within larger, decentralized radiology departments through an ISDN line does not make sense, because of the quantity of data that accumulates. However, the introduction of several teleradiology workstations into a connection that occurs through a local computer network makes direct discussion during complicated examinations possible. Teleradiology might be responsible for increased efficiency in such an instance. Data transfer within the context of scientific cooperation is simplified when teleradiology is used. Furthermore, new means of quality control will develop when image data

that have been acquired no longer need to be sent in cumbersome analog form by using the mail. After our initial experiences, it appears that the notion, much favored by the media, of obtaining an „expert's opinion" by teleradiology is more a construct used to justify this new form of communication than a realistic necessity that occurs on a daily basis.

Results of the Field Test

Between June and December of 1996, the MEDICUS program was accessed nearly 3,000 times. More than 25,000 digital CT and MRI images were imported into the MEDICUS system. Of these, more than 21,000 images in more than 500 packets were transmitted to other medical partners through an ISDN connection. Usually, a packet consists of a single study with several series of images. The average number of images per study was 42. Within the time period of the field test, 10 partners conducted almost 150 teleconferences. A typical conference lasted approximately five minutes. All conferences were less than 10 minutes long. The mean time taken to transmit a study was two minutes. This time was reduced to only a few seconds when a cover letter was not written.

Experiences with MEDICUS

Since December 1995, the system described above has been clinically used in the Division of Oncological Diagnostics and Therapy at the Deutsches Krebsforschungszentrum. Network connections exist to clinics in Heidelberg that regularly refer their patients to the Deutsches Krebsforschungszentrum for

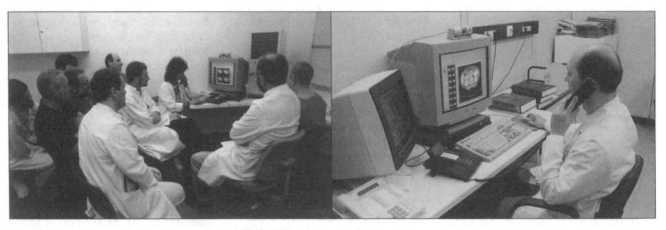

Figs. 69, 70
A teleconference of internists at Salem Hospital in Heidelberg (left photo) with a radiologist at the Center (right photo). The conference participants continuously see the same image. The hands-free talking unit permits the radiologist to simultaneously engage in a discussion with the other participants at the hospital via telephone and to execute certain functions on the computer

CT diagnostics. Furthermore, a connection exists to the Department of Gynecological Radiology at the Clinic of the University of Heidelberg. We conduct teleradiology conferences with these clinics on a regular basis, approximately every other day. The main characteristic of the developed system is its well laid-out usability; this makes it possible for a computer novice to also avail himself of this resource. Aspects of the usability feature that can be mentioned here as an example include the simple transmission of image data to the desired partner and especially the well thought-out design of the so-called user interface.

During clinical use, teleradiology was quickly accepted and integrated into the daily work routine both by the radiologists and also by the participating clinicians. The information flow between the diagnostician and the treating clinician was improved and accelerated. When teleradiology is used, for example, the findings of a small renal carcinoma, obtained by CT in a patient suffering from undefined anemia, can be directly sent to the treating internist after the examination. The subsequent teleconference will include a urologist and the transmitted images will then be discussed together. In this manner, all of this colleague's questions that might arise related to planning the operation can be directly answered and the best therapy for the patient can be immediately discussed and selected together. This entire procedure sometimes takes less time than it does to transport the patient back to the referring clinic; thus, the necessary therapy can be begun immediately in the best possible quality. A second reason for the broad acceptance of teleradiology is found in the possibilities for improving quality. Because of the high sensitivity of modern imaging techniques in oncology, small and still curable tumors can be detect- ed early. However, distinguishing such occurrences from other benign tumors is sometimes difficult. In such a case, it is necessary to use an additional diagnostic procedure. In a CT image, for example, a pancreatic tumor the size of a finger nail can have a very similar appearance to a case of limited pancreatitis. Using so-called endosonography (an ultrasound examination proceeding from the stomach and the duodenum), one can attempt to solve this diagnostic problem. However, localization of the detected change often poses problems since both examination procedures must evaluate the same region. Teleradiology enables the radiologist to comprehensively discuss the anomaly with the internist, so that he can be certain that he has assessed the same area of the organ during the subsequent endosonographic examination. Since reliable findings only become possible in such a manner, this results in an important quality improvement for the patient.

Furthermore, teleradiology creates possibilities for cost reductions in health care, which is becoming increasingly important. Since the treating clinicians often need the images from the radiological examinations, duplicates of the processed films are made available. This has a disadvantage in that it results in significant material costs. With teleradiology these pictures can even be copied and made available several times at a reasonable cost since the only associated expense is for telephone line usage. For a single CT imaging study savings of approximately DM 20.00 can be realized. Additionally, other savings can also be imagined such as those related to patients receiving quicker and more effective treatment which results in their being released from the hospital sooner (so-called shortening of in-hospital admission). Repeated examinations which even today are still sometimes necessary could be avoided or at least significantly reduced by using teleradiology. This shields the patient from additional waiting times and unnecessary stress. However, these effects will not be measurable until teleradiology is used on a broad scale. The actual cost reductions due to teleradiology must still be evaluated and can presently only be estimated in the form of a possible trend. In the near future, teleradiology will also be employed to guarantee quality assurance in radiology. This will entail transmitting radiological images to a central location which would then, if necessary, make concrete recommendations to improve quality. For oncological diagnostics, a certain standardization of the examination procedures could, thereby, be introduced. In the context of possible early detection programs (e.g., the introduction of mammography into the cancer early detection program), teleradiology is, furthermore, a quick and cost-effective transmission method for radiological images that will only be able to realize central quality assurance in the context of screening programs.

Conclusion

MEDICUS represents the development of an easily usable teleradiology system that is based on standards for communication and the exchange of medical images. It fulfills the requirements which radiologists place on such systems. The collected experiences from the testing phase are explicitly positive with respect to the use and functionality of the system as well as the effects on the efficiency and quality of the imaging diagnostics. The improved communication in radiological diagnostics stands out since mutual, speedy discussions between the radiologists and the treating clinicians prove necessary in selecting an individual therapy. Studies that will more precisely evaluate the financial effects on the health care system are currently being conducted.

Outlook

Because of the success of this project, the Steinbeis Transfer Center for Medical Informatics in Heidelberg is presently developing a commercial product called CHILI. This is based on the experiences gathered during the MEDICUS project. CHILI is a completely new concept and program. This product retains the good ideas from MEDICUS and incorporates the features that were requested by the users of MEDICUS. The new system is characterized by being even more DICOM-oriented and also by being expandable. Additional modules, which can even be developed by users of the system, can be seamlessly integrated into the system through an available interface at a later time.

Dr. Uwe Engelmann
Division of Medical and Biological Informatics

Dr. Malte L. Bahner
Division of Oncological Diagnostics and Therapy

Participating staff

Dipl.-Inform. Med. Ulrike Bauer
Irmhild Kocks
Priv.-Doz. Dr. Hans-Peter Meinzer
Henning Müller
Dipl.-Inform. Med. Antje Schroeder
Dipl. Inf. (FH) Andre Schröter
Markus Schwab
Dipl.-Inform. Med. Oliver Werner
Thomas Wolf
Division of Medical and Biological Informatics

Isabell Braun
Prof. Dr. med. Gerhard van Kaick
Division of Oncological Diagnostics and Therapy

Dipl. Ing. (FH) Wilfried Müller
Dipl.-Inf. (FH) Steffen Seeber
Division of Medical Physics

In collaboration with

Prof. Dr. Max Georgi
Dr. Michael Walz
Institute for Clinical Radiology,
Clinics of the City of Mannheim

Dr. Dieter Braus
Central Institute for Mental Health,
Mannheim

Dr. Rolf Rosenthal
Dr. Johannes R. Bayerl
Heinrich Lanz Hospital, Mannheim

Dr. Wolfgang Lederer
Dr. Stefan Schneider
Dr. Wolfgang Wrazidlo
Radiological Group Practice
ATOS Practice Clinics, Heidelberg

Klaus Bredtmann
Annemarie Schmidt
Evangelical Luther Hospital, Essen

Prof. Dr. Dr. Harald Hötzinger
Dr. Stefan Leutzbach
Clinic Niederberg, Velbert
Prof. Dr. Siegfried Hagl
Priv.-Doz Dr. Christian Vahl
Department for Experimental
Heart Surgery,
Surgical Clinic of the University
of Heidelberg

Prof. Dr. Dietrich von Fournier
Dr. Hans Junkermann
Department of Gynecological and Ob-
stetrical Radiology,
Gynecological Clinic of the University of
Heidelberg

Prof. Dr. Helmut Seitz
Prof. Dr. Axel Müller
Department of Internal Medicine,
Evangelical Hospital Salem, Heidelberg

Prof. Dr. Friedrich Willig
Dr. Horst Cornelius
Public Hospital Speyerers Hof,
Heidelberg

Dr. Dr. Reinhard Loose
Institute for Diagnostic and
Interventional Radiology,
Clinic of Nürnberg-Nord, Nürnberg

Selected publications

Baur, H.J., Saurbier, F., Engelmann, U.,
Schröter, A., Baur, U., Meinzer, H.P.: Aspects
of Data Security and Privacy. In: Lemke,
H.U., Vannier, M.W., Inamura, K., Farman,
A.G. (Ed): CAR '96: Computer Assisted Ra-
diology, 10th International Symposium and
Exhibition, Elsevier, Amsterdam, 525–530
(1996)

Engelmann, U., Schröter, A., Baur, U.,
Schroeder, A., Werner, O., Wolsiffer, K.,
Baur, H.J., Göransson, B., Borälv, E., Mein-
zer, H.-P.: Teleradiology System Medicus. In:
Lemke, H.U., Vannier, M.W., Inamura, K.,
Farman, A.G. (Ed): CAR '96: Computer
Assisted Radiology, 10th International Sym-
posium and Exhibition, Elsevier, Amsterdam,
537–542 (1996)

Baur, H.J., Engelmann, U., Saurbier, F.,
Schröter, A., Baur, U., Meinzer, H.P.: How to
deal with Security and Privacy Issues in Teleradiology. Computer Methods and Programs in Biomedicine 53, 1–8 (1997)

Bahner, M.L., Engelmann, U., Meinzer, H.-P.,
van Kaick, G.: Anforderungen an ein Tele-
radiologiesystem – Erfahrungen aus dem ME-
DICUS-2 Feldtest. Radiologe 37, 269–277
(1997)

Engelmann, U., Schröter, A., Baur, U., Wer-
ner, O., Göransson, B., Borälv, E., Schwab,
M., Müller, H., Bahner M.L., Meinzer, H.-P.:
Experiences with the German Teleradiology
System MEDICUS. Computer Methods and
Programs in Biomedicine 54, 131–139
(1997)

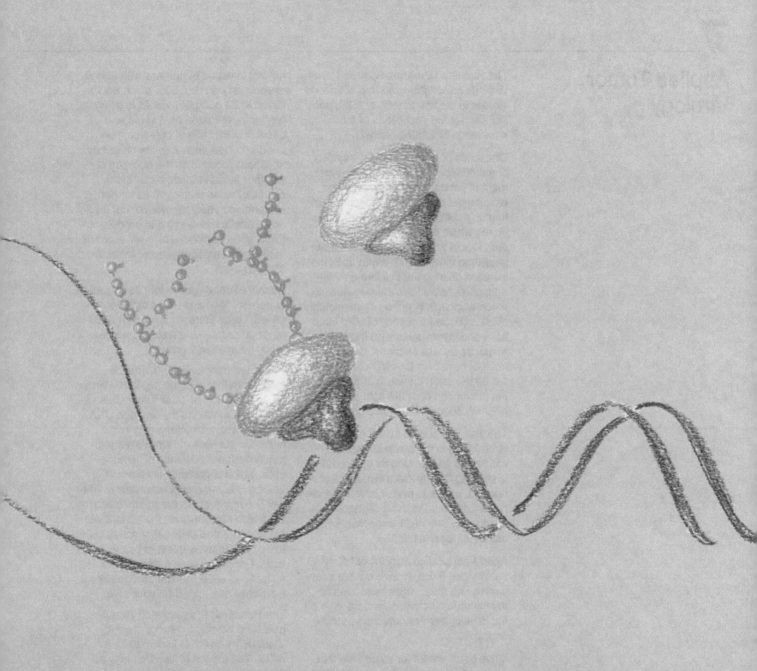

7

Applied Tumor Virology

The Research Program Applied Tumor Virology investigates the role of various viruses in carcinogenesis and the possibilities for the application of this knowledge in fighting cancer.

One focus of work is the investigation of the relationship between development of genital, skin, oral cavity and esophageal cancers and infection with human papilloma viruses (HPV). How do the whole organisms or individual cells reacts to an infection with certain papilloma virus types? When does the infection change the cell into a malignant one? Aside from these questions, much emphasis is put on epidemiologic studies on the frequency of HPV infections and investigations on the immune response as well as on the development of new tools for diagnosis. They will be the basis on which strategies for the prevention of or the fight against HPV infections will be developed.

The vital role played by the hepatitis-B virus (HBV) in the development of liver carcinoma was proven by epidemiologic studies. Researchers investigate certain viral genes to reveal how these viruses contribute to the malignant changes in liver cells, especially by the use of transgenic mice.

Apart from studies on "classic" antiviral substances (such as for example interferons, i.e., messenger molecules of the immune system), scientists work on the development of new therapeutic concepts.

It has been known for some time that the smallest viruses, the parvoviruses, can inhibit cell growth. In epidemiologic studies and with molecular-biological methods the researchers are now attempting to unveil the basic mechanisms of this interaction. In addition, the natural infection of humans with adeno-associated parvoviruses, which are believed to be non-pathogenic, is being further investigated on a virological basis. Another line of research, pursued in cooperation with the university hospitals, focuses on the question of whether these viruses, either themselves or when employed as carrier systems, can help imprive cancer therapy. They are also trying to produce artificial virus particles which will serve as vehicles to introduce genetic information into cells.

Such transfer or genes into cells is a requirement for many forms of the so-called "Gene therapy" for cancer and other diseases, as developed now by many international groups.

The lymphotropic papova virus belongs, together with the papilloma viruses, to the group of small tumor viruses, which contain a double-stranded DNA genome. Experimentally, they can mainly infect cells of Burkitt's lymphoma, a malignant disease of immune cells, which is particularly common among children and adolescents in Africa. The researchers are trying to find out which structures on the surface of the degenerated cells cause these cells to be preferentially infected by the virus. Papova viruses might also be suitable as gene transfer vehicles like the above mentioned parvoviruses.

The Research Program also investigates the Human Immunodeficiency Virus (HIV), which is known to cause AIDS. The stages of infection may be the clue to developing a successful vaccine or therapy. Researchers are therefore investigating the role of the envelope protein in viral infection and cell damage. Using antisense RNA, they are elucidating the function of the various viral genes and attempting to selectively inhibit these genes. This work should be usedful for the development of new forms of antiviral therapy.

Another working group is elucidating the mode of action of gene expression of the human spumaretrovirus (HSRV), which includes the interactions of viral proteins with the host cells and their modifications. In the process, researchers are investigating the functions of the newly found bel genes and identifying the cellular partner molecules. Further research directions include the possible connection between HSRV infections and human diseases, and the development of a retroviral vector system on the basis of HSRV gene expression to be used for gene transfer experiments in the context of gene therapy.

Coordinator of the Research Program:
Prof. Dr. Jean Rommelaere

Divisions and their heads:

Tumor Virology:
Prof. Dr. Jean Rommelaere

Genome Modifications
and Carcinogenesis:
Prof. Dr. Lutz Gissmann

Tumor Virus Immunology:
N. N.

Virus-Host-Interactions:
Prof. Dr. Claus H. Schröder

Characterization of Tumor Viruses:
Priv.-Doz. Dr. Ethel-Michele de Villiers
(D. Sc.)

Retroviral Gene Expression:
Prof. Dr. Rolf Flügel

7.1 Inhibition of PARP: A Possible Approach towards Tumor Cell Sensitization

by Jan-Heiner Küpper

Cells that have been exposed to chemical carcinogens or ionizing radiation often suffer from so called genotoxic stress. This means that there are damages at the coding substance itself, i.e. the DNA which contains all the genetic information of a cell. An immediate reaction of cells to such genotoxic stress is the production of a substance called poly(ADP-ribose) which is a biopolymer like DNA. Poly(ADP-ribose) had been discovered almost thirty years ago. It is synthesized by a cellular enzyme called PARP (this stands for poly[ADP-ribose] polymerase). It is assumed that PARP - together with many other protein factors - has a role in the cellular recovery from DNA damage, in order to avoid cell death, or even tumor development. PARP is an interesting protein not only for scientists investigating the connection between genomic alterations and tumorigenesis. About ten years ago, it has also been discovered that there is a correlation between the amount of poly(ADP-ribose) a cell is able to produce and the longevity of an animal species or the human being: The higher the maximal life span of a species the higher is the capacity of its cells to synthesize poly(ADP-ribose) upon DNA damage. However, the composition of PARP, i.e. the aminoacid sequence, is very similar between all species investigated so far - from man to the fruit fly Drosophila melanogaster. No doubt, PARP has been very conserved during evolution and most likely plays an important role in the cell.

At the Deutsches Krebsforschungszentrum in Heidelberg, we are also interested in PARP since many years. We want to better understand the biological role of PARP in cells, hoping that in future it is possible to apply this knowledge to cancer therapy. Therefore we were looking for a strategy to specifically inhibit the enzyme activity of PARP in cells. There have been chemical inhibitors of PARP used so far, but many laboratories reported also on unspecific effects of those inhibitors on other cellular enzymes. We therefore established a molecular genetic approach at the Center to specifically inhibit PARP. This strategy is based on the genetic information for a truncated PARP that is introduced into a cell. This truncated PARP version still is able to bind to DNA strand breaks but is lacking all the information necessary to synthesize poly(ADP-ribose). If there are many thousands of those truncated PARP molecules in a cell, they should efficiently compete with normal, intact PARP for binding to DNA strand breaks. We call this a dominant negative mutant. In collaboration with Professor Myron K. Jacobson from the University of Kentucky, USA, we could show that introduction of such truncated PARP molecules into a cell indeed causes inhibition of PARP enzyme activity: After treatment of cells with DNA-damaging agents there was no production of poly(ADP-ribose) detectable any longer. We were then intrigued to see what is the biological effect of this kind of PARP inhibition on tumor cells growing in culture. Tumor cells exposed to ionizing radiation are able to repair DNA damages like normal cells, depending on the radiation dose, or they are killed by these damages. This, in fact, is the mechanism by which radiation therapy eliminates tumors. Indeed it is one of the most powerful therapy options to treat many forms of human cancer. Mostly, the desired radiation dose is divided into several fractions which are applied over a time period of several days or weeks. The advantage of this protocol is that side effects on surrounding normal tissues are reduced, but never to zero. Thus, it is desired to kill tumor cells with the lowest possible dose in order to minimize effects on healthy tissues. In collaboration with Dr. Volker Rudat from the Radiological University Clinic Heidelberg we made the interesting observation that the radiation dose required to kill tumor cells can be halved if the PARP function was knocked out by the molecular genetic approach described above, while there is no effect on cells in the absence of DNA damage. In other words, this form of PARP inhibition causes significant radiosensitization. Furthermore, we discovered that there is also drastic sensitization against certain cytostatics.

We see now the chance to combine conventional radiation- and chemotherapy with this novel molecular genetic approach in order to make therapy more efficient. Before this novel combination treatment can be tested at cancer patients we have to solve a very difficult problem, i.e. to find a strategy to introduce truncated PARP molecules in as many cells of a tumor as possible. In collaboration with Dr. Jürgen Kleinschmidt from the Research Program Applied Tumor Virology in the Center we are planning to transfer the genetic information for truncated PARP molecules with the aid of viral vectors. In a recombinant virus, coding sequences of the wildtype virus have been exchanged by foreign sequences, e.g. the sequence coding for the truncated PARP. We are particularly interested in vectors that were derived from Adeno-associated virus (AAV) which seems not to be pathogenic for man. AAV is dependent on so called helper viruses,

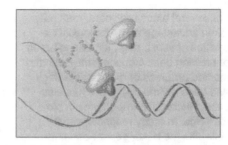

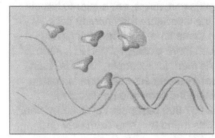

Figs. 71, 72
PARP molecules recognize damages in the genetic material. Binding to the breaks in the DNA strand is the signal for an enzyme to repair the damages (Fig. 71). PARP molecules that have been shortened by genetic engineering can still bind to the break. However, the intact PARP is displaced from its site of action. The enzyme activity ceases

e.g. adenovirus or herpes viruses, in order to proliferate so that AAV-derived viral vectors are considered to be very safe. Furthermore, AAV has one feature making it especially interesting for our purpose: In the laboratory of Dr. Jörg Schlehofer in the Center it was demonstrated a few years ago that infection of tumor cells by wildtype AAV also causes sensitization to g-irradiation and some cytostatics. We are thus optimistic that the genotoxic stress for a tumor can be further increased if it is infected by recombinant AAV particles carrying the genetic information for truncated PARP molecules.

Dr. Jan-Heiner Küpper
Division of Tumor Virology

Participating scientists

Dr. Alexander Bürkle
Dr. Jürgen Kleinschmidt

In cooperation with

Prof. Dr. Myron K. Jacobson
University of Kentucky, Lexington, U.S.A

Dr. Volker Rudat
Radiological University Clinic, Heidelberg

Selected publications

Berns, K.L., Giraud, C.: Adenovirus and adeno-associated virus as vectors for gene therapy. Ann. N. Y. Acad. Sci. 772, 95–104 (1995)

Küpper, J.-H., Müller, M., Bürkle, A.: Trans-dominant inhibition of poly(ADP-ribosyl)ation. A novel approach toward tumor cell sensitization. In: Reduction of Anticancer Drug Toxicity. Pharmacologic, Biologic, Immunologic and Gene Therapeutic Approaches. Contributions to Oncology. Ed.: Zeller, W.J., Eisenbrand, G., Hellmann, K., Karger Verlag, Basel, 48, 142–147 (1995)

Küpper, J.-H., Müller, M., Jacobson, M.K., Tatsumi-Miyajima, J., Coyle, D.L., Jacobson, E.L., Bürkle, A.: Trans-dominant inhibition of poly(ADP-ribosyl)ation sensitizes cells against γ-irradiation and N-methyl-N'-nitro-N-nitrosoguanidine but does not limit DNA replication of a polyoma virus replicon. Mol. Cell. Biol. 15, 3154–3163 (1995)

7.2 Yeast Systems in Oncology

by Karin Butz and Felix Hoppe-Seyler

For several thousand years, man has taken advantage of the biological capacities of yeast, e. g., for baking bread or brewing beer. Concomitantly with the marked progress of molecular biology and gene technology, yeast has also gained increasing importance in biomedicine. In many respects, yeast cells, like the baker yeast Saccharomyces cerevisiae, are easier to handle in the laboratory than human cells. At the same time, they are biologically much more closely related to human cells than, for example, bacteria. Last year, researchers succeeded in determining the complete genetic code (12 057 500 basepairs) of S. cerevisiae. It was found that approximately one third of the genes in S. cerevisiae are closely related to human genes. Many biochemical pathways are conserved between yeast cells and human cells, i. e., they involve structurally related proteins and similar regulatory circuits.

These similarities between yeast and human cells are the basis for using organisms like the budding yeast, S. cerevisiae, or the fission yeast, Schizosaccharomyces pombe, as potent model systems with medical relevance. In the past few years, molecular analyses in yeast have significantly contributed to the understanding of many biochemical pathways in human cells. For example, the genetic manipulation of yeast cells has identified critical factors, and pathways, involved in cellular growth control (e. g., cell cycle regulation) and has contributed much to our understanding of the corresponding regulatory circuits in human cells. Similarly, our knowledge about the regulation of gene expression in mammalian cells has benefitted substantially from studies of the transcriptional control in yeast.

Besides their benefit for basic biomedical research, yeast has also gained importance under more applied aspects. Genetically manipulated yeast strains are used as reactors for the synthesis of biomolecules. For example, yeast cells generate enzymes used in clinical diagnosis (e. g., hexokinase for the determination of blood glucose levels) and can be instructed to synthesize vaccines, such as the vaccine against Hepatitis B virus infection. This genetically engineered Hepatitis B virus vaccine is now in use worldwide and, when compared to earlier vaccines derived from human plasma, has a much higher medical safety.

Yeast cells also have the potential to be valuable model systems for the development and analysis of novel therapeutic agents. For example, immunosuppressants, such as cyclosporin A and rapamycin, target similar regulatory pathways in yeast and human cells. Because of this similarity, yeast cells may be employed to isolate novel immunosuppressant substances. S. cerevisiae has also been used to identify molecules which can specifically inhibit particular enzymes, whose functions are conserved between yeast and human cells (e. g., blockers of the cyclic nucleotide phosphodiesterase which pos-

Fig. 73
With the imprint of a culture dish on sterile velvet, yeast colonies can, in an identical arrangement, be "stamped" onto new culture media. In this manner, identical copies of the original dish can easily be made

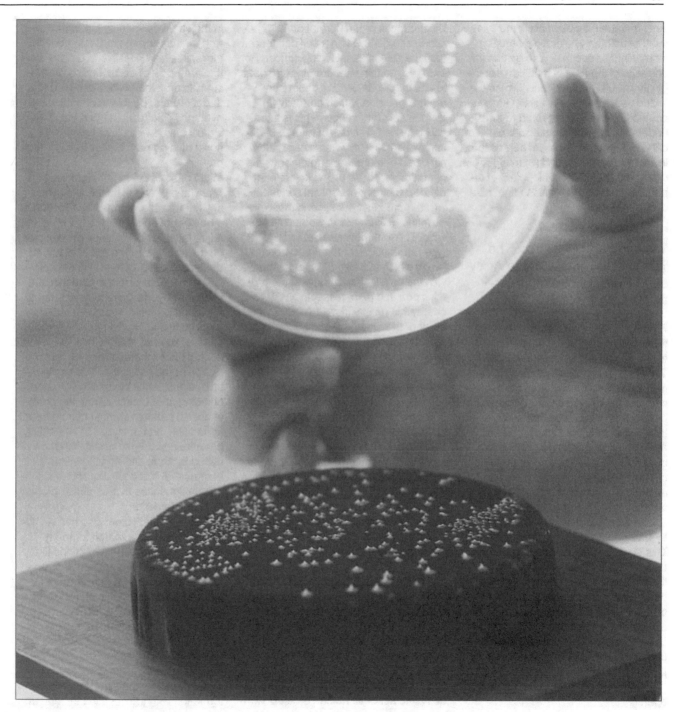

sess therapeutic potential for the treatment of asthma or clotting disorders). Increasingly, yeast has also gained importance in the field of medical oncology. In the following, we will discuss selected yeast systems which: (1) have contributed in basic research to the understanding of the molecular basis of cancer, (2) represent novel approaches in cancer diagnosis, and (3) may provide a basis for the development of future therapeutic strategies to fight cancer.

Yeast in Basic Research: The Two Hybrid System for the Analysis of Protein-Protein-Interactions.

Protein-protein-interactions play a fundamental role for the regulation of biochemical pathways within the cell. Growth factor receptors transmit external signals into the inside of the cell by complex protein cascades, enzymes bind to their substrates, transcription factors build multiprotein complexes to regulate gene expression, antibodies bind to foreign proteins. In order to coordinate these processes, proteins must be able to recognize their binding partners with high specificity which guarantees that they only interact with their physiological binding partner(s). This specificity is achieved by the fact that the three-dimensional structures of the binding partners exactly fit to each other. The great chemist Emil Fischer created, on the basis of the binding of an enzyme to its substrate, the picture of a key fitting into a lock: only when the three-dimensional structures of the partners correspond to each other will the key fit into the lock and be able to open it.

Disturbances of the normal protein-protein-interactions within a cell can lead to many diseases, including cancer. For example, certain viral proteins can bind to and inactivate cellular tumor suppressor proteins, which normally protect the cell from cancer. This is exemplified by certain types of human papillomaviruses (HPVs) which can cause cancer in humans. Among other malignant tumors, HPVs play a key role for the development of cervical cancer, which represents the second most common malignancy in women worldwide. These tumor-associated HPV types synthesize a number of proteins, two of which (E6 and E7) can interact with the cellular tumor suppressor proteins p53 and pRb, respectively. In both cases, this results in the functional inhibition of the tumor suppressor protein: the interaction with E6 leads to the degradation of p53, the binding of E7 displaces the physiological interaction partners from pRb and also degrades it.

In regard to the central role of tumor suppressor proteins as cellular defense factors against the development of cancer, it is of greatest biomedical interest to identifiy proteins which can bind to them and modulate their function. As an experimental approach to analyze protein-protein-interactions, Stanley Fields and coworkers developed the „yeast two hybrid system". This system allows the isolation of proteins which can interact with a given target protein. In a first step, the target protein, which can be derived from humans, is synthesized in yeast cells. Concomitantly, a human gene library (representing all genes expressed in a human cell) is introduced into the yeast. This, theoretically, results in the production of the complete set of all human proteins within

in the yeast cell population, together with the target protein. Using genetic tricks, it is now possible to isolate, from the large pool of cellular proteins, the specific protein(s) which can bind to the target protein. By this approach, it is even possible to identify, as yet, completely unknown cellular proteins as novel binding partners for a given target protein.

In the case of the tumor suppressor proteins p53 and pRb, the two hybrid system has allowed the identification of a number of interacting cellular proteins. Much work currently concentrates on the analysis of the potential effects of these binding partners on the activities of p53 and pRb. Beyond this, the yeast two hybrid system already led to the identification of many other proteins participating in crucial regulatory processes, such as factors involved in the control of cell metabolism or in the regulation of the cell cycle. This assay has, thus, significantly increased our understanding about many fundamental biochemical pathways within human cells. In addition, fine analyses of interacting partners can be performed with the two hybrid system, allowing the elucidation of structural prerequisites and functional consequences of a particular protein-protein-interaction.

The two hybrid system also has significance in cancer research for many other protein-protein-interactions than those involving tumor suppressor proteins. For example, it can be employed to identify factors which interact with (cancer-causing) oncoproteins, which bind to factors critical for cell cycle control, participate in protein cascades involved in signal transduction from the outside into the inside of the cell, or regulate gene expression by complex formation with transcription factors. In

Yeast in Cancer Diagnosis: A System to Detect Mutations of the p53 Tumor Suppressor Protein.

Mutations of the p53 tumor suppressor protein are detectable in approximately 50% of all human cancers and represent the most common known genetic alteration in human tumors. For some tumor forms, the p53 status may be of prognostic value. For example, it appears that patients with cancer of the lung, colon, or breast, have a worse prognosis when their tumors contain p53 mutations. If p53 indeed turns out to be a clinically useful prognostic marker, the analysis of the p53 status within the patient's tumor may eventually influence therapeutic strategies. In addition, there is evidence of a possible correlation between the p53 status and the therapeutic response of certain cancers, suggesting that tumors with mutant p53 are more resistant to cytotoxic treatment regimens, such as radio- or chemotherapy.

Several diagnostic techniques are employed to detect p53 mutations in patient material. In many cases, laboratories rely on screening tests since the complete sequencing of the p53 gene is beyond the capacity of most diagnostic facilities. Immunohistochemistry is such a screening test in which elevated p53 protein levels in tumor cells are detected with p53-specific antibodies. This method is based on the observation that many mutations of the p53 protein result in metabolic stabilization and, thus, lead to elevated protein concentrations within the cell. This method, however, has the disadvantage that some p53 mutations do not result in the elevation of p53 protein levels and, on

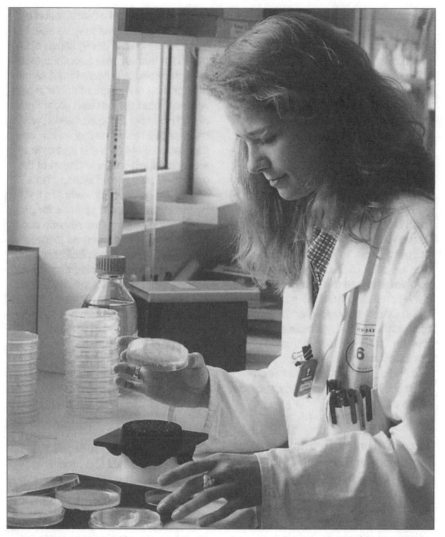

Fig. 74
The yeast colonies can now be examined simultaneously on different culture media. By changing the chemical composition of the culture media, yeast colonies with certain metabolic defects can be identified

addition, several related experimental systems have been developed, including the „one hybrid" system to analyze protein-DNA-interactions, the „three hybrid" system to analyze protein-RNA-interactions, or the „reverse two hybrid" (see below) and the „reverse one hybrid" system to screen for inhibitors of protein-protein- and protein-DNA-interactions, respectively.

the other hand, that normal cells can exhibit increased p53 concentrations under certain conditions which are not due to p53 mutations. These observations can result in false negative or false positive results, respectively. An alternative screening method relies on the detection of p53 mutations on the DNA level. In this method, called SSCP (single strand conformation polymorphismus), fragments of the patients p53 gene are separated by gel electrophoresis. DNA fragments with mutations exhibit altered migration patterns in the gel when compared with control fragments derived from an intact p53 gene. For technical reasons, however, SSCP analysis is often performed for investigating only the most commonly mutated portions of the p53 gene and mutations outside these regions are not detected. In addition, the SSCP method is not able to discriminate between functionally relevant and functionally irrelevant sequence deviations within the p53 DNA (e. g., gene polymorphisms which occur in the population).

Richard Iggo and coworkers developed an alternative screening strategy which is based on the observation that functional active human p53 can be expressed in yeast cells. One of the key functions of p53 is its ability to work as a transcriptional activator, resulting in the stimulation of the expression of certain cellular target genes. Mutant p53 proteins usually are devoid of this function, both in human and yeast cells. This biological difference between normal and mutant p53 is the basis for the yeast assay. A genetically manipulated yeast strain was constructed in which growth is dependent on the ability of the introduced p53 to function as a transcriptional activator.

The p53 gene from the patient can be introduced by relatively simple methods into this test strain, resulting in the production of the patient's p53 protein. If the patient's material contains functional p53, the yeast cells will grow normally, typically forming big white colonies on their solid growth medium. In contrast, yeast cells containing mutant p53 protein will exhibit strongly reduced growth due to the lack of p53 transactivation function. In addition, in this yeast strain the expression of mutant p53 protein results in a red pigment by accumulating an pigmented intermediate of a particular metabolic pathway. Thus, in this assay, the size and the color of the respective yeast colonies indicate the status of the p53 gene originating from the patient's material. One of the advantages of this technically relatively simple assay is the fact that it allows conclusion about the functional potential of the p53 protein and can differentiate between functionally relevant or silent mutations of the p53 gene.

Yeast in Tumor Therapy: Screening Systems to Identify Molecules with Therapeutic Potential

Mutations of the human Ras protein are detectable in approximately 20-30% of all malignant tumors. They induce a deregulated growth stimulation of the cell. Based on the similarity between the human and yeast Ras proteins, S. cerevisiae has been developed as a screening system for inhibitors of Ras function. For its growth stimulatory activity, the Ras protein must be enzymatically modified (a process called farnesylation). S. cerevisiae can be used to screen for molecules which can

inhibit this enzymatic modification of Ras. Such molecules may be able to block Ras-induced deregulation of cell growth in human cells and, thus, possess therapeutic potential for a significant portion of malignant tumor in man. A novel yeast system with great therapeutic potential is the so-called „yeast reverse two hybrid" assay, which was developed by Marc Vidal and coworkers, and represents a variation of the traditional „two hybrid system" (see above). In contrast, however, to the two hybrid system, which screens for protein-protein-binding, the reverse two hybrid system was developed to identify molecules which can specifically inhibit particular protein-protein-interactions. Among other potential therapeutic applications, specific inhibitors of protein-protein interactions have a great potential for the treatment of cancer. In the example of the human papillomaviruses, it could be attempted to screen for molecules, which can selectively inhibit the interaction of the viral E6 and E7 oncoproteins with the cellular tumor suppressor protein p53 and pRb, respectively. The introduction of such inhibitory molecules in HPV-positive cancer cells may result in a functional reconstitution of the cellular tumor suppressor proteins and result in cellular growth arrest or elimination of the tumor cells. Similar experimental approaches are principally possible for many other protein-protein-interactions, which contribute to cancer and, beyond this, to many other human diseases. Thus, the reverse two hybrid system represents an exciting novel screening system for the isolation of a new generation of therapeutic molecules which can specifically attack protein-protein-interactions with pathological relevance.

Dr. Karin Butz
Priv.-Doz. Dr. Felix Hoppe-Seyler
Division of Virus-Host-Interactions

Participating staff

Angela Ullmann
Renata Zucic

Selected publications

Schafer, W. R., Kim, R., Sterne, R., Thorner, J., Kim, S.-H., Rine, J.: Genetic and pharmacological suppression of oncogenic mutations in RAS genes of yeasts and humans. Science 245, 379–385 (1989)

Fields, S., Sternglanz, R.: The two hybrid system: an assay for protein-protein-interactions. Trends Genet. 10, 286–292 (1994)

Flaman, J.-M., Frebourg, T., Moreau, V., Charbonnier, F., Martin, C., Chappuis, P., Sappino, A.-P., Limacher, J.-M., Bron, L., Benhattar, J., Tada, M., van Meir, E. G., Estreicher, A., Iggo, R. D.: A simple functional assay for screening cell lines, blood and tumors. Proc. Natl. Acad. Sci. USA 92, 3963–3967 (1995)

Hoppe-Seyler, F., Butz, K.: Molecular mechanisms of virus-induced carcinogenesis: the interaction of viral factors with cellular tumor suppressor proteins. J. Mol. Med. 73, 529–538 (1995)

Vidal, M., Brachmann, R. K., Fattaey, A., Harlow, E., Boeke, J. D.: Reverse two-hybrid and one-hybrid systems to detect dissociation of protein-protein and DNA-protein interactions. Proc. Natl. Acad. Sci. USA 93, 10315–10320 (1996)

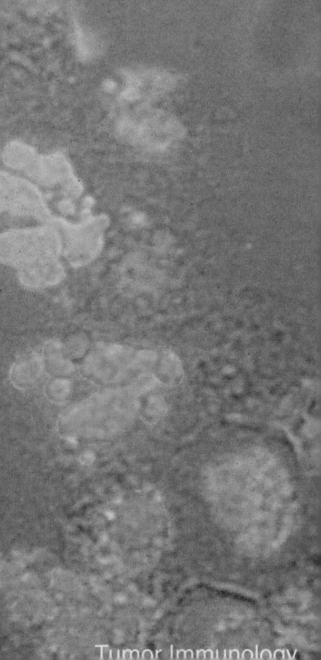

8

Tumor Immunology

The work of the Research Program is concentrated on new immunological methods of tumor diagnostics as well as on immunological concepts for tumor therapy and the investigation of the biological mechanisms underlying processes of cellular interaction and metastatic spreading.

The priorities are in the following fields:

- Manufacturing of monoclonal mono- and bispecific antibodies against tumor associated antigens and differentiation antigens for diagnosis and therapy of tumors.

- Expression of membrane antigens on cells and the development of tumor vaccines. In this context, not only tumor specific antigens, but also viral antigens and mainly histocompatibility genes are investigated. In particular, their role is being explored in the immunological struggle between the host and the tumor.

- Regulation of the immune system. This includes the investigation of immunoregulatory products of tumor cells, the identification and biochemical characterization of lymphokines, biochemical aspects of the activation and regulation of T-lymphocytes under normal and pathological conditions, investigations of mutagenized tumor cell lines as well as the structure of antigens and lymphokine receptors.

- Analysis of the pathogenetic mechanisms involved in cachexia (wasting of the body) and immune deficiency, in cancer and HIV infection, as well as in the aging process and other diseases associated with muscle weakness and wasting of skeletal muscles.

- In addition, the research program investigates the programmed cell death (apoptosis) and its significance in tumor research and in the immune system.

- Auto-immune disease models and immunological tumor models have been established in transgenic mice with histocompatible and other genes. These give important insights into the mechanisms of regulation and pathogenesis.

- Another focus of research is concerned with the mechanisms of tumor invasion and the development of metastases.

The development of new therapeutic concepts with an immunological basis is an important objective of research which is being worked on along various lines in all divisions. These investigations take into account that tumor cells are recognized by the immune system in many cases and also that they can potentially be eliminated. On the other hand, currently unknown regulatory mechanisms prevent resistance in terms of transplant rejection.

Coordinator of the Research Program:
Prof. Dr. Peter H. Krammer

Divisions and their heads:

Cellular Immunology:
Prof. Dr. Volker Schirrmacher

Immunochemistry:
Prof. Dr. Wulf Dröge

Immunogenetics:
Prof. Dr. Peter H. Krammer

Molecular Immunology:
Prof. Dr. Günter Hämmerling

8.1 FLICE:
The Unusual Story
of the Cloning of an
Extraordinary Protein

by Marcus E. Peter
and Peter H. Krammer

Apoptosis, or programmed cell death, has attracted great interest in recent years. Mainly the discovery of specialized cell surface receptors that induce apoptosis on a variety of different cell types has underlined the importance of this process and has made it accessible for molecular investigation. One of these death receptors is CD95 (APO-1/Fas). Like all cell surface receptors CD95 acts as a transducer of a signal which is generated outside of a cell the inside of the cell.

In principle apoptosis is different from any other cellular process and it affects almost all cell components. The apoptotic process first affects the cell sur-

Fig. 75

In programmed cell death, the genetic material is split by a certain enzyme at a defined location. Experimentally, this is seen as a "DNA primer" (right). The genetic material from a cell that has not undergone apoptosis and, therefore, remains unsplit serves as a control. It can be seen on the left

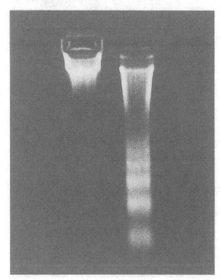

face membrane which starts to bleb. This process is also called zeiosis. Subsequently, a number of essential macromolecules such as components of the cytoskeleton, enzymes, ribosomal RNA, and chromosomal DNA are cleaved. This process involves activation of specific endonucleases which cleave DNA into 200 bp fragments and multiples of it. The resulting DNA cleavage pattern (the so called „DNA ladder") can be visualized on agarose gels and is one of the hallmarks of apoptosis.

During the last three years a lot of emphasis has been put on the elucidation of the apoptosis signaling pathways. Early reports suggested that classical signaling pathways might be involved. We, however, expected a novel signaling pathway that could explain some of the unique features of apoptotic processes. In 1995 it became clear that in most cases the execution of the apoptotic signal involved a certain group of protein cleaving enzymes, the ICE proteases. However, a direct link of these proteases to CD95 had not been established.

In the spring of 1995, using classical biochemical methods, we detected a complex of proteins that specifically associated with CD95 after it had been activated and had received a death signal. We called this complex the death-inducing signaling complex (DISC). The DISC comprises the oligomerized CD95 receptor and at least 4 „cytotoxicity-dependent APO-1-associated proteins" (CAP1-4). CAP1 and 2 were identified as two serine phosphorylated forms of a protein that had been cloned earlier by two different groups. Vishva Dixit's group in Ann Arbor, Michigan (USA) called it FADD and David

155

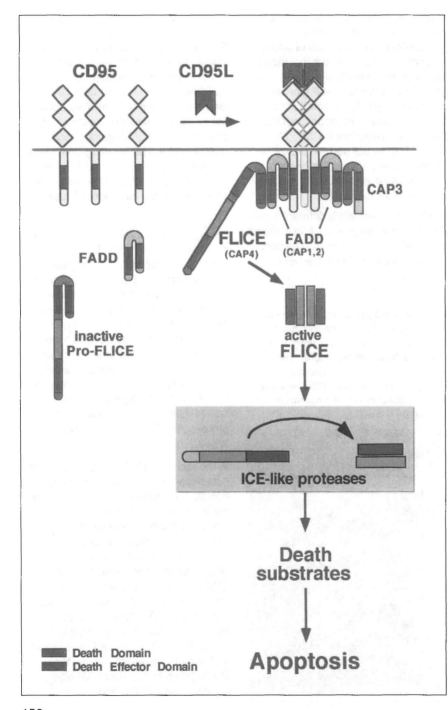

Fig. 76
The process of communicating the "death message" into the interior of the cell: The "death ligand" CD95L binds to the death receptor CD95. To convey the message into the cell, signal molecules that combine to form a complex on the cell membrane (CAP 1 to 4) are used. An active enzyme forms initiating a cascade of enzymes (proteases) that destroy the cellular structures

Wallachs's group in Rehovot called it MORT1. FADD was a good candidate for a cell death-mediating signaling molecule since it induced apoptosis when ectopically expressed in a number of different cells. Yet, the underlying mechanism for its cytotoxic activity remained unknown. The FADD primary structure did not provide any clues to solve this question. In collaboration with Dixit's group we identified two different domains in this molecule. The FADD C-terminal half binds in a ligand dependent fashion to CD95. This interaction is facilitated by a special structure called the death domain present in both FADD and CD95. The FADD N-terminal half contained the part of the molecule that could induce a cytotoxic signal. It was, therefore, termed the death effector domain (DED). It turned out that CAP3 and 4 both required the DED to be recruited to the activated CD95 receptor. CAP3 and 4 therefore likely represented the effector molecules that transduce the death signal into the cell. We therefore wanted to isolate CAP3 and 4 in quantities sufficient to obtain sequence information for cloning. However, that seemed to be an impossible task as both proteins could only be isolated in very small quantities indirectly associated with CD95. After preliminary experiments we estimated that it would take approximately 1000 liters of cell culture to isolate enough protein for protein sequencing using conventional techniques. It became increasingly clear that this was not feasible and if it was only for financial reasons. Hence, the small amount of CAP4 isolated by Frank Kischkel from our laboratory was frozen and stored. CAP4 could only be seen as a faint silver stained spot on an analytical 2D gel.

We began to seek alternatives to characterize CAP3 and 4. In the fall of 1995 we learned from a short report in the journal „Science" that Matthias Mann at the EMBL in Heidelberg was sequencing proteins directly from 2D gels in combination with and using a special data base. We decided to talk to him about the possibility to finally identify CAP3 and 4.

The appointment with him was made for February 1996. At the very day we were about to meet with Matthias Mann we came across a publication in which he and his group demonstrated for the first time that is was possible to get sequence information form very small quantities of proteins from silver stained gels. The technique that had been refined by Matthias Mann and his coworkers is called nanoeletrospray tandem mass spectrometry. We grabbed a copy of the paper and went up to the EMBL.

We got Matthias Mann and his group interested in our project and it turned out that they were indeed looking for opportunities to further demonstrate the potential of there new method. It was March 1996 when we gave them the CAP4 protein that had been stored frozen for more than 8 month at that time. Now we could only wait.

In April 1996 we learned that a group in Israel had cloned two CD95 interacting proteins that had a molecular weight strikingly similar to our CAP3 and our CAP4 protein. We called Matthias Mann and learned that they had just managed to get sequence information of 4 tryptic peptides of our CAP4 spot. A search gave a match of one of the peptides with an EST fragment in a data base that, at the time, contained about 500,000 human „Expressed sequence tags" (ESTs) (representing about 60 % of all expressed human genes). The EST data base at the NIH in Washington (D.C.) that can be accessed worldwide through the Internet is part of the so called human genome project, a scientific project to sequence the entire human genome. The EST clone had been downloaded with the remark „unknown human ICE homologue". This information itself caused a lot of excitement since we now already knew that CAP4 represented an apoptosis protease that directly associated with CD95. In the same night we sent an e-mail message to Vishva Dixit in Ann Arbor (USA) to see whether he could help us to quickly obtain the full length clone. Shortly thereafter, he called and told us that he had access to the private data base of the company Human Genome Sciences (HGS) and that this data base contained already about 80 % of all expressed human cDNAs. Three weeks earlier HGS had sent them a strange clone with an ICE protease domain of unknown function. Could that clone be our CAP4? In this case it had to contain all the peptides sequenced by Matthias Mann. To find out we sent Vishva Dixit a four amino acid sequence of one of the peptides. He promised to call back. Waiting. Then his answer, it was 1:30 am: Our four

amino acids were present in the clone from HGS. To be sure that his clone would code for our CAP4 he asked us for two more tetrapeptides for comparison. We transmitted the sequences. Waiting. Then his call. An obviously relaxed Dr. Dixit announced that the sequences of those peptides were present in his clone, too. Finally we sent him the sequence of all our peptides as an e-mail. All were found in the clone of unknown function. This clone coded for a protein that contained an ICE protease like domain at its C-terminus and two domains at its N-terminus that were homologues to the DED of FADD. We, therefore, called the protein FLICE (for FADD-like ICE). We agreed to publish all data together. Our target journal was Cell. In the following days the necessary functional data were generated. One week after the first contact to Dr. Dixit's group we began to write the manuscript together with the groups at the EMBL and in Ann Arbor. Not only the way FLICE identified was novel for us but also the way this manuscript was generated since it was done through the Internet. Only the Internet made it possible that two investigators at the EMBL, three at the DKFZ, and two in Ann Arbor could work at the same manuscript simultaneously. The drafts of the different sections of the manuscript were sent back and forth by e-mail. Figures were done in the same way. Andrej Shevshenko from Matthias Mann's group would send us a mass spectrum; we would integrate it into one of the final figures and then forward it to Ann Arbor for final print out. The following morning after 30 hours of work and a sleepless night the manuscript was complete. At 7 am CET Arul Chinnaiyan from Dixit's group boarded a plane bound for Boston where he delivered

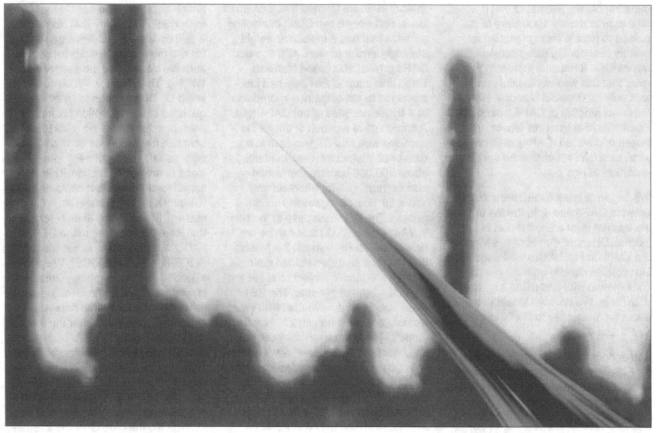

Fig. 77
Nano-electrospray ionization enables one to analyze quantities of proteins that are one hundred-fold smaller than previously possible. In this procedure, one microliter of a peptide mixture flows through a metal needle to which a high voltage is applied. The charged liquid disperses at the point of the capillary and evaporates. The peptide ions collide with gas atoms in the mass spectrometer and disintegrate. The order of the amino acids can be directly read from the mass spectrum of these fragments

the manuscript directly to the editorial office of Cell.

After submission of the manuscript Andrej Shevshenko succeeded to get sequence information of CAP3. CAP3 contained the two DEDs of FLICE. This information as also sent to Cell. A week after submission we presented our results at the 6th TNF Congress on

Rhodes. It was there that we learned that Cell had accepted our manuscript for publication.

For the first time the identification of FLICE linked two different levels in the apoptosis pathway: the level of the death receptors with the level of the ICE-like proteases. The article was released on June 14, 1996 head to head

with a paper describing the cloning of the same protein by David Wallach's group in Israel. They called it MACH. In the meantime we could show that, physiologically, FLICE is activated by the CD95 DISC.

One of the objectives of our work is to sensitize apoptosis resistant cells (e.g., leukemias) or to reduce apoptosis rates

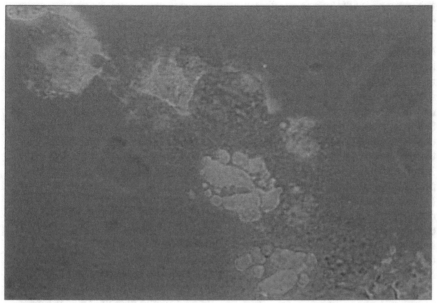

Fig. 78
Cancer drugs can trigger programmed cell death. The cell nuclei (orange) disintegrate and the cell dies

Selected publications

Kischkel, F.C., Hellbardt, S., Behrmann, I., Germer, M., Pawlita, M., Krammer, P.H., Peter, M.E.: Cytotoxicity-dependent APO-1(Fas/CD95)-associated Proteins Form a Death-inducing Signalling Complex (DISC) with the Receptor. EMBO J. 14, 5579–5588 (1995)

Boldin, M. P., Goncharov, T. M., Goltsev, Y. V., Wallach, D.: Involvement of MACH, a novel MORT1/FADD-interacting protease, in Fas/APO-1- and TNF receptor-induced cell death. Cell 85, 803-815 (1996)

Muzio, M., Chinnaiyan, A.M., Kischkel, F.C., O' Rourke, K., Shevchenko, A., Scaffidi, C., Zhang, M., Ni, J., Gentz, R., Mann, M., Krammer, P.H., Peter, M.E., Dixit, V.M.: FLICE, a Novel FADD-homologous ICE/CED-3-like Protease, Is Recruited to the CD95 (Fas/APO-1) Death-Inducing Signaling Complex (DISC). Cell 85, 817-827 (1996)

which are too high as they are found in AIDS. The future will show whether FLICE can serve as a target for drugs to regulate apoptosis.

The editorial staff of the journal Science selected the elucidation of the signaling pathway initiated by FLICE and the TNF receptor involving FLICE among the 10 most important discoveries in natural science in 1996.

Dr. Marcus E. Peter
Prof. Dr. Peter H. Krammer
Division of Immunogenetics

Participating scientists

Frank Kischkel
Carsten Scaffidi

In cooperation with

Prof. Dr. Vishva Dixit
Arul Chinnaiyan
Dr. Marta Muzio
Department of Pathology,
University of Michigan Medical School,
Ann Arbor, Michigan, U.S.A

Matthias Mann
Andrej Shevchenko
Protein & Peptide Group,
European Molecular
Biology Laboratory,
Heidelberg

8.2 Role of Cysteine and Glutathione in AIDS and Several Unrelated Diseases Associated with Cachexia and Immunodeficiencies

by Wulf Dröge

The number of HIV infected patients has increased worldwide to more than 30 million, and there is still no cure. New and more efficient antiviral drugs have brought considerable progress in the treatment of infected patients but are obviously not the final solution to the AIDS problem. The new protease inhibitors cannot remove integrated copies of the virus genome. Some patients develop resistance, and most patients cannot afford to pay the high price for these drugs. In this context, the HIV project of the Division of Immunochemistry has been dealing with the pathogenetic mechanisms of this disease with the aim to develop a more effective and less expensive type of treatment.

The basis of this project was the discover in 1987 and 1988 of our PhD student Hans-Peter Eck that HIV infected persons and SIV infected rhesus macaques express abnormally low plasma cysteine, cystine and intracellular glutathione levels. Cysteine and cystine, are amino acids, i.e., building blocks of protein. Glutathione is a molecule consisting of the three amino acids cysteine, glutamate, and glycine. Glutathione was known for quite some time to be particularly important for the function of the immune system. We, therefore, proposed already in 1988 to consider a cysteine derivative such as N-acetyl-cysteine (NAC) for the treatment of HIV infected patients. Several preliminary studies in different countries have already yielded promising results. Two studies with individually designed doses of NAC are presently being performed in the Division of Immunochemistry in collaboration with the Medical Hospital in Mannheim. In addition, our HIV project has shown that cysteine

and glutathione play an important role not only in the immune system but also in the regulation of the nitrogen balance and the maintenance of body cell mass. The results may contribute to a better understanding of the wasting process not only of HIV infected patients but also in old age and of patients with cancer, sepsis, trauma, and other diseases. These include diseases with unknown etiology such as Crohn's disease and colitis ulcerosa.

The Discovery of a „Low CG Syndrome" in Several Diseases with Unrelated Etiology

Comparative studies have led to the surprising finding that several diseases with unrelated etiology show a similar pattern of biochemical and immunological dysfunctions. This pattern, which we tentatively described as the „low CG-syndrome", is characterized by abnormally low plasma cystine and glutamine levels, progressive loss of skeletal muscle mass or muscle fatigue, abnormally high rate of urea production, and immunological dysfunctions. Abnormally low plasma cystine and glutamine levels have been found in the late asymptomatic stage of HIV infection and in SIV infected rhesus macaques, in patients with sepsis, major injury, Crohn's disease and ulcerative colitis, in some patients with cancer, and in the chronic fatigue syndrome.

The most striking dysfunction in the low „CG-syndrome" is the abnormally low activity of the natural killer cells (NK-cells). The opportunistic infections which are commonly associated with these immunological dysfunctions are in most cases not life-threatening. However, even a temporary decrease in

NK-cell function may have disasterous consequences in the case of HIV infected patients, because NK-cells play a decisive role in the control of virus infections and produce the immunologically important hormone-like factor g-interferon. It is known that primary infection with HIV is typically followed by massive virus replication, but most of the resulting virus particles are subsequently eliminated by the immune system. Subsequently, the HIV infected person can live for many months or even years without symptoms, because his/her immune system can successfully control the virus. Sooner or later, the immune system suddenly fails to control the virus and allows the virus load to increase enormously. This leads eventually to disease progression. Because the studies in our HIV project have shown that the decrease of plasma cystine levels coincides with the massive decrease of CD4+ T cells numbers, it seems that the development of the „low CG-syndrome" including the decrease of NK-cell activity is the decisive event that allows the virus to multiply and to trigger disease progression.

Mechanisms Responsible for Negative Nitrogen Bilance and Wasting

Amongst others, this HIV project has led to the conclusion that cysteine and glutathione play an important role in the maintenance of body cell mass. First, it was noted that all manifestations of the „low CG-syndrome" are associated with a loss of skeletal mass or muscle fatigue. In the case of malignant diseases, the skeletal muscle wasting (cachexia) is correlated directly with survival, and the associated multiple organ dysfunctions may be considered as the most common cause of death among cancer patients.

Earlier studies have shown that the skeletal muscle wasting is in most instances not simply the consequence of inadequate food intake, but rather the manifestation of a biochemical dysregulation. In the context of this dysregulation, an abnormally large amount of amino acid nitrogen is converted in the liver into urea and eventually excreted by the kidneys. Ultimately, the excessive urea production leads to loss of protein and negative nitrogen balance. It was also known that the urea production rate in the liver is strongly influenced by proton generating processes because the ammonium ions in the liver can be converted alternatively into urea or glutamine. Urea production means excretion and irreversible loss of nitrogen, whereas glutamine production means that the nitrogen is maintained in the amino acid reservoir of the body. In contrast to glutamine biosynthesis, urea biosynthesis produces protons because the biosynthesis of carbamoyl-phosphate in the first and rate limiting step of urea biosynthesis consumes hydrogen carbonate anions (HCO_3-). By consuming HCO_3-, proton-generating processes favor glutamine production and inhibit the excretion of nitrogen as urea.

A series of studies in our division suggests collectively that the cysteine catabolism into sulfate and protons (i.e., into sulfuric acid) may play a decisive role in the regulation of urea production and that the dysregulation in certain diseases and conditions with skeletal muscle wasting may result from an inadequate availability of cysteine. Our

Diseases and conditions associated with low plasma cystine and glutamine levels

	Cystine	Glutamine	Glutamate	urea production	immunological functions	
HIV-Infection, late asymptomatic state	↓↓	↓↓	↑	↑	NK-cell-activity	↓↓
Sepsis, multiple trauma	↓↓	↓↓	↑	↑↑	NK-cell-activity	↓↓
Bronchial carcinoma	↓↓	↓↓	↑	↑↑	NK-cell-activity	↓↓
Crohn's disease	↓↓	↓	(↑)	↑↑	NK-cell-activity	↓↓
Ulcerative colitis	↓↓	↓	(↑)	↑↑	NK-cell-activity	↓↓
Excessive exercise (Survival training)	n.d.	↓	↑	↑	NK-cell-activity O.I.	↓↓
"Chronic fatigue syndrome"	↓↓	↓↓	n.d.	n.d.	NK-cell-activity	↓↓
Starvation	↓↓	n.d.	n.d.	↓↓	immunodeficiency; opportunistic infections	↓

n.d. = not determined; NK-cells: natural killer cells

studies, therefore, suggest a cause and effect relationship between the decrease of plasma cystine and glutamine levels, excessive urea production, and skeletal muscle wasting or skeletal muscle fatigue in the „low CG-syndrome". Abnormally low plasma cystine levels were found to be associated with elevated urea concentrations and decreased intracellular sulfate levels in the liver of SIV infected rhesus macaques and tumor-bearing mice. Repeated treatment of tumor bearing mice with cysteine reversed not only the decrease of the hepatic sulfate level but also the increase of the urea concentration to practically normal levels. Changes similar to those found in tumor bearing mice were also found in healthy mice after treatment with the hormone-like cytokine interleukin-6, suggesting that interleukin-6 may play an important role in the development of the „low CG-syndrome". Elevated levels of interleukin-6 have indeed been found in tumor bearing mice as well as in HIV infected patients.

A collaborative study of our division in cooperation with the Dept. of Sports Medicine of the University of Heidelberg suggested finally that the linkage between plasma cystine level and loss of skeletal mass may not be limited to diseases with „low CG-syndrome" but may also apply to healthy human subjects. Healthy subjects with relatively low plasma cystine and glutamine levels showed during a subsequent observation period of 5-8 weeks a striking loss of body cell mass. The lower the plasma cystine and glutamine levels at baseline examination, the larger was the loss of body cell mass. A double blind, placebo controlled study showed, moreover, that the loss of skeletal mus-

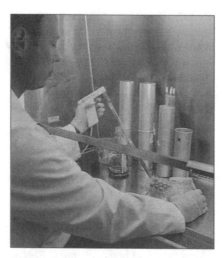

Fig. 79
Cell cultures are applied on the sterile workbench

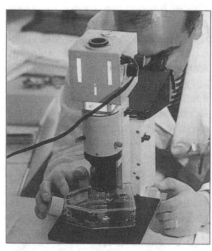

Fig. 80
Various types of cells can be distinguished from one another underneath the light microscope

cle mass was ameliorated by treatment of the subjects with the cysteine-containing drug N-acetyl-cysteine (NAC). Whether NAC may also be used successfully to ameliorate the loss of body cell mass in cancer patients and HIV infected persons is subject of current investigations.

In addition to the available evidence for the role of cysteine in the regulation body cell mass, there are reasons to believe that the regulation of body cell mass is also influenced by the glycolytic activity and lactate production in the skeletal muscle tissue. In several diseases and conditions associated with skeletal muscle wasting, the muscle tissue was previously found to express abnormally high glycolytic activity and lactate production. Importantly, the phenomenon has been seen already in well-nourished cancer patients. It is to be expected that the abnormally high

rate of lactate production is relevant for the regulation of urea production because lactate is converted in the liver into glucose in a process that consumes not only energy but also protons. An abnormally high rate of lactate production in the skeletal muscle tissue is, therefore, expected to antagonize the consequences of the proton generating cysteine catabolism in the liver. Studies with healthy human volunteers in the context of a program of extensive anaerobic exercise yielded results compatible with this interpretation.

Studies on the Regulation and Dysregulation of the Plasma Cystine Level

In view of the abnormally low plasma cystine and glutamine levels in the „low CG-syndrome", we have also investigated the regulation of the plasma cys-

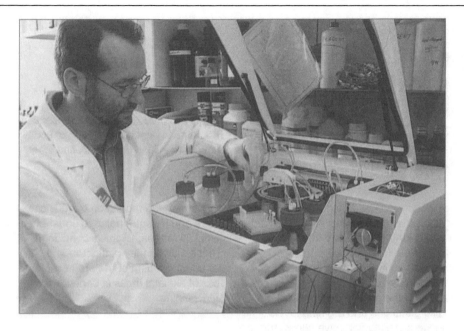

Fig. 81
Working with the amino acid analyzer is an important element in clinical studies that examine the role of cysteine in the organism

tine level in healthy human subjects. Several different methological approaches consistently showed that the plasma cystine level is normally regulated by a controlled adaptive muscular protein catabolism in the postabsorptive period. Taken together, these studies suggest that the plasma cystine level may be part of a regulatory circuit. If at any time the rate of urea production and loss of nitrogen are abnormally high and plasma amino acids accordingly low, a temporary controlled protein catabolism in the skeletal muscle tissue is being induced which leads to the export of cystine, increase of plasma cystine level and ultimately to a downregulation of urea production in the liver. This process may prevent a further loss of amino acids. It is believed that the results of these studies may lead to a more detailed understanding of the wasting process and to new therapeutic strategies for HIV infection, cancer,

sepsis, trauma, and chronic inflammatory bowel diseases.

Skeletal muscle wasting is also commonly seen in the course of senescence and may give rise to severe debilitation, psychological stress, and socio-economical costs. We, therefore, also studied age dependent biological changes. Among other things it was found that the regulatory network and notably the plasma cystine level is substantially altered in elderly persons. Again, it is hoped that this approach may lead to new therapeutic strategies.

The Decrease of the Glutathione Level in the Skeletal Muscle Tissue

The intracellular glutathione level in the liver of SIV infected macaques was essentially normal and in the liver of

tumor bearing mice even moderately increased. The intracellular glutathione level in the skeletal muscle tissue, in contrast, was markedly decreased in these two disease conditions. The more detailed analysis of this phenomenon revealed that the decrease of intracellular glutathione levels was associated with a decreased transport of glutamate into the skeletal muscle tissue and may result directly from a decreased intracellular glutamate concentration. The decreased glutamate transport activity into the skeletal muscle tissue leads to a strong increase of the plasma glutamate level. A study on lung cancer patients in collaboration with the Thorax-Hospital in Heidelberg-Rohrbach revealed that the increase of the plasma glutamate level was strongly correlated with the decrease of immunologically reactivity. In addition, the glutamate level was inversely correlated with the survival time.

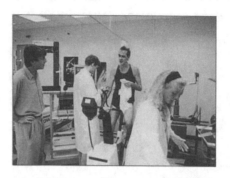

Fig. 82
Sports medicine can make important contributions to our understanding of bodily deterioration in cancer, AIDS, and other diseases

Treatment with N-Acetyl-cysteine (NAC) or Other Cysteine Derivatives

Taken together, the results of these investigations suggest that every substantial decrease of the plasma cystine and glutamine levels may deserve therapeutic intervention irrespective of the etiology of the corresponding disease or condition. Treatment should aim primarily at increasing the cystine and glutamine concentrations to normal levels. On the basis of our first promising observations on NAC-treated HIV infected patients in Heidelberg in 1988, we have recommended to consider routine treatment of these patients with NAC. Two studies with patients in the early and advanced state of the disease, respectively, are presently being performed in collaboration with the University Hospital in Mannheim.

A placebo controlled, double blind study in collaboration with the Dept. of Sports Medicine of the University of Heidelberg with healthy volunteers who happened to have relatively low mean plasma cystine and glutamine levels has shown already that NAC treatment can ameliorate the loss of body cell mass that is typically associated and correlated with low plasma cystine and

glutamine levels. Since April 1988, we also collected longitudinal data on individual NAC-treated HIV infected persons for a time period up to 5 years. These longitudinal data showed that NAC-treatment increases as expected not only the plasma cystine level but also glutamine and arginine levels. The longitudinal studies have shown furthermore that an uncontrolled treatment with NAC can lead to abnormally high plasma cystine and cysteine levels. The dose required to reconstitute essentially normal plasma cystine and glutamine levels was found to vary even at different time points within one and the same patient in the course of the disease. In the current studies we, therefore, try to improve the therapeutic efficacy of NAC by adjusting the dose of NAC to the individual needs. The NAC treatment may also be successful in the treatment of other diseases with skeletal muscle wasting and immunodeficiency such as malignant diseases. The success of this approach will depend on whether the negative effects of lactate production on the rate of urea production can be ameliorated or not.

Apart from the therapeutic approach to several presently uncurable diseases, our studies have revealed detailed information on biological mechanisms

concerning the regulation of body cell mass and nitrogen balance under physiological and pathological conditions. These studies may contribute to a better understanding of the progressive loss of skeletal mass in senescence and wasting.

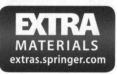

Prof. Dr. Wulf Dröge
Division of Immunochemistry

Participating scientists

Dr. Volker Hack
Dr. Raoul Breitkreutz
Dr. Ralf Kinscherf
Alexander Babylon

In cooperation with

Prof. Dr. Eggert Holm
Medical Hospital Mannheim

Priv.-Doz. Dr. Michael Quintel
Department of Anaesthesiology
and Intensive Care Medicine,
Mannheim Hospital

Dr. Bernd Sido
Department of Surgery,
University Clinic of Heidelberg

Dr. Friedemann Taut
Prof. Dr. Johann Motsch
Dept. of Anesthesiology,
University Clinic of Heidelberg

Prof. Dr. Detlef Petzold
Dr. Helmut Näher
Dr. Martin Hartmann
Department of Dermatology,
University Clinic of Heidelberg

Prof. Dr. Peter Bärtsch
Dr. Claus Weiss
Department of Sports Medicine,
University of Heidelberg

Selected publications

Eck, H.-P., Stahl-Hennig, C., Hunsmann, G., Dröge, W.: Metabolic disorder as an early consequence of simian immunodeficiency virus infection in rhesus macaques. Lancet 338, 346–347 (1991)

Dröge, W., Eck, H.-P., Mihm, S.: HIV-induced cysteine deficiency and T-cell dysfunction – a rationale for treatment with N-acetyl-cysteine. Immunol. Today 13, 211–214 (1992)

Groß, A., Hack, V., Stahl-Hennig, C., Dröge, W.: Elevated hepatic γ-glutamylcysteine synthetase activity and abnormal sulfate levels in liver and muscle tissue may explain abnormal cysteine and glutathione levels in SIV-infected rhesus macaques. AIDS Res. and Human Retroviruses 12,1639–1641 (1996)

Hack, V., Groß, A., Kinscherf, R., Bockstette, M., Fiers, W., Berke, G., Dröge, W.: Abnormal glutathione and sulfate levels after interleukin-6 treatment and in tumor-induced cachexia. FASEB J. 10, 1219–1226 (1996)

Kinscherf, R., Hack, V., Fischbach, T., Friedmann, B., Weiss, C., Edler, L., Bärtsch, P., Dröge, W.: Low plasma glutamine in combination with high glutamate levels indicate risk for loss of body cell mass in healthy individuals: the effect of N-acetyl-cysteine. J. Mol. Med. 74, 393–400 (1996)

Hack, V., Schmid, D., Breitkreutz, R., Stahl-Hennig, C., Drings, P., Kinscherf, R., Taut, F., Holm, E., Dröge, W.: Cystine levels, cystine flux and protein catabolism in cancer cachexia, HIV/SIV infection and senescence. FASEB J. 11, 84–92 (1997)

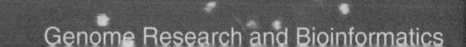

Genome Research and Bioinformatics

The whole of the genetic information encoded in our hereditary material is called the human genome. The rapid advancement of molecular genetics over the past few years has enabled us to analyze and understand the causes of disease on a molecular level. In particular, we have learned that cancer is closely associated with modifications in the genome. We also know that the human genome has a length of 3 billion molecular building blocks and is divided into 44 autosomes (chromosomes that are not linked to the sex) and two sex chromosomes. In view of the wealth of highly complex data accumulated in the process of genome analysis, biologists and geneticists working in this Research Program cooperate closely with computer scientists and mathematicians. With the help of the computer they not only store the deciphered sections of the genome, but also try to assemble from the jigsaw pieces the correct „whole picture" of the individual chromosomes. On the other hand, they use biophysical methods to model and analyze the spatial structure and biological function of the individual genes. Since the gene products, or protein molecules, have a well-defined and functionally optimized spatial structure according to an exact blueprint determined by nature, a defect in the genomic sequence of building blocks is naturally also reflected in the structure of the derived gene product. The knowledge of the effects of such structural defects is particularly important if the defective protein happens to be responsible for cancer suppressing or cancer promoting functions within the body.

Whether and at what rate cells multiply, depends on the interplay of numerous factors. Only if all parts of the machinery engage correctly, or at least the repair mechanisms function properly, can a cell aggregate develop correctly. Otherwise, cancer can be a possible result. Applying mathematical and statistical methods to the data obtained in experimental cancer research, even if they are incomplete, scientists are trying to analyze and simulate the growth of normal and malignant cell populations. In doing so, one of their main objectives is to gain a better understanding of the role of the various internal and external factors.

The central task of experimental molecular genome analysis is to identify specific regions (genes) in the genome, where modifications (mutations) can cause hereditary diseases. To this end, we need, in particular, new techniques facilitating and accelerating the identification of such genes and allowing researchers to isolate functional sequences from larger genomic regions. An important step to understanding the structure and function of the human genome is to analyze the 2- and 3-dimensional structures of complex genomes. Research in this field focuses on genes whose products have regulatory functions and which are considered likely candidates for playing a role in the process of cancer. Through a chromosomal localization of such genes in normal cells and on abnormal chromosomes of tumor cells, scientists hope to gain further insights into their cancer causing (oncogenic) potential. Alongside these structural aspects, another important factor are changes in the biochemistry of the gene functions, which represent the focus of research carried out in classical and molecular cytogenetics.

Coordinator of the Research Program:
Priv.-Doz. Dr. Sandor Suhai

Medical and Biological Informatics:
N.N.

Molecular Biophysics:
Dr. Martin Vingron

Cytogenetics:
Prof. Dr. Manfred Schwab

Biophysics of Macromolecules:
Prof. Dr. Jörg Langowski

Organization of Complex Genomes:
Priv.-Doz. Dr. Peter Lichter

Molecular Genome Analysis:
Prof. Dr. Annemarie Poustka

9.1 Genes, Chromosomes and Cancer: New Techniques in Tumor Diagnosis

by Ruthild Weber and Peter Lichter

Classification of human tumors is presently performed on the basis of morphological criteria by analyzing stained tissue sections through a light microscope. Thus, the diagnosis of tumors is based mainly on the shape of cells and cell nuclei. During the last few decades, however, techniques were developed which allow the individual components within a cell to be examined more closely.

Among these components is DNA, the molecular basis of heredity, which is localized in the cell nucleus in most phases of the cell cycle and must be distributed equally to the daughter cells during cell division to enable controlled cell growth and differentiation. During cell division the DNA is condensed into structures designated as chromosomes. When chromosomes were first analyzed

it became apparent that in tumor cells chromosomal abnormalities may occur. These chromosomal changes may already be contained in precursor lesions of tumors. An accumulation of such genetic alterations seems to be the basis for the aberrant growth of tumor cells. Thus, present efforts to characterize tumors should be supplemented by the systematic analysis of chromosomal abnormalities in different tumor types and stages. This could lead to a better understanding of tumor development and progression and improve tumor diagnosis.

Conventional tumor cytogenetics is a method in which chromosomes are prepared from tumor cells and analyzed by banding techniques. However, it is nei-

Fig. 83
In order to acquire genetic material from tumor cells, scientists "scratch" tumor cells from a tissue sample underneath the microscope and enzymatically remove the hereditary substance

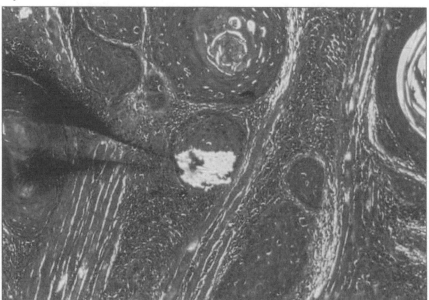

ther easy to induce cell division in cultures of tumor cells nor to produce chromosomes of sufficient quality. In addition, cell culture may change the characteristics of tumor cells and lead to artifactual results.

To screen tumors for chromosomal changes without being confronted by these methodological difficulties a new technique called comparative genomic hybridization (CGH) was developed. In this technique, chromosomes from blood lymphocytes of a normal individual are used which can be prepared more easily than tumor cell chromosomes. The normal chromosomes represent targets of a hybridization experiment in which all tumor DNA fragments bind to their respective „matching" chromosome locus. As a control, DNA fragments derived from normal cells are hybridized simultaneously and at equal amounts to the normal chromosomes. Subsequently, a ratio of the hybridization of tumor and control DNA fragments can be determined. Tumor and control DNA fragments are detected by different fluorescent dyes. With the aid of an epifluorescence microscope, a sensitive camera (CCD camera), and a computer based image analysis system, the intensity of the green and red fluorochromes is measured along the chromosomes, normalized and a ratio is calculated. If this ratio diverges from a normal value beyond upper or lower thresholds this indicates gains or losses of chromosomal material in the tumor versus the control DNA. These measurements allow the identification of chromosomal regions which are deleted (i.e., lost), dublicated or amplified, (i.e. gained) in the tumor. As the chromosomal regions, thus, determined contain genes which are thought to play a role in the development of the analyzed tumors, research projects are subsequently started to identify the particular genes involved.

Thus, only tumor DNA and no tumor chromosomes are required to identify regions which are over- or underrepresented in a tumor by CGH. The required tumor DNA can be extracted from fresh or frozen tumor material but also from archival material which is stored in great numbers in pathology institutes. If the latter is done, it is possible to correlate the determined chromosomal alterations with data on the clinical course of the respective patients. Thus, information on the prognosis of a tumor containing certain chromosomal anomalies is obtained. In ad-

Fig. 84
The new method of "comparative genomic hybridization" permits the comprehensive detection of genomic gains and losses in tumor cells by means of a single experiment. Thereby, it has become an important instrument in tumor genetics. The genomic DNA from tumor cells is hybridized with the chromosomes from a normal cell and, for example, is detected through a green fluorescent dye. Simultaneously, the DNA from normal cells is co-hybridized and is detected by means of a red fluorescent dye. After an overlapping of the signals, mixed colors are formed (lower left). A stronger proportion of green shows those chromosome regions that are overrepresented in the tumor, while regions with a strong red component are underrepresented in the tumor. The right half of the picture shows an analytical evaluation of the image of the identical metaphase cell: Gains from genome regions appear in green and losses in red, while balanced chromosome regions are shown in yellow. The figure stems from the examination of a colon carcinoma

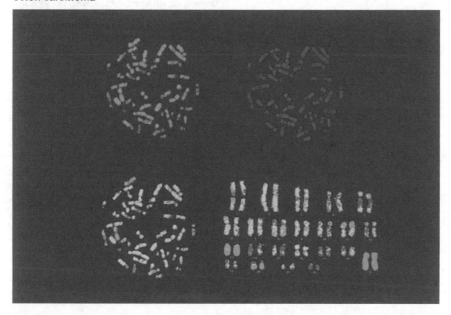

dition, DNA can be selectively extracted from certain cell groups within a tumor or from cells representing precursor lesions of tumors to analyze chromosomal alterations within defined cells. This is done under an inverted microscope with a fine glas capillary which is precisely moved with the aid of a micromanipulator. To obtain sufficient amounts of DNA for the subsequent CGH analysis the DNA from the microscopically small tissue areas is universally amplified by a special procedure termed polymerase chain reaction (PCR).

CGH allows the identification of chromosomal alterations in tumor DNA in a more comprehensive and fast manner than conventional methods. Our laboratory is among the groups which developed and refined the protocol for this technique and use it for the investigation of various tumor types and stages. Thus we find ourselves at the transition from a tumor analysis based purely on cellular findings to a new concept which includes genetic alterations identified within tumor cells. The results thus obtained help to gain a better understanding of the development and progression of tumors and their precursor lesions and to improve tumor diagnosis.

Dr. Ruthild Weber
Priv.-Doz. Dr. Peter Lichter

Participating scientists

Dr. Stefan Joos
Dr. Sabina Solinas-Toldo

In cooperation with

Prof. Dr. Thomas Cremer
Institute of Anthropology and Human Genetics, University of Munich

Prof. Dr. Magnus von Knebel-Doeberitz
Division of General Surgery, Accident Surgery and Outpatient Clinic,
Surgical University Clinic Heidelberg

Priv.-Doz. Dr. Martin Bentz
Priv.-Doz. Dr. Hartmut Döhner
University Clinic and Outpatient Clinic, University of Heidelberg

Selected publications

Bentz, M., Schröder, M., Herz, M., Stilgenbauer, S., Lichter, P., Döhner, H.: Detection of trisomy 8 on blood smears using fluorescence in situ hybridization. Leukemia 7, 752–757 (1993)

Joos, S., Scherthan, H., Speicher, M. R., Schlegel, J., Cremer, T., Lichter, P.: Detection of amplified genomic sequences by reverse chromosome painting using genomic tumor DNA as probe. Hum. Genet. 90, 584–589 (1993)

Du Manoir, S., Schröck, E., Bentz, M., Speicher, M. R., Joos, S., Ried, T., Lichter, P., Cremer, T.: Quantitative analysis of comparative genomic hybridization. Cytometry 19, 27–41 (1995)

Lichter, P., Bentz, M., Joos, S.: Detection of chromosomal aberrations by means of molecular cytogenetics: Painting of chromosomes and chromosomal subregions and comparative genomic hybridization. Methods Enzym. 254, 334–359 (1995)

Joos, S., Bergerheim, U. S. R., Pan, Y., Matsuyama, H., Bentz, M., du Manoir, S., Lichter, P.: Mapping of chromosomal gains and losses in prostate cancer by comparative genomic hybridization. Genes Chromosom. Cancer 14, 167–276 (1995)

Joos, S., Otano-Joos, M. I., Ziegler, S., Brüderlein, S., du Manoir, S., Bentz, M., Möller, P., Lichter, P.: Primary mediastinal (thymic) B-cell lymphoma is characterized by gains of chromosomal material including 9p and of the REL gene. Blood 87, 1571–1578 (1996)

Bentz, M., Werner, C. A., Döhner, H., Joos, S., Barth, T. F. E., Siebert, R., Schröder, M., Stilgenbauer, S., Fischer, K., Möller, P., Lichter, P.: High incidences of chromosomal imbalances and gene amplifications in the classical follicular variant of follicle center lymphoma. Blood 88, 1437–1444 (1996)

Weber, R. G., Sabel, M., Reifenberger, J., Sommer, C., Oberstrass, J., Reifenberger, G., Kiessling, M., Cremer, T.: Characterization of genomic alterations associated with glioma progression by comparative genomic hybridization. Oncogene 13, 983–994 (1996)

Solinas-Toldo, S., Dürst, M., Lichter, P.: Specific chromosomal imbalances in human papillomavirus transfected cells during progressions towards immortality. Proc. Natl. Acad. Sci. USA 94, 3854–3859 (1997)

9.2 Human Genome Project and Resource Center

by Petra Kioschis

The Human Genotype

A human being consists of trillions of cells that are organized into different tissues and organs and which compose the human body. These tissues with specialized functions have formed because of an orderly differentiation of individual cells during the embryonic development of a human being. All these cells have a cell nucleus that contains the genetic material (deoxynucleic acid, DNA) which is the code of life. DNA is constructed from four different components, which because of the double-stranded structure of the DNA helix, are arranged in so-called base pairs. The human genotype contains approximately three billion base pairs which are arranged in a specific order (sequence) in 24 different entities called chromosomes.

The Human Genome Project

Decoding the human genotype is the objective of a worldwide scientific project that officially began in 1990 and is called the "Human Genome Project". The research groups participating in this project hope to decipher the three billion building blocks of the human genome by the year 2005. Parallel to researching the structure and the sequence of the human genome, special attention should be paid to systematically identifying and elucidating the structure, function, and regulation of the estimated 50,000 to 100,000 human genes. An organization (Human Genome Organization, HUGO) working at the international level conducts the worldwide coordination of this project, organizes international collaborations, and initiates new research programs.

The total analysis of the human genotype is the prerequisite for attaining a better understanding of many disease processes; it will lead to a new level of basic knowledge in both biology and medicine.

It follows that the possibilities for diagnosing, preventing and, in initial attempts, treating diseases increase significantly and beyond the deep understanding of human biology.

Current Status of Human Genome Research

Until now impressive advances in discovering the structure and function of the human genome have been attained mainly in the context of national human genome research projects in the USA, France, and Great Britain. The topographic map of the genome has for the most part been constructed. Additionally, researchers were able to trace the causes of almost 4,000 hereditary diseases to a single defective gene; these are the so-called monogenic hereditary diseases. Also, the causes of diseases that are initiated by several factors, so-called multifactorial diseases (e.g., myocardial infarction, cancer, high blood pressure, rheumatism, allergies, diabetes), should be explainable with the new knowledge obtained about the human genotype.

The systematic determination of each of the three billion base pairs of the human genome currently lies at only one percent. By using comprehensive automated processes, improved sequencing technologies and accelerated data processing, it is planned that during the next several years 500 million building blocks of the human code will be read annually on a worldwide basis. The systematic identification of the 50,000 to 100,000 genes, which com-

Fig. 85
The Fugu fish is an important object of study for molecular biologists since it possesses an easily comprehensible genome

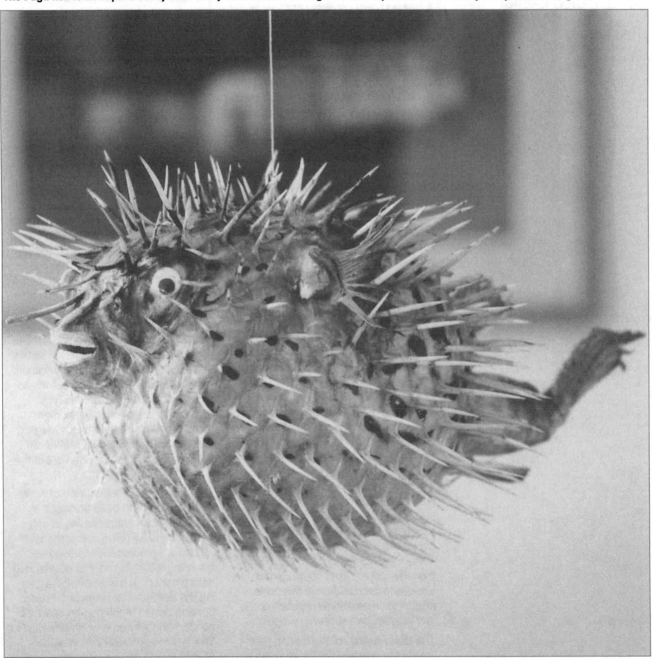

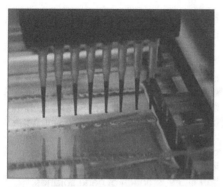
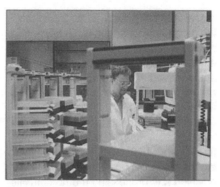
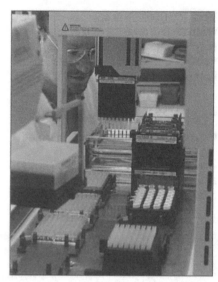

Figs. 86 a, b, c
The automation of procedures such as the polymerase chain reaction or sequencing, which is the analysis of the base order of certain segments of the hereditary material, significantly accelerates the process of deciphering the human genome. The loading of a gel occurs automatically (a). Employees of the Resource Center in Heidelberg monitor the tasks performed by the robots (b and c)

prise only about three to five percent of the total genome, is also very far advanced. Researchers have already attained partial knowledge of between 30 and 50 percent of these genes.

Model Organisms

Not only the human genotype, but also the genomes of other organisms are being simultaneously analyzed to attain a better understanding of gene function and gene regulation. Organisms included: mouse, rat, Zebra fish, Drosophila (fruit fly), Fugu fish, Schizosaccharomyces pombe (backer's yeast), Caenorhabditis elegans (roundworm), chicken, Xenopus, sea urchin and a variety of plant species such as Arabidopsis and rice. These model organisms are characterized by well-defined genetics, well-researched embryology or a small genome, and are very important to genome research for these reasons. Their genes often differ from humans by far less than external appearances

would lead one to believe. In 1996 sequencing of the entire yeast genome was completed and large sections of the genetic code of the roundworm (Caenorhabditis elegans) have also been read. Comparative analyses have already been able to point to specific genes in the human genotype that are important for the regulation of cell division. Additional comparisons between human and animal genes also lead to a better understanding of fundamental life mechanisms; human evolution is an example of this.

Human Genome Research in Germany

In 1996, a common initiative between the German Federal Ministry for Education, Science, Research, and Technology (BMBF) and the German Research Association (DFG) officially created the Research and Support Project for Human Genome Research. Its declared

objective is the systematic identification and clarification of the structure, function, and regulation of human genes, especially those that have medical relevance.

The core of the research concept, human genome research, is formed by central research facilities, independent working groups, and the resource center which all in a manner akin to a division of labor cooperate and work together. This central area is characterized by a large degree of thematic, structural and organizational integration, the effective and cost-effective use of common resources, and the coordination by a scientific coordination committee.

During the next three years, 29 research projects will be supported in the human research program to the tune of 77 million DM. This includes regional areas of concentration such as Berlin, Heidelberg, and Munich. In order to support these planned research projects, the BMBF has sponsored the development of a resource center at the Max Planck Institute for Molecular Genetics in Berlin and at the Deutsches Krebsforschungszentrum in Heidelberg.

The Resource Center in the German Human Genome Project

The resource center is a service entity and an important component of the infrastructure which enables a complex research project such as the deciphering of the human genotype to become a reality. Establishing the center allows extremely large quantities of basic, standardized experimental materials to be prepared; they are obtained with integrated and highly automated methods (e.g., clone libraries, hybridization filters). This uncomplicated access to different gene libraries and characterized clones along with standardized data acquisition and processing methods fulfills a major requirement for being able to realize the objectives of the research program.

At the Max Planck Institute for Molecular Genetics in Berlin and at the Deutsches Krebsforschungszentrum in Heidelberg, the seven scientific and technical areas of responsibility into which the resource center is divided can be seen: primary database, distribution of biological materials, production of hybridization filters, creation of gene libraries, quality control of the produced biologi-

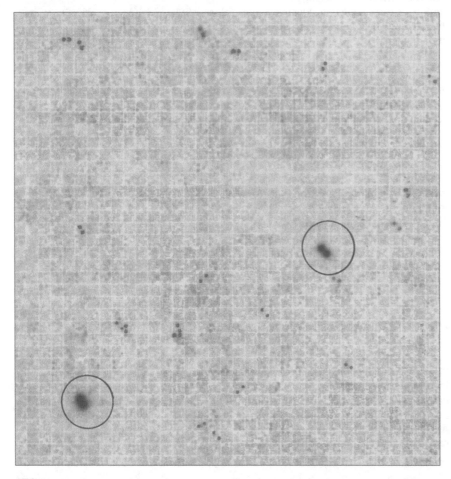

Fig. 87
Autoradiography of a high density hybridization filter of a gene library. A multitude of clones are systematically arranged in a very small space. This keeps the acquisition of data and filing simple. DNA samples that have a corresponding counterpart in the clone library, exhibit a clear signal (circles) after a hybridization. In order to retain a control for the results, each clone is applied twice. Research groups can request identified clones from the Resource Center

cal materials, administration and distribution of gene libraries, screening center.

Dr. Annemarie Poustka (Deutsches Krebsforschungszentrum, Heidelberg), Dr. Hans Lehrach, and Dr. Günther Zehetner (Max Planck Institute for Molecular Genetics, Berlin) are responsible for the scientific management of the resource center. Dr. Rolf Zettl (Berlin) is responsible the administrative management of the resource center.

The Central Service Unit of the Resource Center

In order to support the activities of the research groups participating in the human genome project in a focused manner, the 62 employees of the resource center are engaged in copying, archiving, and distributing available and creating new previously unavailable clone libraries of the human genome and of a variety of different model genomes (e.g., mouse, rat, dog, pig, sea urchin, Fugu fish, yeast, Zebra fish, Drosophila). Additionally, nylon membranes are produced upon which the individual clones from these libraries are applied at a distance of up to 0.1 millimeter and at a density of up to 150 clones per square centimeter. The main advantage of these hybridization filters can be found not only in the large number of clones that are bound to a filter, but also in the fact that the clones are applied in a specific order. Thereby, every clone receives a defined position. This enables data from all experiments conducted with a particular hybridization filter to be collected in a standardized manner.

The employees of the resource center have highly specialized robots available

for their use so that these materials can be produced in sufficient quantities and in reproducible quality. Four specialized „picking" and „spotting" robots collect and transfer 3,000 clones into microtiter plates or onto nylon membranes every hour; these clones are arranged in a regular grid pattern of high density. In this manner matrices are formed on which the DNA from individual clones of a specific genome is bound, so-called hybridization filters. The individual clones of the created gene libraries are stored in microtiter plates at minus 80 (C and are forwarded to the users of the resource center upon request. A replication robot copies approximately 100 of these microtiter plates every day. An additional, highly automated machine can conduct 50,000 PCR (PCR stands for "polymerase chain reaction," the enzymatic replication of genotype segments) experiments at the same time. All of these materials that are classified as resources are made available to all the research groups participating in the human genome project. Within the Heidelberg division of the resource center, a screening center which will provide a screening service is additionally being established. Instructions are also given to scientists and technical personnel concerning the proper way to work with hybridization filters and gene libraries.

The research groups send the primary data collected during the analysis of materials back to the resource center. Data are documented in a database specifically created for this purpose (primary database of the resource center) and are made available to the public. This not only allows all groups to have access to essential experimental material, but especially also leads to a

standardized comparison of the research results obtained with this material.

Upon assuming its duties in July 1995, the resource center had 110 users in Germany and 980 in the rest of the world. In January 1996, these numbers had increased to 151 users in Germany compared to 1,103 international users. By July 1996, there were 229 German users and 1,269 worldwide. In December 1996 the number of German research groups that availed themselves of the resource center's offerings was 510, almost a fivefold increase. International interest reached the level of 1,492. This development demonstrates that the resource center is an important part of the infrastructure of the human genome research program and that it has, furthermore, also established itself on an international basis.

Dr. Petra Kioschis
Division of Molecular Genome Analysis

Participating scientists

Dr. Bernhard Korn
Prof. Dr. Annemarie Poustka
Resource Center in the German
Human Genome Project

Heidelberg Components:

Deutsches Krebsforschungszentrum
Division of Molecular
Genome Analysis

Berlin Components:

Max Planck Institute for
Molecular Genetics

Selected publications

Meier-Ewert, S., Maier, E., Ahmadi, A., Curtis, J., Lehrach, H.: An automated approach to generating expressed sequence catalogues. Nature 361, 375–376 (1993)

Zehetner, G., Lehrach, H.: The Reference Library System - sharing biological material and experimental data. Nature 367, 489–491 (1994)

Chumakov, I.M., Rigault, Ph., Le Gall, I., Cohen, D. et al.: A YAC contig map of the human genome. Nature, 377 (Supp.) 175–299 (1995)

Dib, C., Fauré, S., Fizames, C., Weissenbach, J. et al.: A comprehensive genetic map of the human genome based on 5264 microsatellites. Nature 380, 152–154 (1996)

Goffeau, A., Barell, B.G., Bussey, H., Oliver, S.G. et al.: Life with 6000 genes. Science 274, 546–567 (1996)

Heiss, N.S., Rogner, U.C., Kioschis, P., Korn, B., Poustka, A.: Transcriptional mapping in a 700 kb region around the DXS52 locus in Xq28: isolation of six novel transcripts and a novel ATPase isoform (hPMCA5). Genome Res. 6, 478–491 (1996)

Kahn, P.: German genome program. The right mix of form and function. Science 273, 570–571 (1996)

Kioschis, P., Rogner, U.C., Pick, E., Klauck, S.M., Heiss, N., Siebenhaar, R., Korn, B., Coy, J.F., Laporte, J., Liechti-Gallati, S., Poustka, A.: A 900 kb cosmid contig and eleven new transcripts within the candiadte region for myotubular myopathy (MTM1). Genomics 33, 365–373 (1996)

Group 1: Laporte, J., Hu, L.J., Kretz, C, and Mandel, J.L. Group 2: Kioschis, P., Coy, J.F., Klauck, S.M., and Poustka, A. Group 3: Dahl, N.: A gene mutated in X-linked myotubular myopathy defines a new putative tyrosine phosphatase family conserved in yeast. Nat. Genet. 13, 175–182 (1996)

Miklos. G.L., Rubin, G.M.: The role of the genome project in determining gene function: insights from model organisms. Cell. 86, 521–529 (1996)

Rogner, U.C., Heiss, N.S., Kioschis, P., Wiemann, S., Korn, B., Poustka, A.: Transcriptional analysis of the candidate region for incontinentia pigmenti (IP2) in Xq28. Genome Research 6, 922–934 (1996)

Schuler, G.D., Boguski, M.S., Stewart, E.A., Hudson, T.J. et al.: A gene map of the human genome. Science 274, 540–546 (1996)

9.3 Spatial Organization of Large Genome Segments

by Jörg Langowski

The analysis of the structure of the human genome is one of the pivot topics of modern molecular biology. More and more evidence is accumulating for a genetic etiology of a variety of diseases; in particular cancer is directly related to modifications in the genetic material. Knowledge of the molecular structure of the genome is, therefore, a determining factor for understanding the causes of cancerogenesis and to find ways of cancer prevention and therapy. It is against this background that one has to see the broad public support for the analysis of the sequence and structure of the human genome.

The genetic material of the human cell - deoxyribonucleic acid (DNA) - is organized into 46 chromosomes, each of which contains exactly one molecule of DNA. The genetic information is encoded in the base sequence of the DNA; together all forty-six chromosomes contain six billion bases. Since the distance between two bases is one third of a billionth of a meter (0.34 nm), the total length of the DNA in each individual cell is about two meters (six feet). This thin long 'string' has to be packed into the nucleus which is only ten millionth of a meter in diameter, and this must be done in such a way that the genetic information is accessible rapidly and without error at any time. Moreover, depending on cell type and state of development only a fraction of the 80 000 genes in the human genome is transcribed at any particular time and translated into proteins. The three-dimensional organization of the DNA in the nucleus is important for determining which genes are active at a given moment.

Central cell functions such as differentiation into a variety of cell types and growth control require a finely tuned control of genetic activity; misregulation may be a cause of tumor diseases. This regulation is generally performed by transcription factors. These are proteins that bind to a specific recognition sequence on the DNA, the enhancer, which can be located several hundreds or thousands of base pairs away from the starting point of the gene, the promoter. After binding to the enhancer the transcription factor will contact the promoter-bound RNA polymerase which then starts transcribing the gene. The contact necessitates a DNA loop between enhancer and promoter. The spatial organization of the genome in the nucleus plays a decisive role in determining such long-range contacts within large DNA molecules and in guiding protein factors to their specific recognition sites.

Research Goals

Our research goal is to understand the spatial organization of the genome in the nucleus at its various states of compaction - from DNA to chromatin to entire chromosomes - and to develop models which can deliver a theoretical description of the three-dimensional genome structure. Using such models we can then quantitatively predict possible mechanisms of gene regulation, chromosome organization and genetic damage.

The Genome as an Elastic String

The fundamental properties of the three-dimensional structure of the genome can be understood independently from the atomic properties of the DNA.

If local effects such as base-specific recognition of particular DNA sequences are not taken into account, the DNA can be described as an elastic filament whose behavior - similar to that of a piece of rubber tubing - is determined by its thickness and elasticity. These properties are known for DNA from experiments and can be directly used in computer models.

Of course, DNA is not present in the living cell as a free filament. To a large extent it is bound to histones; these are proteins that package the DNA string into the more compact chromatin fiber. The structural details of that fiber are not very well known yet and are one of the focal points of current genome research. On the other hand, the diameter and elasticity of the chromatin fiber are quite well known, so that it may be described theoretically using similar models as for free DNA.

Modeling of 'Naked' DNA

But many aspects of genome structure may be explained with smaller model systems. As an example, the interaction of a transcription factor with a promoter that was mentioned above depends on the structure of the intervening DNA; it is known that the binding of DNA bending proteins between enhancer and promoter can strongly influence gene activity. This effect may be explained by computer modeling: our computations show that the presence of a bend can enhance the activity of a gene by as much as one thousand-fold.

Another factor that influences gene activity is the global folding of DNA. In the nucleus DNA is strongly entangled with itself and bound to protein structures; therefore, the ends of sone arbitrary

segment of the genome cannot freely rotate against each other. However, when DNA is replicated or genes are transcribed, the DNA filament must rotate along its axis and, therefore, accumulates torsional stress. This stress induces the molecule to wind around itself and assume a more compact structure, also called a superhelix. Superhelicity influences the activity of many genes.

Model calculations show that the interaction between distant positions on the DNA depends strongly on superhelicity; compared to an unstressed, linear DNA it is enhanced about one hundred times in a superhelix and another ten to one hundred times if a DNA bending protein is bound in the middle between the two interacting sites. The activity of a gene that is regulated by the 'looping' mechanism is increased accordingly.

Chromatin

As outlined above, histones and other proteins package nuclear DNA into a compact chromatin fiber. The building blocks of this fiber are the nucleosomes, spherical particles in which the DNA is wound one and three quarters of a turn around the histon 'core', and 'linker DNA' segments which connect the nucleosomes. How exactly this 'string of beads' forms the compact chromatin fiber is being studied by many research groups around the world, because the type of packaging can greatly influence gene activity.

Packing of the nucleosome chain into a chromatin fiber may be described by a model quite similar to that for the folding of 'naked' DNA. Nucleosomes are modeled by globules that are attached

at regular intervals to the elastic DNA filament. Such a simple description allows one to compute the speed of chromatin folding and the resulting compact structure and to cross-check the theory by comparison with experimental data. In a further development of the model we plan to study the influence of environmental conditions on the packing of the chromatin fiber.

Chromosomes and Chromosome Territories

For a long time chromosomes could only be seen during cell division as compact 'sausages' under the microscope, but not in the period called the interphase between cell divisions. From polymer physics it was known that long filamentous molecules like DNA or the chromatin fiber will assume a random coil structure. Therefore, one assumed that during interphase the chromatin fibers of all forty-six chromosomes were intermingled in a random way. Using modern techniques like fluorescence in situ hybridization (FISH) – which for instance are performed at the Deutsches Krebsforschungszentrum by Peter Lichter – one could show that this is not the case: each single chromosome occupies a well-deliminated 'territory' in the nucleus. Genes which are transcribed are rather at the periphery of such territories, and it is supposed that the transcribed messenger RNA and other macromolecules are transported in the space between territories.

For verifying and expanding such hypotheses, computer models can be of great help. On the other hand, the structure of the nucleus is very complex and modeling without continuous comparison against experimental data

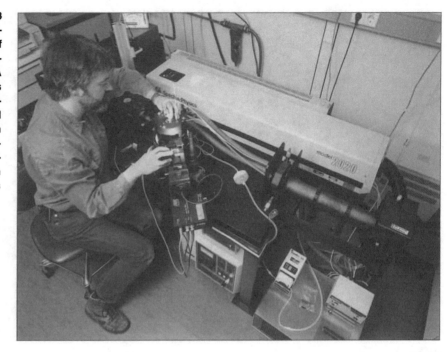

Fig. 88
Internal movements of the genetic material can be measured with the assistance of dynamic light scattering. In this procedure, a laser beam passes through a DNA sample in a cuvette. The laser light is scattered by the DNA. Based on the intensity of the scattered light and additional characteristics, scientists deduce certain qualities of the genetic material. Such experiments contribute to a better understanding of the interactions of genes in cells

would be 'floating in the air' and had no practical value for our understanding of the structure and function of the genome. The division Biophysics of Macromolecules is, therefore, applying a whole set of modern biophysical techniques such as light scattering, ultracentrifugation, scanning force microscopy or fluorescence correlation spectroscopy to examine the structure of DNA molecules or chromatin segments. New microscopy techniques also allow to study the motion of single molecules; these will be used to investigate the migration of proteins and nucleic acids in the nucleus, in order to develop a dynamical picture of the channels between chromosome territories. In a joint project on 'three-dimensional mapping of the human genome' funded through the German human genome in-

itiative, other groups are also participating in related research: Peter Lichter at the Krebsforschungszentrum and Thomas Cremer at the University of Munich determine the position of genes in the nucleus through FISH techniques, Christoph Cremer at the Institute for applied physics of the University of Heidelberg and Ernst Stelzer at the European Molecular Biology Laboratory are developing ultra-high resolution light microscopy techniques, and Willi Jäger at the Interdisciplinary center for scientific computation (IWR) of the University of Heidelberg is advancing modern image processing methods with which the microscopy data are treated and analyzed.

Today such techniques allow one to display individual gene segments of

chromosomes in the nucleus in different colors. By computer modeling we can reproduce the significant properties of those measured structures and – by comparison with experiments – discriminate between different alternatives of chromatin organization. The distances between pairs of genes as measured under the microscope for a great number of nuclei depending on their separation in the DNA base sequence in a characteristic manner. These experimental data can be well reproduced by the model, if certain presumptions are made about the folding of the chromatin fiber. The best agreement with the measured distances is given by a structure model in which chromatin is folded into loops of approximately 100 000 base pairs. Several of these loops are combined into 'compartments' which

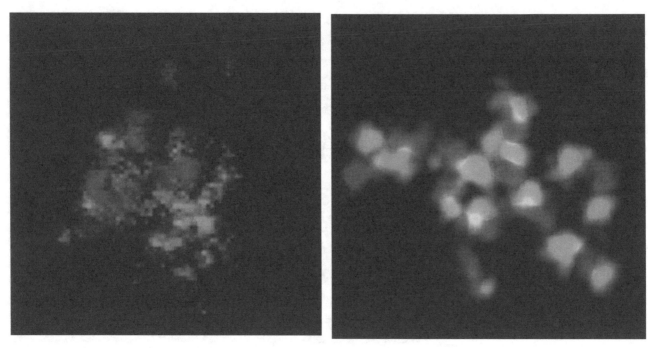

Fig. 89
An example of the good agreement between the simulation of a decondensed chromosome and experimental findings. Red marks the early replicating, active and green the late replicating, inactive regions

correspond in size exactly the active and inactive regions of the chromatin. Microscope images simulated from these models are very similar to the experimental ones. The compartments do not overlap; in a way they represent structurally independent parts of the genome. One possible mechanism for the activation and inactivation of genome segments could be to change the packing of the chromatin fiber in individual compartments.

Chromosome Damages by Ionizing Radiation

It is well known that ionizing radiation such as X-rays or radioactivity can damage the genome and thereby cause cell death, cancer or permanent genetic change. Leukemia, a typical 'radiation cancer' is often induced by chromosome breaks where parts of one chromosome are exchanged with another one. According to the territory model such genetic exchanges should depend on a direct proximity of the corresponding chromosomes in the interphase nucleus. The probability of a radiation induced chromosome exchange

modeled according to this hypothesis depends characteristically on the chromosome size. The same dependence is found in a genetic analysis of a series of leukemia cases in Hiroshima survivors. Our models can also help to answer questions like whether of not a threshold dose exists or why certain genes are particularly susceptible to radiation damage.

Technical Requirements

Modern high performance computers are necessary to model the genome structure of a cell. The demands on computing power are even such that the simulations can be performed in a reasonable time only on parallel machines, where different parts of the model are computed simultaneously by separate processing units. At the Krebsforschungszentrum an IBM SP2 is available for such calculations; it consists of 54 processors each of which can perform up to 500 million arithmetic operations per second. Another machine of similarly high performance is the Parsytec Power GC of the IWR, where 192 computing units work in parallel. Even such powerful machines have to work days and weeks to compute only a few thousandths of a second of the dynamics of the genome. However, the expected results – a three-dimensional 'map' of the nucleus which represents the spatial arrangement of individual genes – largely justify the computational effort.

The long-range goal of our research is a description of the structure and dynamics of the complete genomic material in the human nucleus to better understand the interactions of genes in healthy and diseased cells and point out ways to new therapeutic approaches.

Prof. Dr. Jörg Langowski
Division of Biophysics
of Macromolecules

Participating scientists

Dipl.-Phys. Markus Hammermann
Dr. Konstantin Klenin
Dr. Christian Münkel
Dr. Karsten Rippe
Dipl.-Phys. Michael Tewes
Dr. Katalin Tóth
Dr. Waldemar Waldeck
Dipl.-Phys. Gero Wedemann

In cooperation with

Dr. Giuseppe Chirico
Institute of Solid-State Physics,
University of Milano, Italy

Dipl.-Phys. Lutz Ehrlich
European Molecular
Biology Laboratory,
Heidelberg

Selected publications

Klenin, K., Frank-Kamenetskii, M. D., Langowski, J.: Modulation of intramolecular interactions in superhelical DNA by curved sequences: a Monte-Carlo simulation study. Biophys. J., 68, 81–88 (1995)

Rippe, K., Hippel, P. H. v., Langowski, J.: Action at a distance: the effect of DNA looping on the local protein concentration. Trends-Biochem.Sci. 20, 500–506 (1995)

Chirico, G., Langowski, J.: Brownian dynamics simulations of supercoiled DNA with bent sequences. Biophys. J., 71, 955–971 (1996)

Cremer, C., Münkel, C., Granzow, M., Jauch, A., Dietzel, S., Eils, R., Guan, X.-Y., Meltzer, P.S., Trent, J.M., Langowski, J., Cremer, T.: Nuclear architecture and the induction of chromosomal aberrations. Mutation Res. 366, 97–116 (1996)

Ehrlich, L., Münkel, C., Chirico, G., Langowski, J.: A Brownian dynamics model for the chromatin fiber. CABIOS 13, 271–279 (1997)

9.4 DNA-Chip Technology as a Tool for Gene Expression Studies

by Nicole Hauser, Marcel Scheideler and Jörg D. Hoheisel

The main emphasis of current genome analysis work is still the deciphering of the basic sequence information of both the coding and non-coding regions of genomic DNA. However, technology development has already moved on to experimental analysis procedures on the cellular effects and consequences of the DNA encoded information. For many such studies the inherent function of nucleic acids is utilizing the fact that single-stranded molecules of complementary sequence form a duplex structure in a highly specific manner. The selectivity of this hybridisation process allows for the conception of various, rather complex analysis procedures.

In recent years, DNA-chip technology has emerged as a prime candidate for the performance of many such analyses even on a routine basis. One of the technology's main features is the high degree of parallelism, making a large throughput possible. On a chip, sensor molecules made of single-stranded DNA of known sequence or even of synthetic origin are located, and attached to the surface in an ordered manner so that each sequence is correlated with a given grid position. A nucleic acid of interest is then hybridized onto the chip. For detection, the probe must be labelled with a fluorescence dye or other identifiable substances. The occurrence of hybridization is scored by detecting signal position and intensity generated by this reporter molecule on the chip.

The basic methodological arrangement could be adapted to serve as an analytical tool in a variety of different applications. The emphasis of our work is twofold, the sequence analysis based on hybridization (SBH) and the profiling of expression patterns on all genes of an organism. The arrays could be very small indeed. The smallest being used to date contains several thousand different DNA spots on an area of about a square inch. Thus, the intentions are to design a relatively compact device that could be used in hospitals or even individual surgeries.

The parallel determination of the activity of all genes of an organism is important both for basic and applied science. From each gene an RNA-copy is produced that in case of mRNA is used for the synthesis of a protein. This protein expression is regulated by a variation of the transcription rate, besides other mechanisms. If certain proteins are needed during a specific period of existence of a cell, the transcription rate of the relevant genes usually increases, while in the opposite case the transcription can even come to a stop entirely. The transcription rate is, therefore, an immediate reporter on the cell status. The expression of all genes of an organism is regulated in an interrelated, network-like process in such a way that transcription of one gene may influence the activity of others. For the understanding of the complex regulative mechanisms and the investigation of the cellular control management, a parallel determination of the expression of all genes under various growth conditions is prerequisite.

With the completion in the spring of 1996 of the sequencing of the entire genome of the yeast Saccharomyces. cerevisiae, the entire set of about 6000 genes of this organism is known and easily accessible. This set of genes resembles to quite an extent the minimal gene set that is essential for the existence of a higher (eukaryotic) cell. The relatively small number – 6000 instead of the estimated 80,000 genes in man – will make the unravelling of the basic processes of expression control in a eukaryotic and especially a human cell much easier or even at all possible. Since there exists a surprising degree of structural and partially even functional homology between some human (disease and cancer) genes and their yeast equivalents, an analysis of the expression patterns of this complete gene set is not only very informative for the analysis of yeast gene expression and regulation itself but also has much relevance in the understanding of such mechanisms in higher eukaryotes.

Funded by the German Ministry of Education, Science, Research and Technology (BMBF) and within two network projects supported by the European Union, technical aspects of the above analysis approach are being developed. The data generated during this process are directly correlated to biochemical and physiological findings that are resulting from the experiments of other groups from within the networks. For the analysis, PCR-products and, although on a smaller scale so far, oligonucleotides that represent each gene of yeast were selected and attached to or directly synthesised on a solid support medium. Since the genomic sequence is known, oligomers can be chosen by length and sequence that should be similar in their duplex stability, which is prerequisite for specific hybridization under one set of conditions. In ongoing studies, total RNA from cells of a distinct state of cell growth and various growth conditions is isolated, labeled and hybridized on to the grids. The signal intensity obtained at each grid position indicates how frequently each of the potentially 6000 different RNA-molecules was present in the cells,

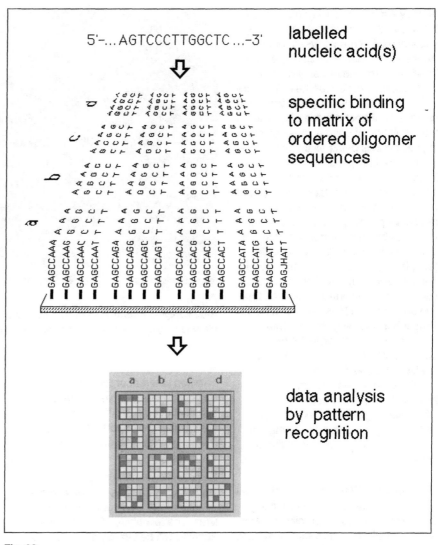

Fig. 90
Fundamental structure of DNA chip analysis: Information about the genetic contents of the sample material is obtained from the unknown DNA sample's binding behavior (position and signal strength) to many chip-bound sensor molecules

hence, how strongly the respective genes were expressed. By growing yeast cultures at various conditions, the adaptation of the gene expression pattern to the environmental conditions is been detected and potential regulative factors of the transcription rates of other genes are identified.

Already experiments with „normal" cultures revealed pseudogenes – coding sequences that are not used for protein synthesis – or house-keeping genes – genes that encode proteins which are continuously needed for the cell metabolism. Isolating RNA from synchronized cultures at distinct periods of growth, the regulation of gene expression during cell cycle is being examined. These studies are indispensable for a molecular understanding of cancer, a disease which is caused by a lack of cell growth regulation. Also from such experiments, regulative pathways and cascades of transcription that occur as the result of a sudden change in growth conditions (e.g., heat shock, toxic or carcinogenic agents, radiation) are definable. Using exon-specific oligonucleotides, alternative splicing of RNA is being examined although the yeast genome contains only few and mostly short intron sequences. Much more significant are analyses on knock-out mutants for the identification of gene complementarity in the cell, especially in combination with physiological and biochemical results that are obtained on the mutant strains by the other groups of the network projects.

Ultimately, the DNA-chip technology will be used as a system to test routinely the biological effect or toxicity of many and especially carcinogenic substances on a molecular basis. Thereby, a wide field of applications in molecular medicine and environmental analyses will be opened. On the basis of the ongoing yeast analyses, similar procedures will be established for the analysis of gene expression in man, especially studies on the variations in expression patterns correlated to the onset of cancer in individual patience. Comparative analyses

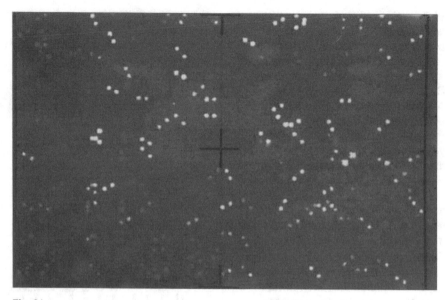

Fig. 91
After applying a color-tagged sample to a DNA screen, this photo clearly shows that binding only occurs at specific positions of the screen (light points)

between different organisms will produce important information on functional homologies and differences and studies that are important to developmental biology and, thus, again to cancer therapy.

Besides the human component of the work, important benefits are also expected for the study of micro-organisms. The technique of transcription analysis will be directly applicable to genomic libraries of short clones of 1 to 3 kb in length, which that were ordered by a mapping technique developed in the group for low-redundancy sequencing. Due to the high gene density in micro-organisms and the lack of intron sequences, each such clone should contain at least part of a gene. Therefore, a minimal set of clones spanning the entire genome represents a normalized gene library although individual genes are neither localized nor characterized. However, on such a DNA-substrate transcriptional analysis will define genes and the corresponding genomic regions of interest. By this approach, functional analyses on an entire organism will precede its sequencing or even limit the still rather laborious sequence analysis to specific areas of the genome that are found to be interesting on the basis of the transcriptional analysis.

Nicole Hauser
Marcel Scheideler
Dr. Jörg D. Hoheisel
Division of Organization of Complex Genomes

Participating scientists

Dr. Jan Weiler
Dr. Patrik Scholler

In cooperation with

Dr. Thomas Gress
Medical University Clinic,
University Clinic,
Ulm

Prof. Albert Hinnen
Hans Knoll Institute,
Jena

Prof. Bernard Dujon
Institut Pasteur,
Paris, France

Dr. Michel Rossignol
Ecole Nationale Supérieure Agrono-
mique de Montpellier,
Montpellier, France

Dr. Johannes Hegemann
University of Giessen

Dr. Mark Johnston
Washington University, St. Louis,
U.S.A

Selected publications

Gress, T.M., Hoheisel, J.D., Lennon, G.G., Zehetner, G., Lehrach, H.: Hybridisation fingerprinting of high density cDNA-library arrays with cDNA pools derived from whole tissues. Mamm. Genomes 3, 609–619 (1992)

Hoheisel, J.D.: Application of hybridization techniques to genome mapping and sequencing. Trends Genet. 10, 79–83 (1994)

Goffeau, A., Barrell, B.G., Bussey, H., Davis, R.W., Dujon, B., Feldmann, H., Galibert, F., Hoheisel, J.D., Jacq, C., Johnston, M., Louis, E.J., Mewes, H.W., Murakami, Y., Philippsen, P., Tettelin, H., Oliver, S.G.: Life with 6000 genes. Science 274, 546–567 (1996)

Hoheisel, J.D.: Sequence-independent and linear variation of oligonucleotide DNA-binding stabilities. Nucleic Acids Res. 24, 430–432 (1996)

Weiler, J., Hauser, N., Hoheisel, J.D.: New developments in oligomer array technologies. Nucl. & Nucl. 16, 777–780(1997)

Weiler, J., Hoheisel, J.D.: Combining the preparation of oligonucleotide arrays and synthesis of high quality primers. Anal. Biochem. 243, 218–227 (1996)

Hoheisel, J.D.: Oligomer chip technology Trends Biotechnol. 15, 465–469 (1997)

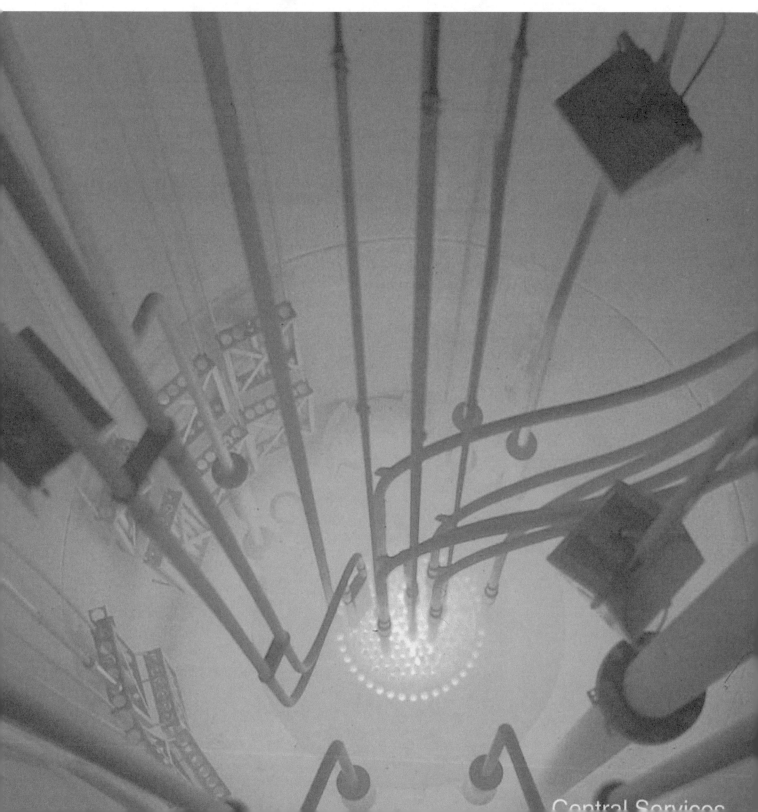

Central Services

Central Services

Central Library

It is the task of the Central Library to collect, develop, and make available scientific literature that is relevant for the Deutsches Krebsforschungszentrum – German Cancer Research Center. Additionally, it is in charge of

A selection of the bibliographic databases, electronic reference books, laboratory handbooks, works detailing methodology, and monographs offered by the library through the Center's computer network

Bibliographic Databases and Monographs

Bioethicsline Plus
BIOSIS/Genetic References
BookFinder (available English language literature)
Cancerlit
CDMARC (collection of the Library of Congress since 1969)
Current Contents (life sciences and chemical and physical sciences)
DKFZ Online Catalog (literature until 1995 under "Access", after 1996 under "Horizon")
IARC Monographs on the Evaluation of Carcinogenic Risks to Humans (available as full text)
Medline Express
Science Citation Index
Toxline Plus
Catalog of Available Books [Verzeichnis lieferbarer Bücher / VLB] (available German language literature)

Reference Books

Cancer Incidence in Five Continents
Collier's Encyclopedia
Duden Rechtschreibung
Encyclopedia of Virology Plus
European Research and Development Database
Hazardous Substances Data Bank (HSDB)
Journal Citation Reports
Material Safety Data Sheets (MSDS)
Pschyrembel: Dictionary of Clinical Medicine [Pschyrembel Klinisches Wörterbuch]
Registry of Toxic Effects of Chemical Substances (RTECS)
Who Delivers What? [Wer liefert was?]

Works Detailing Methodology and Laboratory Handbooks

Current Protocols in Molecular Biology
Immunology Methods Manual
Methods in Enzymology / Recombinant DNA

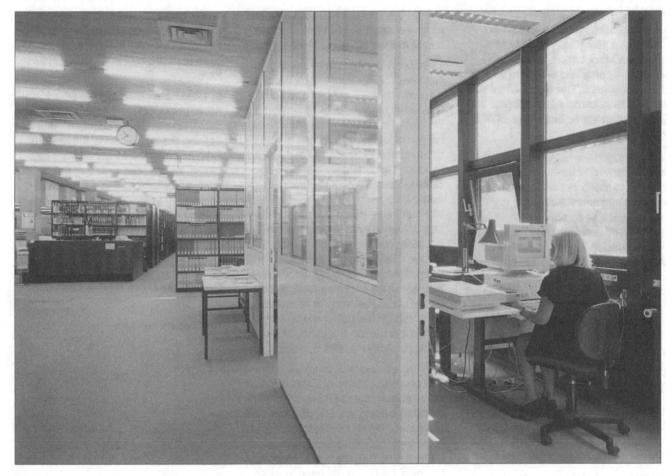

Fig. 92
Electronic search facility for users of the Central Library

the eight decentralized libraries that are assigned to the main areas of research.

In addition to staff members of the Center, guests also have access to the library. Because of its location on the campus of natural science and medical institutes and its close proximity to uni-versity clinics, the library is also heavily used by members of the University of Heidelberg, especially by physicians and students of the medical and natural science faculties. Because of their comprehensiveness and in the context of cooperation with the University of Heidelberg, the services provided for the Tumor Center Heidelberg/Mannheim as well as for the Cancer Information Service (CIS) are especially worth mentioning.

Corresponding to the areas of research conducted at the Center, the library's collection has particular strengths in literature about tumor biology, mechanisms of cancer development, carcino-

191

genic factors, cancer prevention, as well as research in diagnostics and therapy. In 1996 the holdings of the Central Library encompassed some 75,000 volumes and 870 journals that are kept current. The eight decentralized libraries contain an additional 300 journals and approximately 16,000 monographs.

The arrangement of the holdings according to subject area (separated according to monographs, journals, and abstracting journals) allows many individuals seeking specific literature to directly orient themselves in the stacks without needing to use the catalogs. Approximately 80 percent of the literature is available to both staff members of the Center and external users on an unrestricted basis in the reading room. Only the older literature is stored. The library has working space for 80 people. In consideration of the research responsibilities of the Center, the library is, with certain exceptions, a reference library. Within the Center itself, books may be checked out. Journals may not be checked out; however, five photocopiers (two of which are coin operated) are available.

In the context of the rapid development of information technology, supplementing the usual tasks of the library by offering electronic services and expanding the facility to an electronic library has become of ever increasing importance. This initially affects the offerings of bibliographic databases, electronic reference books, laboratory handbooks and monographs. Presently, the library offers more than 30 databases of this sort in compact disk form (CD-ROM) that contain approximately 20 gigabytes of information. They are available to scientists seeking information on a self-service basis by accessing the internal computer network (IBM and Mac platforms) at the Krebsforschungszentrum.

Overall this provides the following advantages for literature-based tasks and for research itself: subject and author-specific inquiries of publications on a worldwide basis and at any time; a high degree of topicality; avoiding the duplication of previously conducted research by means of constantly available specialized literature on a worldwide basis over a time period of 30 years; a nearly one hundred percent and prompt display of journal articles produced in-house; in contrast to the Internet, high technical reliability and acceptable computer response times; availability throughout the entire network of the Center; statistical support of evaluations through the possibility of determining the citation frequency of authors, publications, and journals.

Offering an electronic journal system that meets the needs of users and that would contain the most important periodicals including articles, pictures, and graphical images in full text form, is still in the very early stages of development. It is our objective to prepare highly topical full text information that can be accessed by PC directly at the staff member's workplace. Presently, the following online journals are available on the Internet: Experimental Biology, Journal of Biological Chemistry, Journal of Clinical Investigation, Journal of Molecular Biology, Medical Tribune, Nucleic Acids Research, Science, Structure, and 29 Current Opinion journals such as Current Opinion in Cell Biology or in Oncology.

Because of the usually inadequate response times on the Internet, the practical use of the preceding is still limited and is generally reduced to accessing the newest issues of, for example, American journals that have not yet been received by the library in printed form.

In 1996 a new EDP system called „Horizon" (manufacturer: Ameritech Library Services) was finally acquired. After finalizing the adaptation of the system (with its components acquisition, cataloging, journal management, public access, and check out) to the organization of the library, it provides services in holdings' management and as a user instrument to quickly find and check out any printed literature held in-house.

Head:
Dr. Horst Metzler

Deputy:
Rolf-Peter Kraft, M.A.

Central Animal Laboratory

Health, quality of life, and life expectancy of human beings and animals stand in direct relationship with the development of biomedical research. Despite the development of surrogate and supplementary methods for animal experimentation, the use of animal models in classical medical disciplines still remains indispensable (see the appropriate memorandum of the German Science Foundation issued in 1993). In this context, the use of animals is limited to a level that proves to be absolutely essential. It can be demonstrated that animal experiments have contributed to an increased knowledge about interrelationships in the biomedical sciences and also to an understanding of the very complex processes that participate in the development of cancer. Animal experiments that still prove necessary are found to an extent of 60 percent in the disciplines of basic research. These experiments are also concerned with developing methods that can provide an improved diagnosis and therapy of tumors as well as acquiring knowledge about the possibilities of cancer prevention.

The Central Animal Laboratory (or better still, Centralized Animal Laboratory consists of five stocks of animals held in barriers, two isolator stations that are subdivided into seven units, and a conventionally held (open, half open) stock of animals that is becoming less important. Among other responsibilities, the basic obligation of this central facility is to provide modern accommodations, animal keeping, care, and medical supervision to all animal species (mice, rats; a limited number of rabbits, guinea pigs, chickens, various amphibians)

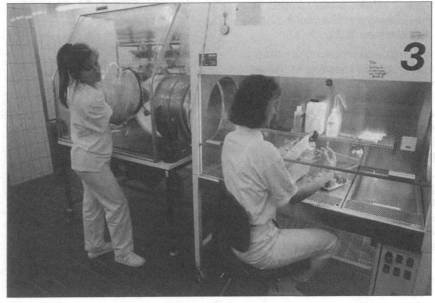

Fig. 93a
Trained staff working at a sterile bench examine animals for changes in their condition

used in scientific research (focus is on: animal protection and animal behavior). In general, breeding is not conducted. Whenever possible, needs for the various animal species are met through purchases from selected and reliable breeders.

With respect to carrying out all aspects of personal and industrial hygiene as well as laboratory animal science, the management of the Animal Laboratory has the authority to give instructions to its users. The Laboratory is a professionally managed and operated facility. In it the following individuals may be found: veterinarians with specialist training in laboratory animal science and microbiology, veterinarians (in postgraduate training to become specialists in veterinary medicine), administrative employees, diagnostic/technical staff members, and almost exclu-

sively at our own facility, trained laboratory animal technicians (total of 30, both male and female) and workers (8).

The head of the Central Animal Laboratory and his deputy fall directly under the authority of the foundation directorate and are personally responsible for observing and carrying out all valid national and international laws, ordinances and regulations that apply to the keeping of laboratory animals. The same holds true for the just amended, internal regulations governing use of the facility that define the rights and responsibilities of both the operating authority and the users. In addition to keeping and supervising the general stock of animals, the staff members of the Animal Laboratory provide advice and information about the characteristics of certain species of laboratory animals and suitable laboratory animal models. They also actively participate in the planning and technical execution of animal experiments.

The Central Animal Laboratory has the important duty of imparting fundamental knowledge and capabilities in laboratory animal science and animal experimentation. To this purpose, we have since 1990 offered an, „Introductory Course in Conducting Research with Laboratory Animals" for diploma and doctoral candidates in the fields of biology, veterinary medicine, and medicine. Participation in this course is the requirement for gaining admission to the CAL and being able to begin one's own research. In 1996 this course was adapted to conform to the corresponding EU guideline (86/609 EEC, Art. 14, Category B) and now consists of 40 instructional hours overall.

Additionally, the Animal Laboratory has since 1989 been a training institution for veterinarians pursuing specialist postgraduate training in the disciplines of laboratory animal science and/or microbiology.

Animal experiments that require authorization or that must be reported can fundamentally only be conducted after appropriate applications have successfully passed through a comprehensive internal and external (executive committee of the government of Karlsruhe) process of evaluation and approval. This takes approximately one to three months.

The Central Biostatistics Unit will usually develop a supplemental biometric research plan to accompany individual applications. This forms the basis for the subsequent, concrete, statistical evaluation of the experimental results. The Internal Commission for Animal Protection (founded in 1985) will conduct an

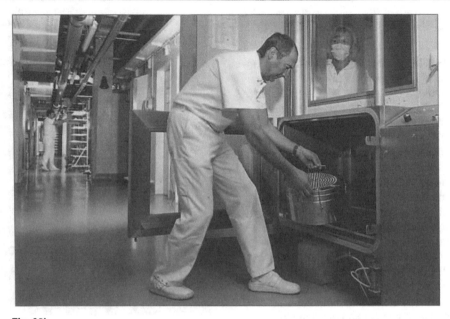

Fig. 93b
Used animal cages are cleaned in a chemical disinfection installation

internal evaluation of the scientific relevance of a planned experiment. All stages of an animal experiment (from completing the application to obtain authorization to the end of the observation period of the laboratory animals used in the experiment) are accompanied in an advisory and supervisory capacity by animal protection officers (veterinarians, physicians, biologists) who do not have a duty to comply with instructions in the performance of their official duties. The divisions that conduct animal experiments are in each case assigned to a single sphere of responsibility that may have up to six (three from the Central Animal Laboratory) part-time animal protection officers.

Many environmental factors can affect the biology and the physiology and, thereby, also the reactivity of our laboratory animals. Therefore, to properly standardize the laboratory animal

„measurement system" it is of decisive importance to reduce the fluctuations of the animals' physiological characteristics from the norm to an absolute minimum by maintaining constant and precisely defined environmental conditions. Only in this manner can relevant experimental results be obtained that use an absolute minimum number of laboratory animals; unnecessary repeat experiments can also be avoided. Costly construction and expensive technical equipment in the animal laboratories guarantee that a climate appropriate for a particular animal species is maintained. Regular illumination that is independent of external conditions for the most part minimizes significant daily or seasonal fluctuations that occur in the world outside. Uniform environmental conditions have to a great extent been achieved by giving the animals balanced diets that are particularly suited to the energy requirements of the specific animal species and by providing very important care in the form of trained personnel (the exclusive use of trained laboratory animal technicians). In addition to the standardization of the laboratory environment and the genetic standardization provided by the breeder of laboratory animals, microbiological and parasitological standardization is very important. Infectious agents that have once taken hold in a stock of laboratory animals can spread and, thereby, affect many animals. Therefore, it is our constant goal to keep away all microorganisms that can affect the health of animals (or staff members taking care of them), their life span or physiological characteristics. Our animals should not just be healthy. We additionally strive to attain the goal that they also be free of any infectious agents that may influence experiments conducted with them although these agents may not make the animals sick in a recognizable manner. For this reason, we, as far as possible, keep only so-called „specified pathogen free" (SPF) animals. This term signifies that the animals were shown to be free of infectious agents (microorganisms as well as macroorganisms) that can make the animals ill or can interfere with experimental results. Just like human beings, animals of this status possess a normal, physiological bacterial flora. In monitoring this high standard (SPF), it is not sufficient for the animals to merely be examined for the absence of clinical symptoms. The desired germ status, absence of individual named infectious agents, is assured by means of regular examinations that use sensitive laboratory methods. In order to avoid individual infections as well as infections of entire animal stocks, the introduction of infectious agents into the individual areas where animals are kept must be avoided. This forms the first line of defense. Therefore, purchased animals and all biological substrates that cannot be disinfected and which may pose a potential risk of infection (e.g., tumors, sera) are examined for the absence of undesirable infectious agents. Furthermore, we have also developed an examination program that through the regular examination of a sufficiently large number of so-called search or monitor animals (spot check) with suitable methods can at an early stage detect infectious agents that have unexpectedly managed to enter the animal stocks. This permanent monitoring of infections is conducted in our own laboratory that employs modern diagnostic methods to directly or indirectly detect infectious agents such as bacteria, viruses, and parasites. Therefore, the microbiological status of all animals is known all the time, is documented, and can even be considered subsequently during the evaluation and interpretation of the animal experiments.

The reason underlying the measures taken in 1987/1988 to transform the still open animal stocks into closed (standardized) laboratory animal stocks was the objective of minimizing the variability of physiological and pathophysiological measurements conducted on laboratory animals and, thereby, to increase the informative value of animal experiments. It can be shown that the overall number of required animals was reduced to less than a third of the previously used animal numbers (reduction of the animal stocks by approximately 50,000 to 20,000 animals). Financial and personnel requirements for the keeping of specified pathogen free animals are significant, but they are absolutely necessary from a scientific viewpoint and also for reasons of animal protection.

The scientific staff members of the Central Animal Laboratory conduct the following scientific programs (or significantly participate in them):

– Microbiological diagnostics in laboratory animals and the effect of infectious agents on animal experiments (Dr. Werner Nicklas)

– Use of carrier-bound fluorescent dyes in the laser-induced fluorescent depiction of malignant gliomas in the rat brain model - Improvement of intraoperative tumor preparation of the glioblastoma in humans (Dr. Uwe Zillmann, Dr. Paul Kremer*, Andreas Wunder, Markus Reinwald, Dr. Hannsjörg Sinn)

– Fluorescence diagnostics and photodynamic therapy:

Fluorescence diagnostics and photodynamic therapy of squamous cell carcinoma (mouse model) occurring in the oropharynx (Dr. Uwe Zillmann, Dr. Dr. Alexander Kübler*)

Intraoperative, adjuvant, photodynamic therapy (PDT) of colon carcinomas and sarcomas (mouse model) (Dr. Johannes Gahlen*, Dr. Uwe Zillmann)

– Activity of antineoplastically effective alkylphosphocholine compounds and metal complexes against medically significant African (and South American) trypanosomes (Prof. Martin R. Berger, Dr. Uwe Zillmann)

Head:
Dr. med. vet. Uwe Zillmann

Deputy:
Dr. med. vet. Werner Nicklas

---

* University of Heidelberg

Central Spectroscopy

The Central Spectroscopy has been organized as a central facility for complex analytical techniques which require sizable investments and special expertise and are therefore impractical to install and operate in individual departments. With our instrumentation a wide variety of analytical services can be offered to all departments within the Deutsches Krebsforschungszentrum. In addition to carrying out the daily service work, the members of our Department are engaged in a number of long-term cooperative research projects, in which the available spectroscopic techniques are further developed and applied in a problem-oriented manner to various areas of cancer research. The particular strengths of spectroscopic methods lie, on the one hand, in their high sensitivity (trace analysis) and, on the other hand, in the detailed structural information obtained at the molecular and atomic level.

The most important analytical methods of the Central Spectroscopy are nuclear magnetic resonance (NMR) spectroscopy and mass spectrometry (MS). Optical techniques such as infrared (IR) and ultraviolet (UV) spectroscopy are also available.

Complementary to our experimental methods, are our activities in the area of computer-assisted molecular modeling, which makes it possible via mathematical simulation to investigate and visualize the structural and dynamic properties of individual molecules or the interactions between molecules on the computer display monitor.

Analytical Service and Nuclear Magnetic Resonance:
Dr. William E. Hull

Mass Spectrometry:
Prof. Dr. Wolf-Dieter Lehmann

Molecular Modelling:
Dr. Claus-Wilhelm von der Lieth

Radiation Protection and Dosimetry

The diverse research projects conducted at the Deutsches Krebsforschungszentrum require the use of many radioactive labeled compounds and equipment for therapeutic irradiation with ionizing radiation as well as large equipment for the production of radioactive substances. For this purpose, use and operating permits are required by law. The Central Service for Radiation Protection and Dosimetry with its skilled staff members concerns itself with obtaining the necessary permits and guaranteeing that radiation protection regulations are fulfilled in the various areas. These areas include the various radionuclide laboratories in the individual departments that comprise seven major areas of research, the experimental and clinical radiotherapy equipment, the cyclotron facility and the research reactor.

According to the Strahlenschutzverordnung (Radiation Protection Ordinance), use and operating permits are granted by the Staatliches Gewerbeaufsichtsamt (State Trade Supervisory Office) Mannheim. The Atomgesetz (Atomic Energy Act) specifies that the operating permit for the research reactor falls under the authority of the Ministry for

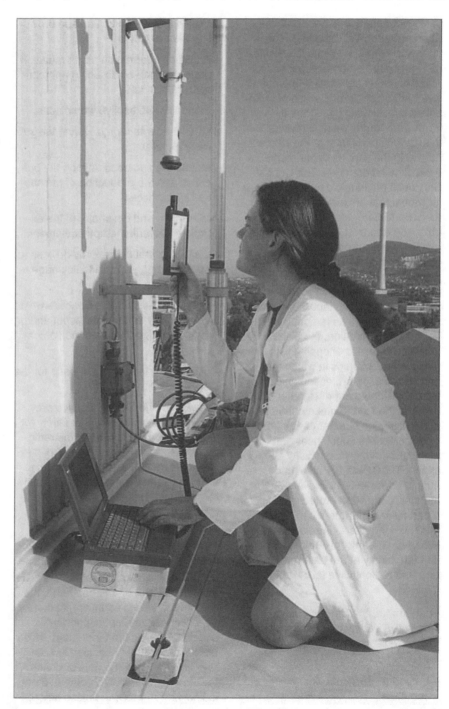

Fig. 94
Above the roofs of Heidelberg, on the building of the Deutsches Krebsforschungszentrum, a dose-rate meter continually records the radioactivity as part of the program for monitoring the surroundings

the Environment and Transport of the State of Baden-Württemberg. These agencies are also responsible for appropriate governmental supervision. The Center possesses a comprehensive authorization for the use of radioactive substances; this forms the framework for the many individual authorizations pertaining to the work conducted in the various departmental radionuclide laboratories. The Central Service is responsible for issuing these individual authorizations, for keeping them up-to-date, and in each case for obtaining approval from the governmental agency. Each individual permission for a department lists the radiation protection officers responsible, the maximum allowable use of radioactive substances, and the laboratory rooms that are equipped as radionuclide laboratories. In addition, the Central Service also compiles shopping lists for radioactive substances in which the named radiation protection officers of the departments are designated as being authorized to make purchases and which also enumerate the authorized radioactive substances and the maximum permissible activity per purchase. These lists are also made available to the selected suppliers. In this manner, a radiation protection officer in a particular department can directly purchase the needed radioactive substances. Thereby, maintaining an unneeded supply of radioactive substances in the radionuclide laboratories is avoided.

Furthermore, the Central Service also conducts a variety of routine tasks relevant to radiation protection that include the following:

– Personnel dosimetry with official dosemeters,

– Monitoring the workplace and providing relevant advice,

– Providing information about radiation protection and establishing appropriate regulations,

– Equipping radioactive workplaces,

– Measurements for monitoring the surrounding areas,

– Monitoring and documenting the purchase and the production of radioactive substances,

– Monitoring and dosimetry of the experimental radiotherapy equipment,

– Quality control of the x-ray devices for medical radiography and its image processing,

– Central collection of radioactive waste and delivery to the state depot and/or to governmentally approved companies,

– Conducting the various reports for the agency.

The work of the Central Service provides an important margin of safety for those individuals working in the radionuclide laboratories. Furthermore, it relieves the departments from having to fulfill requirements that are not directly related to the research-work and facilitates research with radionuclides and ionizing radiation.

The most important radionuclides used in experiments conducted in the molecular biological/biochemical radionuclide laboratories are, on the one hand, the beta emitters such as tritium, carbon-14, phosphorus-32, phosphorus-33, and sulfur-35, on the other hand, those radionuclides that in addition to beta rays also emit gamma rays or characteristic x-rays such as chromium-51 or iodine-125. Annual purchases amount

to between 100 and 120 Gigabecquerels (GBq) of activity. Applications in nuclear medicine mainly use technetium-99m, indium-111, iodine-131, and gallium-67. The yearly activities used of the generator nuclide, technetium-99m, are approximately 1,000 GBq and approximately 200 GBq overall for the additionally named radionuclides.

The Central Service is also responsible for the monitoring and the dosimetry of the three experimental radiotherapy units in which the sources of radiation contain cesium-137. Along with medical physicists, the Central Service is additionally in charge of the radiotherapy equipment GammatronS (source of radiation contains cobalt-60) that is currently being used for the irradiation of patients as well as for experimental irradiations. Furthermore, the Central Service must prepare the annual testing of the therapy equipment by the manufacturers and a governmentally approved expert. The radiotherapy equipment for treating patients with fast neutrons has not been used since 1994; it was shut-down in 1995 and was subsequently disassembled. The non-radioactive parts were sold as scrap metal and the remaining generator tubes were delivered to the state depot. The radioprotective housing for the generator tube that weighs approximately eight tons was placed in the control area of the cyclotron for the decay of the remaining activity (due mainly to manganese-54 and slightly to cobalt-60). The decay period was set at five years; afterwards, these metal parts can be released and sold as scrap. These tasks were completed in cooperation with an external company.

The cyclotron is used to produce the short-lived positron emitters such as carbon-11, nitrogen-13, oxygen-15, and especially fluorine-18 for examinations in nuclear medicine that employ positron emission tomography (PET). Fast neutrons for radiobiological research are also produced. The activities of the short-lived positron emitters that are produced daily amount to between 50 and 100 GBq. The calculations and measurements pertinent to radiation protection in the running of a PET unit were conducted by staff members of the Service and the Research Program Radiological Diagnostics and Therapy. With respect to the local doses in the surrounding areas, the results obtained are applicable to PET facilities in general and have been published. These findings may be used to determine the radiation exposure of individuals working near the PET and to arrive at necessary protective measures.

Neutrons from the research reactor TRIGA HD II can be used to produce individual radionuclides and entire radionuclide groups, for example, for radiochemistry and trace element detection. The neutrons can also be directly used in quality control and in calibration of detectors to measure the neutron flux density. The Central Service has to ensure that the radiological safety of the facility is guaranteed and that the activity of the radionuclides that are produced lie within the permissible range. Moreover, it must regularly report the results of radiation protection measurements to the responsible agency and conduct the required repeat evaluations of the comprehensive set of instruments used in radiation protection in the presence of independent experts. The head of the Central Service of Radiation Protection and Dosimetry is a member of the Working Group on Op-

eration and Safety of Research Reactors in the German Atomic Forum and its Working Group on Decommissioning of Research Reactors. He is also a member of the Working Group on the Fuel Cycle of Research Reactors, of the Federal Research Ministry.

Six staff members work in this unit. One male and one female member are participating in a dual training program for three years that combines practice and theory that will result in their qualifying as radiation protection engineers.

Head and Radiation
Protection Officer:
Dipl.-Phys. Otto Krauss

Deputy:
Dipl.-Phys. Dr. Wolfgang Kübler

Research Reactor TRIGA Heidelberg II

The research reactor TRIGA Heidelberg II in the Deutsches Krebsforschungszentrum is a swimming pool reactor with a thermal power of 250 kW. It is a very reliable and safe neutron irradiation source and is mainly used in the following research activities:

– Neutron activation analyses of biological material in medical research;

– Production of radionuclides for labeling experiments in radiochemistry;

– Production of special radioactive tracers for diagnostics and therapy in nuclear medicine;

– Production of radionuclides and the performance of activation analyses for guests from other research facilities;

– Irradiation for industry and other facilities.

The TRIGA reactor is an inherently safe unit; this is a consequence of the nuclear physical qualities of its uranium zirconium hydride fuel elements. These elements possess a prompt negative temperature coefficient that limits the power of the reactor and automatically returns the unit to normal operating power. This explains why TRIGA may be operated on a university campus or in a densely populated area.

The reactor has a maximum neutron flux of 1×10^{13} neutrons per second and cm^2 at a continuous power of 250 kW.

The reactor has been in operation since August 1966. It was located in the first building of the Center and was subsequently moved to its present location

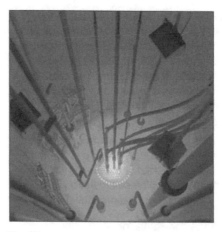

Fig. 95
The view into the research reactor with the characteristic Cerenkov radiation of a swimming-pool reactor

where it has again been in operation since February 28, 1978 after a reconstruction period of about 10 months. Since 1966, more than 13,000 experiments and approximately 3,000 samples annually have been performed. During this time period, the energy output amounted to approximately 9MW days. An rotary rack for samples with 40 positions is available for irradiation and five in-core positions with a higher neutron flux are available in the reactor core. The reactor is operated by three technicians in the Research Program Radiological Diagnostics and Therapy. They perform all the experiments and all the inspections and maintenance work in cooperation with the special workshops in their department. The fuel elements of the reactor are presently burned up to an extent of approximately 12 percent and after some additional use and decommissioning of the reactor they will be placed in final storage.

The reactor is regularly inspected by the state regulatory agency and the TÜV (Technischer Überwachungs-Verein – safety and standards authority). There have been no significant disturbances in the past; it is a reliable and safe facility for experimentation in biological research.

Head:
Prof. Dr. Walter J. Lorenz (until 1997)
Dr. Karl-Heinz Hoever

Operating manager:
Dr. Wolfgang Maier-Borst (until 1997)
Dr. Karl-Heinz Hoever
Dr. Jochen Schuhmacher

Cyclotron

The modern variant of diagnostics in nuclear medicine, so-called positron emission tomography (PET), is used by the Department of Radiological Diagnostics and Therapy to quantitatively determine the vitality of tumors before and after therapy in the sense of checking the effectiveness of treatment (therapy monitoring). Radioactively labeled biomolecules whose structure is adapted to the metabolism are used to detect physiological processes. They accumulate more or less strongly in the observed area. Their distribution and kinetics enable the physician to draw conclusions about the growth of the cancerous tumor.

The biochemistry of the marked preparation should not be changed by the coupling of the radioactive „label". Therefore, PET employs „short-lived" „brothers" of those elements that physiologically occur in tissues, carbon (C), nitrogen (N) and oxygen (O), namely C 11, N 13 or O 15 and, lacking a short-lived hydrogen isotope, the nuclide fluorine 18. These radioisotopes decay very rapidly and have a half life that ranges between two and 110 minutes. With the exception of fluorine 18, they cannot be ordered through an external supplier. They must be produced at the

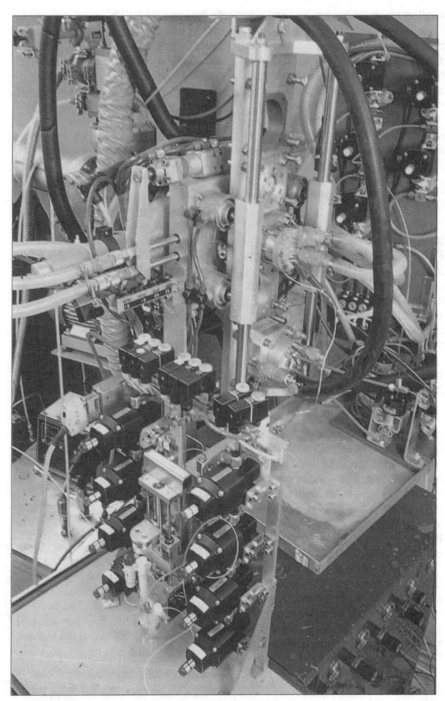

Fig. 96
Use of the cyclotron for producing radioisotopes for diagnostic examinations. In connection with the development of new radiochemical methods, this apparatus for interchanging up to four targets is used to investigate new radioactive substances

location where they are to be used since they would decay during transport. For their production, one requires atomic nuclei that are rich in energy with which one shoots at a stabile substance - a gas, a liquid or a solid - that has been packed into a target station. By means of nuclear transformations, a minimal quantity of the desired radionuclide with respect to its mass is formed in the target. However, after chemical separation from the mother substance, it possesses the highest specific activity.

In the 1995 edition of „Current Cancer Research" we introduced the new particle accelerator, a negative ion cyclotron, that produces the mentioned fast nuclei which in our case are protons and deuterons. It is the first compact cyclotron for use in biomedical research that can accelerate negative ions of light as well as heavy hydrogen (deuterium). Deuterons make possible the production of fluorine 18 in the gas phase; this means in the non-ionic state by way of a nuclear reaction involving the gas Neon 20. In this chemical form, the nuclide opens a wide variety of radiochemical preparations that cannot be attained with the usually used fluorine 18 ion (from the costly form of water (oxygen 18), irradiated with protons). Also the preparation of frequently used oxygen 15 from the ordinary, inexpensive gas, nitrogen 14, succeeds easily with deuterons and results in a large yield. The vast majority of negative ion cyclotrons that are in use throughout the world today exclusively produce protons. The radiochemistry of the radionuclides that are thus produced is, therefore, limited with respect to the possible labeling procedures.

By far, our cyclotron is mainly engaged in the production of the above-named isotopes that partially because of their short half life must be produced „online" and in a reliable manner at the same time that the patient is being examined. The radiopharamaceuticals are mainly used in the PET project of the Research Program Oncological Diagnostics and Therapy at the Center. However, external clinics are also supplied. A preparation that cannot be purchased (18F-Dopa) and is beneficial in brain diagnostics is sent to an institute some 100 km away where it is used to measure the functions of the brain. An additional longer-lived isotope, rubidium 81, is regularly produced in highest possible isotopic purity for the Department of Nuclear Medicine, Radiological Clinic, University of Heidelberg. It decays into a very short-lived noble gas (krypton 81m) that has a half life of only 13 seconds; it is used in the scintigraphic depiction of lung function. This „81rubidium/81mkrypton generator" is four to ten times more powerful than the commercially available product. A special target system and a thereto connected computer-guided apparatus was developed for it.

Apart from direct medical use, the versatility of the cyclotron unit and the good yields obtained during radionuclide production make possible the development of new radiochemical procedures that will expand the spectrum of diagnostic applications for positron emission tomography. This task regularly occupies several doctoral candidates associated with the chemical and pharmaceutical institutes at the University of Heidelberg.

Equipment for the production of fast neutrons that was installed at the cyclo-

tron is especially intended to be used for biological research. Scientific interest has been aroused in research groups both within and outside of the Center with respect to the possibilities of examining complex radiation damage in the macromolecules responsible for heredity and the possibilities of conducting activation analyses with fast and slow neutrons.

After the first years of successful operation, we can state that our cyclotron has not only fulfilled the expectations associated with its construction, but with respect to its effectiveness and reliability has surpassed all expectations. The ideas and needs of the experimenters provide constant incentive to further improve the systems and to rationalize procedures. The capacity of this facility is such that the planned cooperative Heidelberg PET Center can also be supplied with radionuclides.

Head:
Prof. Dr. Walter J. Lorenz (until 1997)
Priv.-Doz. Dr. Gunnar Brix

Operating manager:
Dr. Gerd Wolber

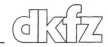

Central Data Processing

Both the need for and the use of information processing has developed much more strongly at the Deutsches Krebsforschungszentrum than at classical research centers of the Hermann von Helmholtz Association. This can be traced to several factors. Especially worth mentioning are the early conversion of the Central Data Processing to an organizational form that uses a distributed computer systems (client/server architecture). This conversion proceeded from one traditional mainframe computer to a large number of dedicated servers with cost-effective processors taken from large-scale production, the concentration on a few, advanced operating systems and a notably user friendly service structure. The transformation from an allocating "computer center" to a center of competence with a pronounced service character for all questions related to information technology has proven decisive for the center's self-image.

Services offered by Central Data Processing can be classified as follows:
– Basic services for the mutual use of large equipment (servers);
– Operating the central computers;
– Access to servers, supercomputers and high performance networks;
– Preserving data, storage, backup and archiving for all computers in the Center.

User Services for Special Peripherals include:
– Digital slide recorder, color and poster printing, list distribution;
– PC lending pool (notebooks and desktop equipment);
– Generally accessible PCs in the training room;

– Hardware and software installation for distributed computers and workstations.

Training and Advice for Hardware and Software include:
– Advice and information in the acquisition of hardware and software;
– Training and advice in the use of PCs, applications, and operating systems:
– Lending instructional videos for PC software:
– Advice concerning all aspects of computer networking.

Access to Computers and Information Services via Networks:
– Worldwide e-mail and data exchange;
– Access to the Internet, news, and the WWW;
– Information services on CD, e.g., timetables and telephone books;
– Internal information services in the intranet.

To make available computer power that is shared by a large user group two super computers have been installed: a parallel computer IBM SP2 with 78 processors (type MPP) and a multiprocessor system HP Convex SPP2000 with 16 processors (type SMP). With their power of 20.8 GFLOPS (= billions of floating point operations per second) and 11.5 GFLOPS, respectively, they are comparable to computers at cancer research centers of the USA and Japan. They process data that are stored on file servers with RAID disks (180 GB) and cartridge robots (5,000 GB) that also contain data from additional computers throughout the Center. Software on the supercomputers mainly stems from applications in the disciplines of bioinformatics, molecular dynamics, quantum chemistry, DNA se-

quence analysis, and the resulting databases for genome data.

User services supports 1,600 registered users at the Center who work on approximately 1,000 personal computers, roughly 180 Macintosh computers and 150 Unix workstations. Almost all of these desktop computers are connected through a structured, local network (ATM, FDDI, fast ethernet, ethernet). They load user software, especially the MS Office package, from a license server running under Novell 4.2. In the context of distributed DP architecture, Central Data Processing additionally supports ten servers running under Novell and in case of problems assists the user in matters that range from the selection of devices to obtaining repairs. This support also includes regular training of staff members in the commonly used software packages. For external communication through computer networks into the German Scientific Network (Wissenschaftsnetz – WiN) and the worldwide Internet with electronic mail (e-mail), data exchange (FTP), discussion and news forums, Central Data Processing operates a high power connection (40 Mbps) with ATM that is provided by the German Research Network (Deutsches Forschungsnetz – DFN e.V.). In this manner, the Center also presents itself in the World Wide Web (WWW) with more than 1,000 pages of information. Parallel to this, a comparable amount of information as well as a comparable communication medium can be found internally in the intranet that is currently under development.

Head:
Dr. Kurt Böhm

Safety

The planning staff of the Safety Unit advises responsible individuals and employees in all matters of occupational safety. It also concerns itself with environmental safety. It answers to the scientific management board. The safety engineer in charge is the waste officer of the center. In this function, he gives advice in matters concerning the disposal of special wastes (especially research-related) and supervises that the strict legal regulations governing waste disposal and the recycling of materials are followed.

Scientific research that involves contact with chemical, biological and infectious materials requires that a multitude of laws, regulations, guidelines and standards be followed. Especially since 1994, a steady increase in regulations has been observed, because of European law. The corresponding translation of guidelines of the European Union (EU) into national law and the adjustment of DIN standards to conform to EU standards requires that additional measures be undertaken both in the laboratory and in attached facilities. Internal directives and rules are necessary for this purpose.

A major area of interest that safety engineering focuses on is advising experimenters during their use of carcinogenic substances and substances that can cause genetic changes. By establishing appropriate safety measures, negative effects upon human beings and the environment are avoided. The same holds true when employing methods that use infectious, biological materials or techniques from genetic engineering. In addition to internally issued operational di-

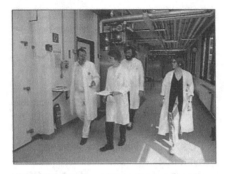

Fig. 97
To check the safety of the equipment and installations, regular inspections are carried out together with representatives of the staff council

rectives, important foundations for optimizing safety include tasks such as advising, monitoring safety facilities and decontamination and disinfection measures.

Important cornerstones upon which safety is built include eliminating defects, ascertaining possible sources of danger, taking measurements at the workplaces as well as developing and testing safety measures. The laboratory of the planning staff for safety is equipped with modern measuring equipment that can measure relevant chemical and physical values. In cooperation with other internal units (e.g., Division of Toxicology and Cancer Risk Factors or Central Spectroscopy) additional analytic methods and other resources can be used. Close cooperation also exists with property management which is responsible for waste disposal and for questions concerning hazardous goods. Main areas of cooperation include chemical waste, determination of important metrological parameters, categorization and declaration of special hazardous waste.

An internal fire department, whose members are specially trained to deal with the specific demands related to scientific research, enables rapid intervention in case of incidents or accidents. This occurs in coordination with the professional fire department.

In all matters relating to safety at work a close collaboration with the facilityis physician and the staff council goes without saying. It is only in joint efforts that comparably low accident rates can be attained; this can be seen at the Center.

The committee for occupational safety, which is mainly composed of scientifically trained safety officers and, among others, representatives from technical fields and radiation protection, regularly discusses safety problems and proposes solutions.

Of special significance is the participation in external committees and bodies such as, for example, insurance associations, Association of German Safety Engineers (VDSI) or the Hermann von Helmholtz Association of German Research Centers.

Head:
Dipl. Ing. Edgar Heuss

Deputies:
Dipl. Ing. Annekathrin Kollenda
Sich. Ing. Mathias Beyer

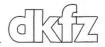

Evaluation of Results and Main Research Objectives

Since 1983, internal presentations of the scientific work within the individual divisions and external assessments of whole research programs with their divisions have alternated at regular intervals. The internal presentations of the research activities take place regularly and are supervised by the Scientific Council, the Coordinators of the research programs, and the Management Board. Here, the researchers from one division report on their work and their results and present concepts and prospects for future research. As a rule, each division presents itself every 2 years to the other staff of the Center and every 5 years to an expert panel consisting of the members of the Scientific Committee of the Board of Trustees and external experts from Germany and abroad. These assessments may result in a redefinition of scientific priorities, a readjustment of resources distributed, an exchange of staff, an increase or reduction of working space, additional investments, or the establishment of special working groups or new divisions. The results of the presentations and the external assessments are discussed within the Scientific Council and implemented in coordination with the Board of Trustees and the Management Board. In the years 1994 to 1996, 5 research programs were subjected to external assessment and 30 internal presentations took place.

In the period of this report, several new divisions have been set up (see next page). In addition to these new divisions established during the years 1994, 1995, and 1996, further research focuses have been defined according to the Center's course of continuous reorientation and have been declared as temporary divisions.

Furthermore, with the arrival of a new generation, several division heads have retired. Their fields of research have been superseded by new scientific challenges.

The appointment procedures for the new clinical cooperation unit "Dermato-Oncology" at Mannheim Hospitals were started in 1995.

Research sponsorship organizations both in Germany and abroad are funding a large number of projects for which scientists at the Deutsches Krebsforschungszentrum have sucessfully applied, having been judged worthy of support by the relevant expert boards. In 1994, 270 projects were approved (DM 29.3 million), in 1995 there were 299 projects (DM 33.3 million), and in 1996 there were 318 projects (DM 36.6 million). Funding by the European Union amounted to DM 7.6 million in 1994, DM 5.5 million in 1995 and DM 6.9 million in 1996.

The publication of the scientific results achieved at the Center in leading specialist journals in Germany and abroad is another element of the continuous evaluation of results.

New Divisions

During the years 1995 and 1996, five new divisions were founded at the Deutsches Krebsforschungszentrum.

Tumor genetics, genome research, and developmental biology of the immune system are the focal areas of the new permanent division "Experimental Therapy of Malignant Tumors". Its head, Prof. Dr. Thomas Boehm, was previously in the department Medicine I at the Albert-Ludwigs University Hospital in Freiburg. Thomas Boehm studies the early phases of maturation of the thymus during development of the immune system. It is in the thymus, located in humans behind the sternum, that certain immune cells, the T-lymphocytes, learn to distinguish between friend and foe. This is an important prerequisite if they are to identify certain cancer cells or cells of the body that are infected with viruses. Boehm has discovered a gene (nude/whn) that is responsible for one of the longest-known immune deficiencies in mice and rats. In animals with a defective whn gene, the thymus does not develop its normal functionality so that immune cells can no longer mature in this organ. Another feature of these animals is that their hair growth is disabled and they have no fur. Scientists are able to implant human tumor tissue into these mice without evoking an immune reaction. This makes it possible, among other things, to test the response of human tumor cells to new cancer drugs in an environment that is broadly similar to that of the human organism, hence, contributing to the development of new treatments.

In order to better understand and model evolutionary processes, Dr. Martin Vin-

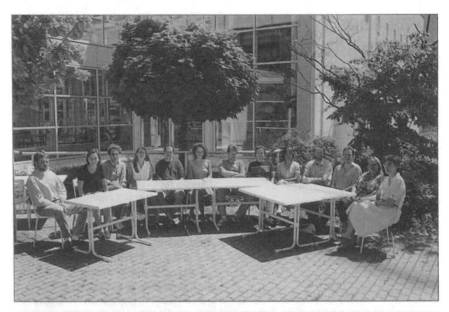

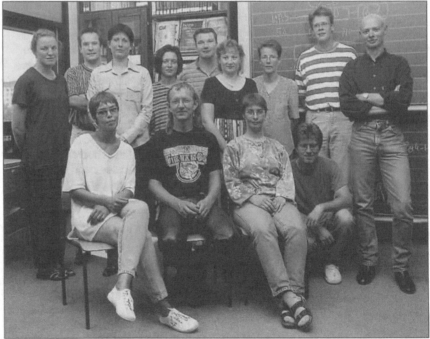

Figs. 98, 99
New divisional heads with their staff: Prof. Dr. Thomas Boehm (fourth from right, Fig. 98), Dr. Peter Angel (far right, Fig. 99)

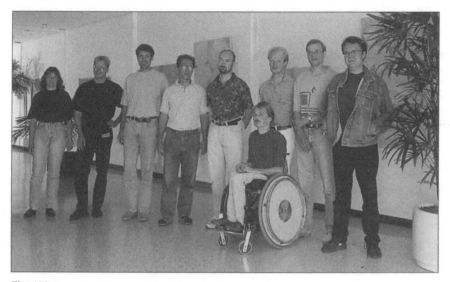

Fig. 100
Dr. Martin Vingron, fourth from left, and his staff

gron, head of the new division "Theoretical Bioinformatics", is developing mathematical procedures and computer programs for the structuring of the evolutionary trees. The enormous amount of data that are generated in connection with the human genome project complement and complete our existing knowledge about aspects such as molecular evolution.

Computer-assisted procedures in oncological radiology are being developed by Prof. Dr. Wolfgang Schlegel in the new division „Medical Physics". Using his previous experience in the division „Biophysics and Medical Radiation Physics", Prof. Schlegel will employ the methods of physics, technology, and modern data processing to further improve procedures of precision radio-

therapy of tumors. In addition to classical radiological treatment, he also intends to pursue new avenues in local tumor therapy. His program will thus in-

clude the application of lasers and the planning of chemotherapeutic intervention, each targeting well-defined tissue regions.

The new division "Signal Transduction and Growth Control" is led by Dr. Peter Angel and addresses the effects of hormones, growth factors, high-energy radiation, and carcinogenic environmental poisons at the molecular-genetic level. The biologist and his staff are investigating the functioning of so-called transcription factors, whose job it is to control the translation of the genetic information into a "transport form" for protein synthesis. Defects in some of these transcription factors are known to play a role in the transformation of a healthy cell into a cancer cell.

The identification of genes responsible for hereditary diseases is the major aim of of the new division "Molecular Genome Analysis" headed by Priv.-Doz. Dr. Annemarie Poustka. A molecular biologist, she previously led a working group in the Research Program "Applied Tumor Virology". Poustka's foremost concern is a region on the human X chromosome which is known to have a particularly high density of "disease genes". She has already gained recognition for her important contribution to the work that identified the gene responsible for Chorea Huntington, located on chromosome 4. Poustka is also attempting to refine procedures of gene mapping for locating defective genes.

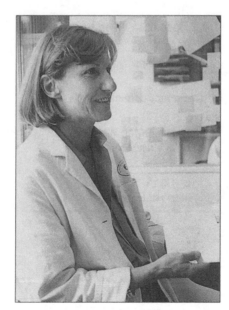

Fig. 101
Priv.-Doz. Dr. Annemarie Poustka at her workplace

Distinctions and Honors

In the years 1994 to 1996, as in the past, numerous scientists and employees at the Deutsches Krebsforschungszentrum received prizes and honors.

1994

Walter Friedrich Prize of the German X-Ray Society	Dr. Peter Bachert
1994 Poster Prizes of the German X-Ray Society	Michael Bock, Boris Krems, Clemens Müller
Gottron-Just Science Prize of the University and the City of Ulm	Dr. Petra Boukamp
Helax Prize of the 11th International Conference on Computers in Radiation Therapy in Manchester	Dr. Thomas Bortfeld
1994 Animal Protection Research Prize of the Federal Ministry of Health	Dr. Harald Enzmann and Prof. Dr. Peter Bannasch
Carl Zeiss Award Lecture of the German Society for Cell Biology	Prof. Dr. Werner Franke
Hans Bloemendahl Prize of the Faculty of Biochemistry of the University of Nijmegen	Prof. Dr. Werner Franke
Falcon Prize of the company Becton-Dickinson	Dr. Jan-Michael Peters
1994 Philips Prize of the German Society for Medical Physics	Katrin Rempp
Poster Prize of the German Society for Nuclear Medicine	Dr. Peter Schmidlin
Research Prize "Smoke-free Living" of the Medical Association "Smoking and Health"	Prof. Dr. Jürgen Wahrendorf and Dr. Heiko Becher
1994 Paul Ehrlich Prize of the Paul Ehrlich and Ludwig Darmstaedter Foundation	Prof. Dr. Dr. h. c. mult. Harald zur Hausen

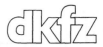

1995	
1995 Journalism Award of the SmithKline Beecham Foundation	Editorial team of „einblick": Susanne Glasmacher, Renate Ries, Dr. Birgitt Sickenberger, Dr. Luise Wagner-Roos, Hilke Stamatiadis-Smidt
1995 German Cancer Award (clinical part) of the German Cancer Society	Prof. Dr. Werner Franke
Feldberg Prize 1995 of the Feldberg Foundation	Prof. Dr. Werner Franke
Poster Prize awarded at the international annual meeting of the German Society for Nuclear Medicine	Dr. Uwe Haberkorn, Iris Morr
1995 DEGUM Dissertation Award of the German Society for Ultrasound in Medicine	Dr. Peter Huber
Poster Prize for tumor diagnostics on the occasion of the Research Symposium of the Tumor Center Heidelberg/Mannheim	Dr. Stefan Joos and other contributors to the prize-winning project
Ernst von Bergmann Badge of the Federal Medical Board of Registration and the German Doctors' Association	Prof. Dr. Gerhard van Kaick
Poster Prize at the Research Symposium of the Tumor Center Heidelberg/Mannheim	Dr. Michael Knopp and other contributors to the prize-winning project
Erna Weber Prize of the German Section of the International Biometrical Society	Dr. Annette Kopp-Schneider
Robert Koch Prize of the Robert Koch Foundation	Prof. Dr. Peter Krammer
1995 Behring Award Lecture of the Philipps University in Marburg, donated by Behringwerke AG	Prof. Dr. Peter Krammer
1995 Philips Prize of the German Society for Medical Physics	Boris Krems
Poster Prize for tumor therapy on the occasion of the Research Symposium of the Tumor Center Heidelberg/Mannheim	Dr. Markus Lindauer and other contributors to the prize-winning project
Hans Popper Sponsorship Prize 1995 on the occasion of the 10th International Liver Symposium	Rosemarie Mayer

1995

Poster Prize on the occasion of the German X-Ray Conference 1995	Martin Mory and other contributors to the prize-winning project
Award of the Society for Research on Laboratory Animals	Dr. Werner Nicklas
1995 Award of the German X-Ray Society; Association for Medical Radiology	Dr. Katrin Rempp and Priv.-Doz. Dr. Gunnar Brix
1995 Walter Friedrich Prize of the German X-Ray Society	Priv.-Doz. Dr. Lothar Schad
Grünenthal Sponsorship Prize "Skin and Environment" (half share)	Dr. Klaus Schulze-Osthoff
Poster Prize awarded at the Research Symposium of the Tumor Center Heidelberg/Mannheim	Simone Seiter and other contributors to the prize-winning project
Award of the Organization of European Cancer Institutes (OECI) for the best lecture held at the Conference on Cancer and Quality of Life	Hilke Stamatiadis-Smidt
Johann Peter Süßmilch Medal of the German Society for Medical Computing, Biometry, and Epidemiology (GDMS)	Dr. Karen Steindorf
Poster Prize on the occasion of the Conference of the European Association of Radiologists	Dr. Gerald Weißler
Research Award of the State of Baden-Württemberg	Prof. Dr. Margot Zöller

1996

Coolidge Award 1996 of General Electric Systems and the German X-Ray Society	Dr. Matthias Bellemann
Gottfried Wilhelm Leibniz Prize of the German Research Association (DFG)	Prof. Dr. Thomas Boehm
Poster Prize awarded at the conference "Environmental UV-Radiation, Risk of Skin Cancer and Primary Prevention"	Dr. Petra Boukamp
EACR Young Cancer Researcher Award Lecture 1996 of the European Association for Cancer Research	Raffaella Corvi

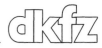

1996

Baltimore Student Award 1996 on the occasion of the 15th Papillomavirus Workshop in Brisbane, Australia	Kerstin Crusius
Four Magellan Stars of the McKinleys Group	Dr. Uwe Engelmann
1996 Mallinckrodt Sponsorship Prize for Nuclear Medicine of the German Society for Nuclear Medicine	Priv.-Doz. Dr. Uwe Haberkorn
1996 Erna Weber Prize of the German Section of the International Biometrical Society	Dr. Carsten Heuer
Poster Prize of the German X-Ray Society	Knut Jöchle
1996 German Cancer Award (experimental part) of the German Cancer Society	Prof. Dr. Peter Krammer
Heinz Ansmann Prize of the Heinz Ansmann Foundation	Prof. Dr. Peter Krammer
Meyenburg Prize of the Wilhelm and Maria Meyenburg Foundation	Prof. Dr. Peter Krammer
Order of Merit, 1st Class, of the Federal Republic of Germany	Prof. Dr. Peter Krammer
Behring Kitasato Award of Hoechst Japan Ltd.	Prof. Dr. Peter Krammer
Award for Creative Work in Organofluorine Chemistry of the Division of Fluorine Chemistry of the American Chemical Society	Dr. Franz Oberdorfer
1996 Paul Ehrlich Prize of the Paul Ehrlich and Ludwig Darmstaedter Foundation	Prof. Dr. Hans-Georg Rammensee
1996 Karl-Heinz Beckurts Prize of the Karl-Heinz Beckurts Foundation	Prof. Dr. Wolfgang Schlegel
GDMS Sponsorship Prize for Students of the German Society for Medical Computing, Biometry and Epidemiology	Silke Schmidt
International Partner Award of the National Cancer Institute/Cancer Information Service, USA	Hilke Stamatiadis-Smidt, Cancer Information Service KID
Order of Merit, 1st Class, of the Federal Republic of Germany	Hilke Stamatiadis-Smidt

1996

Ernst Jung Prize for Medicine of the Jung Foundation for Science and Research, Hamburg	Prof. Dr. Dr. h. c. mult. Harald zur Hausen

1997

Scientific Award for Clinical Research 1997 of the SmithKline Beecham Foundation	Prof. Dr. Klaus-Michael Debatin
2nd Prize of the competition "Medical Software" by Human Interfaces, Lucern	Dr. Uwe Engelmann
Behring Kitasato Award 1997 of the Behring Kitasato Foundation	Prof. Dr. Günter Hämmerling
Poster Prize on the occasion of the European Congress of Radiologists	Dr. Hans Hawighorst
Research Grant of the ECR Research and Education Fund	Priv.-Doz. Dr. Michael Knopp
Poster Prize on the occasion of the European Congress of Radiologists	Priv.-Doz. Dr. Michael Knopp
Poster Prize on the occasion of the annual Meeting of the German Society for Connective Tissue Research	Jan Tuckerman
Poster Prize of the German Society for Nuclear Medicine	Sven Wagner
Carl-Gottfried Schmidt Research Award of Pharmacia & Upjohn	Dr. Bianca Wittig
Jacob Henle Medal of the Georg August University in Göttingen	Prof. Dr. Dr. h. c. mult. Harald zur Hausen

Dr. Lutz Edler was elected Full Member of the International Statistical Institute in 1994 and Vice-President of the International Association for Statistical Computing for the period 1995 to 1997.

Prof. Dr. Norbert Fusenig was elected Honorary Member of the Sky Club for Skin Research in 1995.

Prof. Dr. Ingrid Grummt was appointed to the Foundation German-American Academic Council for the period 1996 to 1997.

Brigitte Hobrecker was appointed to the Senate of the Hermann von Helmholtz Association of National Research Centers (HGF) in 1996.

Dr. Martina Pötschke-Langer was appointed in 1995 as the German representative to the Advisory Board of the European Network on Young People and Tobacco.

Dr. Annemarie Poustka was elected HUGO Council Member in 1995 for three years.

Prof. Dr. Manfred Schwab was elected Vice-President of the Board of the German Cancer Society in 1996.

Hilke Stamatiadis-Smidt was appointed to the European Network for the Prevention of Smoking as representative of the "Coalition Against Smoking" in 1995.

Prof. Dr. Dr. h. c. mult. Harald zur Hausen was awarded an honorary doctorate for medicine in 1995 by the Karls University in Prague. In 1997, he received an honorary doctorate from the University of Salford, England.

Former Divisional Heads

In the years 1994 to 1996, a number of divisional heads left the Deutsches Krebsforschungszentrum due to retirement and the attainment of emeritus status. By the year 2000, nearly all members of the Center's founding generation who, since 1964, have laid the groundwork for, and continuously developed, its research program will have retired.

The years 1994, 1995, and 1996 saw the retirement of Prof. Dr. Gerhard Sauer, head of the division „DNA Tumor Viruses", Prof. Dr. Hans-Christian Kaerner, head of the division „Tumor-Virus Genetics", and Prof. Dr. Erich Hecker, head of the division „Mechanism of Tumorigenesis" and founding director of the former Institute of Biochemistry. Professor Hecker continues to work as the German coordinator of the cooperation program between the Deutsches Krebsforschungszentrum and the Israeli Science Ministry.

Prof. Dr. Claus Köhler, head of the division „Medical and Biological Informatics", retired in 1995. He had been Co-ordinator of the Research Program „Bioinformatics" since 1994.

The aims and tasks of the divisions have been redefined. For some divisions, new divisional heads have already been appointed (see „Evaluation of Results and Main Research Objectives", „New Divisions and Project Groups").

Three divisional heads have been offered professorships at other research institutes. In 1995, Dr. Hans-Georg Kräusslich accepted a C4 professorship at the medical faculty of Hamburg University, where he heads the Division of Cell Biology and Virology of the Heinrich Pette Institute for Experimental Virology.

Prof. Dr. Stefan Meuer, head of the division „Applied Immunology" of the Deutsches Krebsforschungszentrum since 1987, has been appointed Medical Director of the Institute for Immunology of the University of Heidelberg.

In 1996, Prof. Dr. Hans-Georg Rammensee, head of the division „Tumor-Virus Immunology", left the Deutsches Krebsforschungszentrum to take up a C4 professorship in immunology at the University of Tübingen, where he heads the Interfaculty Institute for Cell Biology.

Prizes Awarded by the Deutsches Krebsforschungszentrum

Five prizes for exceptional achievements in the field of cancer research and early detection of cancer are awarded in cooperation with the Deutsches Krebsforschungszentrum.

Since 1981, the Wilhelm und Maria Meyenburg Foundation has awarded the Meyenburg Prize for outstanding accomplishments in cancer research. The prize is endowed with DM 30,000. In addition, the board of the foundation supports research visits by scientists from Germany and abroad to the Deutsches Krebsforschungszentrum as well as research projects of scientists from the Deutsches Krebsforschungszentrum and the facilities cooperating with them.

In 1994, the Meyenburg Prize was awarded to Prof. Dr. med. Gert

Fig. 102
Dr. Marion Meyenburg presents the 1994 Meyenburg Prize to Prof. Dr. Gert Riethmüller, Institute of Immunology of the University of Munich

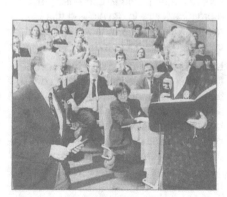

Fig. 103
Prof. Dr. David P. Lane of the University of Dundee, Scotland, (center) receives the 1995 Meyenburg Prize from the Members of the Management Board Prof. Dr. Stefan Meuer (right) and Dr. Wolfgang Henkel

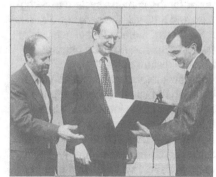

215

Riethmüller, director of the Institute of Immunology of the Ludwig Maximilian University of Munich. He was awarded the prize for his outstanding achievements in cancer research. In an innovative approach using monoclonal antibodies to boost the body's natural immune defense, he was able to significantly prolong the lives of cancer patients. The immune system produces a countless variety of antibodies to fight germs. In a study supported by the German Cancer Aid and carried out at clinics in Munich, Augsburg, Essen, Hamburg, Hannover, and Cologne, 189 patients with intestinal cancer were first treated by surgery to remove the tumor. At the time of the operation the cancer had apparently not yet spread to distant organs; however, nearby lymph nodes were found to contain cancer cells. Then, an antibody taken from mice was repeatedly injected into the bloodstream of 90 of these persons. The patients in the control group were only treated by surgery. All participants in the study were treated between 1985 and 1990. Five years later, 51 percent of the patients in the control group had died, compared to only 36 percent of those treated with antibodies in addition to surgery. The antibody binds to a structure on the surface of cancer cells called 17-1A. This apparently makes it easier for the immune system to recognize, and thus kill, the cancer cells. The antibody can thereby find cancer cells that have spread from the primary tumor to distant parts of the body to form new tumors (metastases), which are often the cause of death in patients with cancer of the intestine. Unlike chemotherapy, which attacks only dividing cells, 17-1A antibodies also mark resting cells. Therefore, Riethmüller intends to develop a combined treatment with antibodies and chemotherapy in the future.

The 1995 Meyenburg Prize was awarded to Prof. David P. Lane from the University of Dundee in Scotland. The Wilhelm and Maria Meyenburg Foundation thereby acknowledged Lane's outstanding contributions to identifying and functionally characterizing the tumor suppressor gene p53 and applying these findings to clinical practice.

More than six million cases of cancer are diagnosed each year. In every second case a defect in the genetic material of a protein called p53 can be found. The task of this protein is to ensure the stability of the human hereditary information. It stops cell growth if, for example, the DNA has been damaged by x-rays or a carcinogenic chemical, thus giving cellular repair mechanisms a chance to mend the defect. If the damage is too great, p53 induces a mechanism called apoptosis, the self-destruction of the cell. However, if p53, the molecular „guardian of the genome", is activated due to a defective modification in its own genetic material or by a cellular or viral carcinogenic protein, i.e., an oncogene, then the cell divides unchecked even if its DNA is defective. This can lead to the formation of a malignant tumor. David P. Lane has played a prominent role in developing this model, which, in the meantime, has become generally accepted.

Lane discovered p53 in the late seventies, when he was doing research on a tumor virus in monkeys called SV40. It was in the context of this research that he observed a close link between this previously unknown 53-kilodalton protein and the large T antigen, an oncogene of the virus. Thus, he was the first to discover a complex of this sort, which, as is known today, forms the basis of the carcinogenic potential of certain tumor viruses.

Lane and his co-workers gained substantial insights into the function of p53 and its appearance in various organ tumors by producing and exactly characterizing monoclonal antibodies. With the help of these highly specific proteins Lane obtained information on the relationship of p53 to DNA and cellular proteins as well as on the structure of intact and transformed p53 molecules. In tumors of the rectum and the breast he observed highly increased levels of p53. His subsequent research revealed that this phenomenon occurs in the majority of human cancers and generally implies a bad prognosis for the patients. Lane and his co-workers at the University of Dundee have also developed various routine immunological tests to examine tumor tissue samples for the presence of p53.

Professor Dr. Peter Krammer, head of the Division of Immunogenetics at the Deutsches Krebsforschungszentrum, was awarded the 1996 Meyenburg Prize. Krammer and his co-workers discovered that cancer cells can induce apoptosis, programmed cell death, in immune cells. In this process, the protein CD95L functions as a „death messenger" by binding to CD95, a particular molecule on the surface of many cells in the body. This triggers a cascade of biochemical processes within the cell, which lead to its death. The scientists found out that certain cancer cells stop producing CD95. Thus, they elude the programmed cell death induced by immune cells. At the same time they produce large quantities of the „death messenger" CD95L. Since activated T lymphocytes, which fight against tumors in the body, have the CD95L molecule on their surface, they are responsive to the deadly message. Thus, cancer cells can turn the tables: Instead of being killed by immune cells, they start attacking them.

The Walther and Christine Richtzenhain Prize is awarded annually by the Deutsches Krebsforschungszentrum for contributions to the field of experimental cancer research. It is awarded alternately to PhD students from research facilities in Heidelberg and to scientists from all over Germany. The prize is financed from the estate of the late husband and wife Walther and Christine Richtzenhain.

The winner of the 1994 prize was Dr. rer. nat. Robert Arch from the Division of Tumor Progression and Immune Defense headed by Prof. Dr. Margot Zöller. The biologist was awarded the prize for his PhD thesis on the topic „Physiological Functions of CD44 Isoforms in the Activation of Lymphocytes as a Key to Metastasis". Robert Arch is examining the question of which characteristics enable a cancer cell to form metastases. To date, this question is still largely unsolved, as is the sequence of events leading to the growth of metastasizing cells in the distant organ. In cooperation with a working group headed by Prof. Dr. Peter Herrlich from the Institute of Genetics at the Karlsruhe Research Center (Forschungszentrum Karlsruhe), the scientists working under Prof. Dr. Margot Zöller detected a molecule called CD44v in metastases of a pancreatic cancer in rats. Under certain circumstances this molecule can also be found on intact white blood cells (lymphocytes). Metastasizing tumor cells seem to be using a program sim-

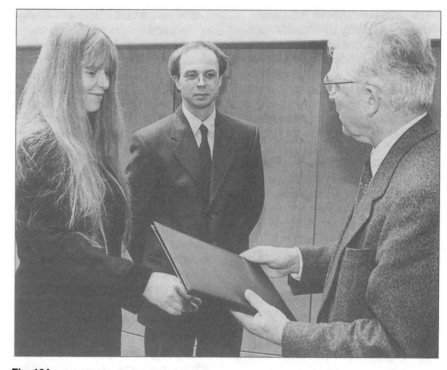

Fig. 104
Dr. Kirsten Falk and Dr. Olaf Rötzschke receive the 1995 Richtzenhain Prize from Prof. Dr. Harald zur Hausen, Scientific Member of the Management Board of the Deutsches Krebsforschungzentrum

ilar to that of the lymphocytes. It is conceivable that they thereby acquire the lymphocytes' ability to travel through tissue and the bloodstream and settle and start multiplying in other organs. The CD44v molecule was not found in the cells of non-metastasizing tumors. CD44v was also found to be expressed in several human tumors including intestinal and gastric cancers. In his PhD thesis, Arch was able to show that CD44v plays an important role in the multiplication both of lymphocytes during immune response and of metastasizing tumor cells. In this process, both cell

types rely on cell-cell interactions with other cell types present in lymph nodes. CD44v not only reinforces the contact between different cells, but also functions as an important link between the surface and the interior of the cell. Studies performed by Robert Arch to block CD44v with an antibody represent a first step towards understanding the molecular basis of the function of this molecule in the complex process of metastasis. Thus, he has provided insights that may serve as a basis for developing new strategies to treat metastasizing tumors and to prevent metastasis.

The 1995 Richtzenhain Prize was shared equally by Dr. Kirsten Falk and Dr. Olaf Rötzschke. The prize, which this time was endowed with DM 20,000, was intended for young scientists who are developing molecular approaches to cancer treatment. In the interior of most cells of the body one finds so-called MHC (major histocompatibility complex) molecules which collect fragments of all proteins and transfer them to the cell surface where they are presented to the immune system as a kind of molecular identity card. Now, if these fragments called peptides stem from proteins that do not belong in the cell (e.g. from a virus or a cancer-specific protein), the cell is recognized as foreign and killed by the immune system. Thus, a potential source of danger is eliminated.

Kirsten Falk and Olaf Rötzschke received the prize for their research work within the group of Prof. Hans-Georg Rammensee, initially at the Max Planck Institute of Biology in Tübingen and from June 1st, 1993 to March 31st, 1996 as head of the Division of Tumor-virus Immunology at the Deutsches Krebsforschungszentrum. The scientists succeeded in isolating these peptides from cells and examining them. They were able to show that the structure of the MHC molecules, which is different in every individual, determines the way in which the fragments are cut for presentation. In addition, they were able to prove that individual families of MHC molecules can only bind peptides with a very characteristic structure. This enabled the two scientists, working together with Prof. Günther Jung from the Institute of Organic Chemistry of the University of Tübingen, to assign specific peptide motifs to every MHC family.

Thanks to these results, vaccine development and tumor immunology took a big step forward: The protein building blocks of pathogens can now specifically be searched for such motifs. Only a vaccine containing motifs that fit for the different MHC families ensures that the immune cells of many patients are sufficiently mobilized against cancer or viruses.

Since 1990, the Deutsches Krebsforschungszentrum has awarded the Ernst von Leyden Prize every two years as an encouragement and a reward for outstanding activities in the field of early cancer detection. The prize, which is donated by the company SKD, is endowed with DM 20,000. Its presentation is supervised by the Press and Public Relations Department of the Deutsches Krebsforschungszentrum.

The physician Ernst von Leyden (1832-1919), after whom the prize is named, was for many years chairman of the German Central Committee for Cancer Research and director of the 1st Clinic for Internal Medicine of the Charité in Berlin. He is regarded as a pioneer of cancer research in Germany.

In 1994, the Ernst von Leyden Prize, which was originally donated by the company Procter & Gamble (formerly Röhm Pharma GmbH, Darmstadt), was awarded for the third time for outstanding contributions to the field of early cancer detection by the German Federal Minister of Health in Bonn. The DM 20,000 prize was shared equally by Dr. med. h.c. Hans Mohl, medical journalist and publicist, and Helga Ebel, head of the cancer advisory and contact center for self-help groups in cancer aftercare of the „Paritätischer Wohlfahrtsverband" (non-denominational welfare organization), regional association of the federal state of North Rhine-Westphalia, and active member of the support group for the Aachen Tumor Center.

Hans Mohl, who headed the section „Health and Nature" of the German TV channel ZDF for 30 years, is regarded as the founder of medical journalism on German television. His program „Gesundheitsmagazin Praxis" was the first scientific TV program in the world and is still the most successful medical broadcast in Germany. Through his work, he has set high standards for medical journalism in Germany and has contributed to educating the public and disseminating critical information about numerous areas of medicine. Within the program „Europe Against Cancer" he played an important role in providing people, through the media, with specific information on the opportunities available in the field of early cancer recognition.

To the present day, early detection as a key instrument in combating cancer has continued to be a focal topic for Hans Mohl and the ZDF. Over the course of many years, millions of television viewers have thus been continuously informed about their own choices and possibilities in relation to cancer.

Helga Ebel was honored for her involvement in the organization and coordination of a citizens' action group sponsored by the support association of the Aachen Tumor Center (Förderkreis des Tumorzentrums Aachen e.V.). The aim of the action group was, on the one hand, to encourage citizens to make use of available early cancer detection measures and, on the other hand, to motivate doctors to offer their patients such examinations. Since the start of the campaign in the summer of 1992, participation in the screening programs in the three quarters evaluated so far has increased by 34.8 percent for men (from 4.19 to 5.65 percent) and by 28.35 percent for women (from 49.05 to 62.96 percent).

In 1996, Prof. Dr. med. Günter Flatten was awarded the Ernst von Leyden Prize for his contribution to a successful implementation of the government screening program aimed at early cancer detection. Dr. Flatten has been Medical Director of the Federal Association of Panel Doctors in Cologne since 1977 and has simultaneously headed the Central Institute for the Provision of Benefits to Panel Doctors in Germany since 1985. In 1994, he was named honorary professor of the University of Cologne.

Günter Flatten was awarded the Ernst von Leyden Prize in appreciation of his exemplary engagement in promoting the acceptance of the government's early cancer diagnosis program in East and West Germany and for his contributions to developing concepts for model projects to ensure the quality of individual early recognition measures.

In 1996, the Dr. Emil Salzer Prize was awarded for the tenth time. This prize is presented by the Deutsches Krebsforschungszentrum on behalf of the Ministry for Science, Research, and Arts of the state of Baden-Württemberg. Its donor, Emil Salzer, was a doctor, scientist, and committed citizen who lived in the Southern German town of Reutlingen. Alongside his work as a practising doctor he was engaged in research on various diseases including tuberculosis and cancer. He died in 1963 aged 81. He entrusted the state of Baden Württemberg with his estate, making it a condition that the revenues be used to support „chemical, physical, and bio-

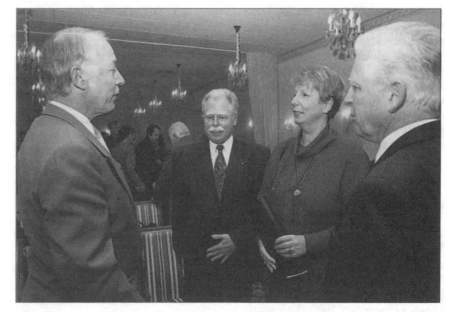

Fig. 105
Prof. Dr. Günter Flatten was awarded the Ernst von Leyden Prize for his contribution to a successful implementation of the government screening program aimed at early cancer detection (from left to right: Dr. Andreas Johnsen, SKD Pharma, the company donating the prize, Prof. Günter Flatten, State Secretary Dr. Sabine Bergmann-Pohl, Federal Ministry of Health, Prof. Harald zur Hausen

logical cancer research". The 1996 Dr. Emil Salzer Prize of the state of Baden-Württemberg was awarded to Priv.-Doz. Dr. med. vet. Wolfgang Hammerschmidt, Institute for Clinical Molecular Biology and Tumor Genetics of the GSF Research Center in Munich, for the experimental elucidation of the molecular mechanism by which the Epstein-Barr virus causes changes in immune cells. The award comprises a cash sum of DM 20,000 and the presentation of a ring which is passed on from one prize winner to the next. Wolfgang Hammerschmidt was awarded the prize for his fundamental research on the Epstein-Barr virus. This virus is

associated with Burkitt's lymphoma, a cancer which occurs mainly in children and young adults in tropical Africa and Asia and usually affects the face or neck. Hammerschmidt was able to show how this virus affects the immune system and how a tumor can develop as a result.

In cooperation with Boehringer Mannheim GmbH, the Deutsches Krebsforschungszentrum offered the Curt Engelhorn Research Grant in 1996. The grant is donated by Boehringer Mannheim with the aim of supporting young scientists in biotechnological research. It is awarded to two to four scientists to

finance research visits to leading onco-
logically oriented international working
groups (for a two-year period each).
The grant is intended for young researchers holding a PhD degree who
are working in the field of molecular oncology. A main objective of this scheme
will be to promote the area of molecular
genetics with a special focus on new
approaches in diagnostics and therapy.

Publications

The scientists from the Deutsches
Krebsforschungszentrum regularly publish their research results in scientific
journals, university publications, and
books. At the end of 1996, the annual
list of publications "Veröffentlichungen"
recorded a total of 13140 publications
by scientists from the Deutsches Krebsforschungszentrum. In the years from
the foundation of the Center until the
end of 1996, these lists recorded 8418
contributions in scientific journals, 1310
diploma theses, doctoral and "Habilitation" theses, as well as 3412 other publications. Out of these, there were 429
books and contributions in handbooks
that appeared during the years 1994 –
1996.

These publications have been supplemented by thousands of lectures held
at scientific conferences and for members of the general public.

The Center's list of publications is compiled annually and can be obtained free
of charge.

The communication of research results
and their relevance for cancer prevention, early diagnosis, and improved
therapies for cancer sufferers to the

general public lies in the hands of the
Press and Public Relations Department, which maintains permanent contacts to the media and the public (see
the acontirbution "Press and Public Relations").

Detailed information on the scientific
activities of the Deutsches Krebsforschungszentrum are contained in the
biannual „Research Report" (German
version: "Wissenschaftlicher Ergebnis-
bericht"). This report presents an overview of the projects carried out at the
Center, their objectives, and results.
The current issue 1994/1995 appeared
in 1996.

12

International and National Collaboration

The integration of the research work of the Deutsches Krebsforschungszentrum into international research concepts is documented by the high percentage (about 50%) of publications that are written jointly with scientists from other German and foreign research institutes. The Center's research program comprises 800 cooperation projects with researchers in Germany and abroad. On the international level, there are working contacts with about 300 universities and other research institutes. The cooperation with the University of Heidelberg is centered around the joint clinical-experimental projects within the Tumor Center Heidelberg/Mannheim and the projects within the framework of the German Genome Project and the Bio-Regio Association. In the field of fundamental research, the collaboration within the special research programs (Sonderforschungsbereiche) of the German Research Association (DFG) deserves special mention. These include, in particular, the special research program Nr. 229 "Molecular mechanisms of gene expression and differentiation".

A testament of the excellent international standing of the Center is the frequency of citations from publications of the Deutsches Krebsforschungszentrum in international specialist journals, as are reports on the Center in the US, French, and Italian specialist press (see article on page xxx).

The long-standing cooperations with scientists in the United States, Japan, Israel, France, and many other countries have been intensified. This fact is also reflected in the high number of visiting researchers who stay for a considerable time at the Center.

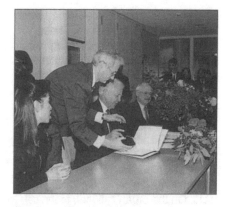

Fig. 106
Signing of a cooperation agreement between the Deutsches Krebsforschungszentrum and the Chulabhorn Research Institute, Thailand, concerning research on cancer risk factors and cancer prevention. From the left: Princess Prof. Chulabhorn Mahidol, Chulabhorn Research Institute, Dr. Norbert Frank, Prof. Harald zur Hausen, Prof. Helmut Bartsch, Deutsches Krebsforschungszentrum

Collaboration on the basis of bilateral agreements with other countries has also been continued intensively. Cooperation with the USA is based on a "Memorandum of Understanding" with the National Cancer Institute (NCI) in Bethesda. An agreement concluded with the National Council of Research and Development (NCRD) in Israel has provided the basis for more than twenty years of highly successful cooperation with researchers from various Israeli research institutes. The Israeli cooperation partners are the Ben Gurion University, the Tel Aviv University, the Hebrew University of Jerusalem, the Weizmann Institute of Science, the Technicon in Haifa, and the Hadassah University Medical Hospital in Jerusalem. Close contacts have also evolved on the administrative level, in particular with the Weizmann Institute. These have led to the dispatch of delegations from both countries and to an intensive exchange of knowledge concerning administrative solutions – a process which is being carried on continuously.

The research program agreed upon with the Tanzania Tumour Centre in Daressalam, now renamed Ocean Road Hospital, comprises molecular-biological, epidemiological, and clinical projects. On the organizational, technical, and humanitarian levels, this cooperation is substantiated and supported by the Tanzania Tumor Aid Association ("Tansania Tumorhilfe") whose members are scientists from the Deutsches Krebsforschungszentrum and other citizens from Heidelberg and the Heidelberg area. The association provides help for the tumor center in Tanzania through regular donations of scientific apparatuses, by providing technical equipment, by training staff at the Deutsches Krebsforschungszentrum, and by collecting goods or money.

The research work continues to be characterized by the personal contact between scientists from different nations. Offical agreements provide particular support in cases where special funds are being used.

International Scientific Exchange

The lifeblood of science is the exchange of ideas, a process which is substantially promoted by research visits of scientists from other institutes. This is true, in particular, for a field such as cancer research, since its problems touch upon almost all areas of medicine as well as numerous disciplines from the natural sciences.

The research visits, which are limited to a certain period of time, enable the guest scientists, on the one hand, to gain insights into particular lines of research and to learn techniques for

Fig. 107
Talk with a foreign guest scientist

which scientists at the Deutsches Krebsforschungszentrum are famous; on the other hand, they help the Krebsforschungszentrum to benefit from the specialist knowledge and experience of the visitors, thus, supplementing the range of scientific activities at the Center in a useful way.

An important aim of international collaboration in the field of cancer research is the development and implementation of joint projects and programs. The figures of the past few years serve as an impressive documentation of the intensity of international and national collaboration at the Deutsches Krebsforschungszentrum: In the years 1994 – 1996, a total of 527 visiting scientists from 52

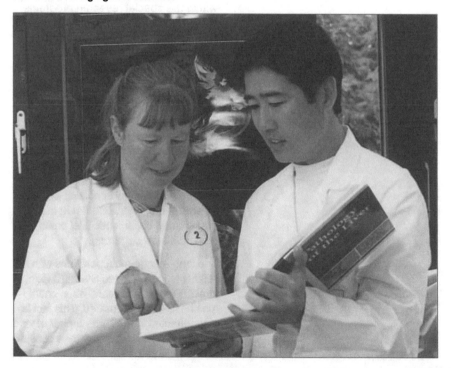

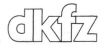

nations worked at the Center. The guest scientists were supported by internal grants and fellowships as well as by external institutions such as the: European Union, German Academic Exchange Service (DAAD), Alexander von Humboldt Foundation, World Health Organization, German Research Association (DFG), Study Foundation of the German Nation, European Molecular Biology Organization (EMBO), NATO, Union International Contre le Cancer, Federal Ministry of Education, Science, Research, and Technology, International Atomic Energy Agency, Boehringer-Ingelheim Fund, Hanns Seidel Foundation, Dr. Mildred Scheel Foundation, Volkswagen Foundation, European Science Foundation, Roland Ernst Foundation, Theo Nasemann Foundation, Associa-

tion for the Promotion of Science and Humanities in Germany, and other foundations, international programs, as well as governments and universities.

In addition, there are numerous national and international collaborations.

To house its guests, the Center has at its disposal 46 fully equipped apartments (with one to three rooms) in three guest houses in Heidelberg. Due to the high level of international contact, the guest houses are fully booked all the time and can thus be maintained on a cost-covering basis.

Cooperation Program with Israel – 20 Years of Successful Research Work

The 7th Workshop („Status seminar") of the cooperation program with Israel took place on March 17th and 18th, 1997 at the Deutsches Krebsforschungszentrum. This program has been pursued since 1976 in close collaboration with scientific institutions in Israel. At the workshop, the scientists in charge of the 14 ongoing cooperation projects reported and discussed their research results, together with technical and other issues arising in the current work of the laboratories involved and in the cooperation as such. These workshops take place every three years and are appreciated by the participating scientists as an important instrument for collaboration and exchange of knowledge and experience.

The Cooperation Program, Its Projects and Their Financing

The program is based on an agreement concluded in 1976 between the Deutsches Krebsforschungszentrum and the Israeli Ministry of Science (MOS) as the two partner organizations. Over the past 20 years, this agreement has been translated into an extremely lively scientific reality. Each project usually consists of one Israeli and one German subproject where the scientists actively collaborate in their research work on a common topic over a three-year term. In rare cases, where it is necessary, an expert partner from outside the Center (e.g. from the University of Heidelberg or some other German university) may also be involved. The program is fi-

Fig. 108
The stays of guest scientists at the Deutsches Krebsforschungszentrum

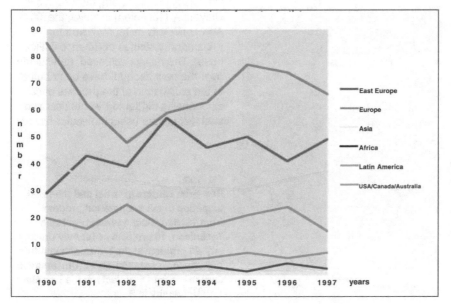

12

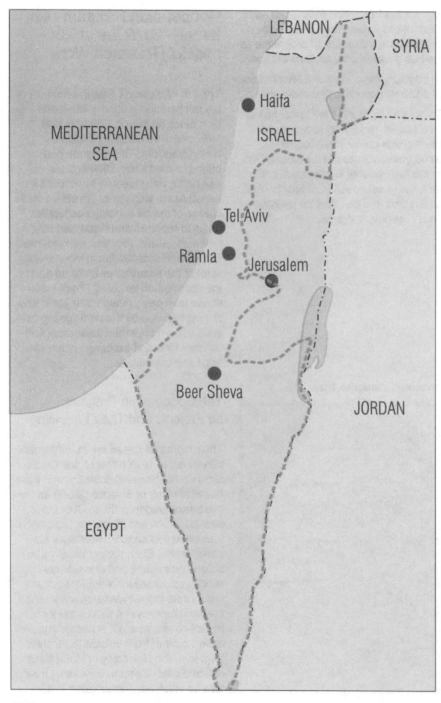

nanced from the budget of the Deutsches Krebsforschungszentrum, which, over the 20 years from 1976 to 1996, has invested a total of 21.6 million DM in the exchange of scientific knowledge with Israel in selected areas of cancer research. Of this sum, 8.6 million DM went into the German subprojects and 13 million DM into the Israeli subprojects. The lifeblood of the cooperation program is the personal contacts between the participating Israeli and German scientists.

The Jubilee Symposium

As a part of the 7th Workshop, the Deutsches Krebsforschungszentrum also critically assessed the scientific collaboration with Israel over the past twenty years. So far, 61 cooperation projects have been successfully carried out. From the Israeli side these involved scientists from the Ben Gurion University in Beer Sheva, the Hebrew University in Jerusalem, the Technical University (Technion) in Haifa, the Tel Aviv University in Tel Aviv, and the Weizmann Institutes of Science in Rehovot. The results achieved, particularly over the past decade, have contributed to the elucidation of the process of carcinogenesis triggered by chemical and viral risk factors using molecular-biolog-

Fig. 109
Research centers in Israel and their participation in the cooperation program from 1976 to 1996: 4 projects at Haifa Technicon, 10 projects at Tel Aviv University, 23 projects at the Weizmann Institute in Rehovot, 18 at the Hebrew University in Jerusalem, and 6 projects at the Ben Gurion University in Beer Sheva

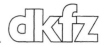

ical methods. This included, for example, an experimental verification of the basic „somatic gene mutation hypothesis of cancer development" postulated almost 70 years ago by the Heidelberg surgeon and initiator of the Deutsches Krebsforschungszentrum Professor Karl Heinrich Bauer. In fact, numerous other laboratories around the world have also demonstrated that the principles of this theory are correct. In addition, the hypothesis was substantially consolidated, further developed, and specified in numerous details within the cooperation program. The fundamentally new findings and molecular-biological techniques involved have already inspired many new approaches to the treatment of cancer patients, which the Krebsforschungszentrum also actively seeks to put into practice.

The Highlight Projects

Within the framework of the Jubilee Symposium, the Management Board of the Deutsches Krebsforschungszentrum especially honored as projects of excellence seven of the 61 finished projects of the cooperation program for the outstanding results achieved. They had been identified and selected on the basis of uniform criteria by the Scientific Program Committee which consists of four Israeli and four German external scientists. These „highlight projects" fall into five of the eight Research Programs of the Deutsches Krebsforschungszentrum. The scientists involved were awarded a certificate of the Deutsches Krebsforschungszentrum.

The Management Board drew special attention to the work of the Scientific Program Committee over the 20 years of the existence of the cooperation program. As a representative of all other members of the Program Committee, the Israeli member Prof. Dr. Michael Schlesinger from the Hadassah Medical School of the Hebrew University in Jerusalem was honored by the Deutsches Krebsforschungszentrum: As an expression of its gratitude, the Management Board invited Prof. Schlesinger to a Meyenburg lecture at the Center. The funds for this event are made available to the Center by the Wilhelm and Maria Meyenburg Foundation, Heidelberg.

Evaluation of the Program

The Federal German Ministry for Education, Science, Research, and Technology together with the Israeli Ministry of Science used the 20th anniversary of the cooperation program as an opportunity to subject the program to a thorough scientific assessment. The international evaluation committee appointed jointly by the two ministries consisted of Prof. Paul Kleihues (chairman), WHO Lyon, Prof. Bernhard Fleckenstein, Virology, Erlangen, and Prof. Leo Sachs, Cell Biology, Rehovot (Israel). Applying common directives of both ministries, the committee assessed and evaluated the activities of the program in the 20 years of its existence and the results of the projects. To this end, the committee visited the participating research institutions in Israel on July 23, 1996 and the Krebsforschungszentrum on November 11, 1996 in order to thoroughly examine a selection of the 61 cooperation projects carried out so far. The results of this international assessment have been positive in all respects.

New Projects

Within the framework of the 7th Workshop, the Scientific Program Committee selected the eight best projects out of a total number of 25 proposals submitted jointly by Israeli and German scientists. The selection process was based on uniform criteria. The projects will start in 1998.

The success of this cooperation program over the past two decades has demonstrated that the mutual stimulation of ideas through national talents, the exchange of new technology and newly developed scientific methods as well as working together in the same place can extend the capabilities of the individual scientist who benefits from the partnership.

Prof. Dr. Erich Hecker

Coordinator of the German-Israeli Cooperation Program and deputy chairman of the Program Committee

Tumor Center Heidelberg/Mannheim

Modern cancer research and the fight against cancer can usually only be pursued effectively within multi- and interdisciplinary approaches. In order to achieve the best possible scientific and clinical performance, the medical and scientific facilities in the area Heidelberg/Mannheim joined forces in 1979 in the form of an interdisciplinary cooperative association, the Tumor Center Heidelberg/Mannheim. The partners that form this association are: the University Hospitals in Heidelberg, the Deutsches Krebsforschungszentrum, the Mannheim City Hospital, and the Thorax Clinic Heidelberg-Rohrbach of the State Insurance Institution, Baden.

Both cancer therapy and cancer research have a long tradition in Heidelberg. As early as the turn of this century, the surgeon Vincenz Czerny introduced intraoperative radiotherapy, and in 1906 Heidelberg was the location of the first international cancer congress, which was also organized by Czerny. He also founded the interdisciplinary cancer research institute, inspired by the similar institutes already existing in Moscow (Morosow Institute) and in Buffalo/USA (Roswell Park Memorial Institute). Finally, K.H. Bauer, director of the Heidelberg University Surgical Hospital from 1941 to 1964, took the initiative in creating the Deutsches Krebsforschungszentrum, a public foundation of the State of Baden Württemberg, and later a National and State Research Center.

The cooperatve association Tumor Center Heidelberg/Mannheim grew out of the Oncological Working Groups founded in 1966 in Heidelberg and in 1973 in Mannheim. The two Oncological Working Groups play an important role in the field of caring for patients with malignant diseases. They form a common forum for the interdisciplinary discussion and cooperation in clinical oncology. They have produced "Empfehlungen für eine standardisierte Diagnostik, Therapie und Nachsorge" (Recommendations for a Standardized Diagnostic, Therapy, and Aftercare) – which are also well-known as the "Grüne Reihe" (green series) of the Tumor Center Heidelberg/Mannheim. Within the Oncological Working Groups Heidelberg and Mannheim, these recommendations are regarded as obligatory. Whether they are observed in individual cases, however, is the responsibility of the doctor concerned. These brochures are made available to all the cooperating doctors and others that are interested, as diagnostic and therapeutic recommendations; they are addressed both to private practitioners and hospital doctors.

One copy of each brochure can be obtained free of charge from the coordination and administrative office of the Tumor Center Heidelberg/Mannheim, Im Neuenheimer Feld 105/110, D-69120 Heidelberg, Germany; Telephone: (++6221) 566557, -8, -9 or 472645; Fax: (++6221) 565094. For additional copies a small fee is charged. When a new brochure appears, the coordination and administrative office automatically sends copies to a wide circle of recipients of the series, located in all parts of Germany and also abroad. The Tumor Center strives to add titles to this series whenever these are required to keep it up to date and revise them when new results make this necessary. The following publications have already appeared in this series, partly in new revised editions:

1. „Das Bronchialkarzinom" (Lung Cancer), 1st edition 1979 – now replaced by No. 8

2. „Gastrointestinale Tumoren" (Gastrointestinal Tumors), 1st edition Jan. 1981 – replaced by Nos. 9, 12, 15, and 17

3. „Malignes Melanom" (Malignant Melanoma), 4th completely revised edition September 1991

4. „Weichteilsarkome im Erwachsenenalter" (Adult Soft Tissue Sarcoma), 4th edition May 1992

5. „Morbus Hodgkin", 3rd revised edition Dec. 1993

6. „Das Mammakarzinom" (Breast Cancer), 4th completely revised edition Jan. 1993

7. „Non-Hodgkin Lymphome" (Non-Hodgkin Lymphoma), 2nd edition July 1985

8. „Die bösartigen Tumoren von Lunge, Pleura und Thymus" (Malignant Tumors of the Lung, Pleura, and Thymus), 2nd revised edition Sept. 1991 – new edition of brochure No. 1

9. „Das Pankreaskarzinom" (Pancreatic Cancer), 2nd edition March 1996

10. „Nierenzellkarzinom" (Renal Cell Cancer), 2nd revised edition June 1991

11. „Das Schilddrüsenkarzinom" (Thyroid Cancer), 2nd completely revised edition May 1993

12. „Das kolorektale Karzinom" (Colorectal Cancer), 1st edition Jan. 1987

13. „Das Sozialrecht in der medizinischen und sozialen Rehabilitation von Krebskranken" (Social Legislation in

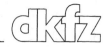

the Medical and Social Rehabilitation of Cancer Patients), 4th revised edition Sept. 1994

14. „Diagnostik und Therapie des Tumorschmerzes" (Diagnosis and Therapy of Tumor-Induced Pain), 2nd revised edition Jan. 1993

15. „Das Magenkarzinom" (Gastric Cancer), 1st edition Jan. 1990

16. „The bösartigen Tumoren der ableitenden Harnwege" (Malignant Tumors of the Urinary Tract Collection System), 1st edition Dec. 1990

17. „Das Oesophaguskarzinom" (Esophageal Cancer), 1st edition Jan. 1991

18. „Die bösartigen Tumoren der männlichen Geschlechtsorgane" (Malignant Tumors of the Male Genitals), 1st edition June 1991

19. „Hausärztliche Mit- und Nachsorge von Tumorpatienten" (Care and Aftercare of Tumor Patients by the Family Doctor), 1st edition Jan. 1992

20. „Die bösartigen Tumoren der Kopfspeicheldrüsen" (Malignant Tumors of the Salivary Glands), 1st edition July 1992

21. „Das Prostatakarzinom" (Prostate Cancer), 1st edition Nov. 1992

22. „Der geriatrische Tumorpatient" (The Geriatric Cancer Patient), 1st edition March 1993

23. „Hypophysentumoren" (Pituitary Tumors), 1st edition June 1995

24. „Früherkennung" (Early Diagnosis), 1st edition Oct. 1995

25. „Die bösartigen Tumoren des Kehlkopfes und des Rachens" (Malignant Tumors of the Larynx and the Pharynx), 1st edition June 1995

26. „Das Ovarialkarzinom" (Ovarian Cancer), 1st edition Sept. 1995.

In the period of this report, a new edition of the brochure on pancreatic cancer appeared, and also new brochures about pituitary tumors, early diagnosis, the malignant tumors of the larynx and pharynx, and ovarian cancer. At present new editions of the brochures on melanoma, colon cancer, and gastric cancer are in preparation. New brochures are being prepared on the subjects of bone tumors, chronic myeloproliferative diseases, and rectal cancer.

The Oncological Working Groups meet regularly. The Oncological Working Group Heidelberg convenes every Wednesday at 4 p.m. in the large lecture theater of the Heidelberg University Surgical Hospital. Following lectures about about topical oncological matters, questions from external colleagues about problematic cases or important oncological cases in the Heidelberg hospitals are addressed. The questions are answered in writing in the form of a recommendation for further diagnostic and therapeutic procedures. The Oncological Working Group Mannheim holds its interdisciplinary case discussions every Tuesday at 4.15 p.m. in the conference room of the Oncological Center in Mannheim and also meets every second Monday for sessions which begin with a lecture.

In addition to its main aim of ensuring a first-rate care of tumor patients at the hospitals in the region, the Tumor Center association also attempts to accelerate the transfer of research results into clinical practice. An instrument for this purpose are interdisciplinary clinical/fundamental-science research projects. In addition the association cooperates with other tumor centers and

specialized oncological institutions in Baden Württemberg. A basis for this was provided by the Cancer Association of Baden Württemberg, which, with its annual conferences (Association of Tumor Centers and Specialist Oncological Institutions, Baden Württemberg – ATO), offered an additional opportunity for the exchange of experience and information.

The running of the Tumor Center Heidelberg/Mannheim is in the hands of the Steering Committee. This comprises 14 members who represent the four contractual partners, along with practicing doctors, and the chairpersons of the Oncological Working Groups Heidelberg and Mannheim. The chairpersons of the Oncological Working Groups and the coordinators of the main research activities of the Tumor Center have advisory roles. The Steering Committee decides upon the main areas of activity of the Tumor Center. The main emphases of the work of the Tumor Center are the following:

1. Clinical Oncology

1.1 Coordination and regulation of the care of cancer patients (in part via the Oncological Working Groups)

1.2 Planning and coordination of continuing and further education

1.3 Coordination of the clinical cancer register of the associated hospitals

2. Planning and organization of collaborative research projects.

The meetings of the Steering Committee are led by the chairperson (until August 1996 Prof. Dr. Christian Herfarth; since Sept. 1996 Prof. Dr. Dr. Michael Wannenmacher), who is also in charge of the coordination and administrative office of the Tumor Center Heidelberg/Mannheim.

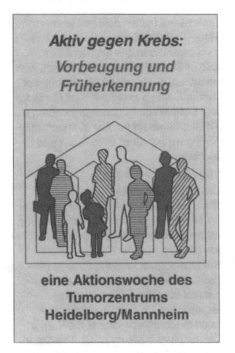

Aktiv gegen Krebs:

Vorbeugung und Früherkennung

eine Aktionswoche des Tumorzentrums Heidelberg/Mannheim

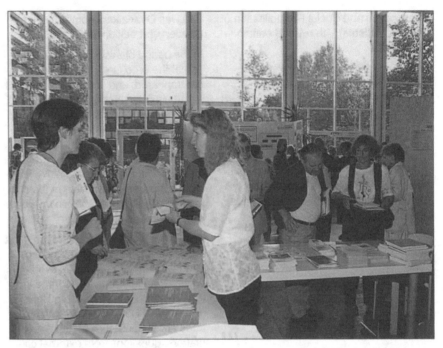

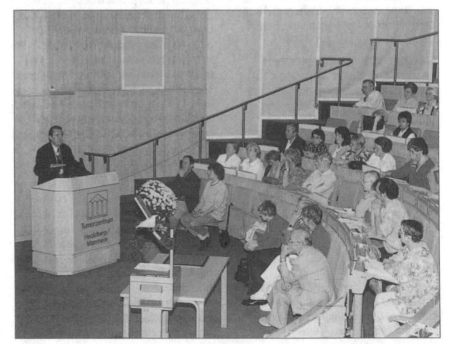

Figs. 110, 111, 112
An initiative for the general public
„Prevention and Early Diagnosis" was
organized by the Tumor Center

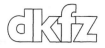

Optimal Care of Tumor Patients

Special oncological units at the hospitals of the Tumor Center form certain crystallization points for particular diagnostic and therapeutic problems. These units are also responsible for a part of the clinical/fundamental-science research coodination. They include:

- the section for Surgical Oncology at the Heidelberg University Surgical Hospital
- the department of Internal Medicine V of the Medical Hospital and Outpatient Clinic of the University of Heidelberg
- the Oncology-Hematology section of the University Pediatric Hospital Heidelberg
- the Orthopedic-Oncology section of the Foundation Orthopedic Hospital of the University of Heidelberg
- the section for Special Oncology of the III Medical Clinic, Oncological Center at the Mannheim University Hospitals, and
- the department of Internal Medicine and Oncology of the Thorax Clinic Heidelberg-Rohrbach of the State Insurance Institution, Baden.

The University Radiological Hospitals in Heidelberg and Mannheim treat almost exclusively tumor patients. Other clinical institutions in Heidelberg and Mannheim which are also concerned with the treatment of cancer patients cooperate via the Oncological Working Groups and through interdisciplinary discussions.

In addition to the Oncological Working Groups in Heidelberg and Mannheim, there are other special facilities for an optimal care of tumor patients. These include the psycho-social aftercare facility and its further education seminars at the Heidelberg University Surgical Hospital – founded in 1979 by the „Deutsche Krebshilfe e.V." (German Cancer Aid Society) and financed, since 1984, by the State of Baden Württemberg. This facility is dedicated to the psycho-social care of cancer patients, in particular those at the University Surgical Hospital, the University Gynecological Hospital, and the Outpatient Clinic in Heidelberg. It is also concerned with the continuing and further education of doctors, nurses, psycho-social health experts, and laypeople, and patient-centered research. Via these facilities, the tumor patients are offered, alongside their medical care, psycho-social support through advice, crisis intervention, and psychotherapy. Furthermore, continuing education is provided for all clinical personnel interested in psycho-social questions. Outpatients, too, can take advantage of the help offered by the psycho-social aftercare facility.

Since the middle of the 1980s continuing and further education for nursing personnel has been offered in Heidelberg. With the support of the Social Welfare Ministry of Baden Württemberg and the Federal Health Ministry, vocational training courses in oncology have been developed for the practicing nursing staff. The professional course on the care of tumor patients and chronically ill patients received government recognition in 1991. The course runs over a period of two years as an accompaniment to normal duties and addresses nursing staff and pediatric nurses with at least two years' professional experience. In May 1992 the first two-year further education course began with 11 participants. The second course was completed in April 1995 with a successful examination.

In Fall 1993, the Hospital Committee of the State of Baden Württemberg approved the concept of „bridging nurses" with the provision of 50 positions for Baden Württemberg. The name „bridging nurses", from which the expression „bridging care team" has also been coined, reveals the main idea of the concept: it is intended that the bridging nurses should create a bridge between the hospital and the home environment.

For the region of the Tumor Center Heidelberg/Mannheim, four positions were approved, three for the Heidelberg area and one for Mannheim. In the meantime the Mannheim hospital has added two further part-time staff to the team. The aim of the bridging care is to avoid the necessity of long hospital stays for tumor patients. The patient, his relatives, the nursing services, and the entire domestic environment should thereby be supported in such a way that it is possible to care for the sick person in his own home to a medical standard equaling that in the hospital. Normal nursing duties, however, are not part of the job of the bridging care team (with the exception of emergencies occurring while they are on call) since the emphasis lies in the organization and coordination of domestic care. This means that the bridging care team ensures that the patient is properly cared for in his home and, where desired, gives appropriate instructions and advice. In the subsequent home visits, the main tasks are to give advice on nursing matters, to assist in questions concerning the further financing of the care, and to ensure that psycho-social support is available to the patients and their relatives.

Cooperative Research Projects of the Tumor Center

The research projects that win support are selected from a large number of applications by an external board of referees. This board comprises experts from the relevant disciplines, who assign financial support and also allocate the equipment and personnel that are foreseen within the research budget. Regular interim reviews decide whether the individual projects should receive further support, so that the efficiency of the research in the Tumor Center Heidelberg/Mannheim is maintained at a high level.

The cooperative research projects of the Tumor Center Heidelberg/Mannheim also exercise an internal self-monitoring; this is guaranteed by the creation of a board of coordinators who sit on the Steering Committee. This board reports regularly on the individual projects and on research symposia in which the results of the projects are presented to the public. Regular research colloquia held by the project leaders began in 1997 and these now supplement the exchange of information achieved in the research symposia.

The research projects of the Tumor Center Heidelberg/Mannheim are marked by the combination of clinical and fundamental research. The projects are led, in general, by one project leader from the field of clinical research and one from fundamental scientific research. The research projects, thus, form axes of research between the hospitals and the Deutsches Krebsforschungszentrum.

In the early years of the Tumor Center individual oncological research projects were supported, but these had no sig-

nificant relationship to one another. In 1983/84 the concept of central projects for particular tumor types was introduced. Examples of central projects were „malignant lymphoma and leukemias", „colorectal carcinoma", „breast cancer", and „lung cancer". Although the work done in these central projects was very fruitful and the development showed that this planning was the right one, research lives from the further evolution of the concepts and from posing new questions. At the beginning of the 1990s, extensive discussions were held at the Tumor Center about placing the emphasis on the various research methods. This idea was also strongly supported by the external referees. Thus, for the years from 1992 the following main research areas were developed, each with one clinical and one fundamental-science coordinator (status 11.02.97):

Research Area I: Immunological and molecular-biological approaches in tumor diagnostics

Coordinators: Priv.-Doz. Dr. Hartmut Döhner, Dr. Gerhard Moldenhauer

Research Area II: Biological response modifiers and molecular therapies

Coordinators: Prof. Dr. Stefan Meuer, Prof. Dr. Peter H. Krammer

Research Area III: Loco-regional tumor therapy – research on radiotherapy including diagnostics

Coordinators: Dr. Dr. Jürgen Debus, Prof. Dr. Gerhard van Kaick

Research Area IV: Tumor cell heterogeneity, metastasis, and resistance

Coordinators: Priv.-Doz. Dr. Thomas Lehnert, Prof. Dr. Werner W. Franke.

The four main research areas each comprise several projects. At present,

the following projects are being supported:

Research Area I:

Group I: Molecular biology and cytogenetics

Project 1: Characterization of unbalanced chromosomal regions in malignant lymphomas and myeloid leukemias, identification of pathogenically relevant genes

Project leaders: Priv.-Doz. Dr. Hartmut Döhner, Priv.-Doz. Dr. Peter Lichter

Project 2: Investigation of chromosome modifications in soft tissue sarcomas by means of modern molecular-cytogenetic methods

Project leader: Dr. Gunhild Mechtersheimer

Project 3: Molecular genetics and expression of tumor-suppressor genes in premenopausal breast cancer: Analysis of the clinical diagnostic significance

Project leaders: Dr. Ute Hamann, Dr. Peter Sinn

Project 4: Immunohistological, electron-microscope, and molecular-biological investigation of apoptosis, apoptosis-relevant genes, and EBV status

Project leaders: Dr. Caroline Verbeke, Priv.-Doz. Dr. Hanswalter Zentgraf

Group 2: Residual disease and micrometastasis

Project 1: Molecular mechanisms and diagnostic detection of the invasion and dissemination of solid tumors

Project leaders: Prof. Dr. Margot Zöller, Prof. Dr. Magnus von Knebel Doeberitz

Project 2: Tumor cell detection in bone marrow, peripheral blood, and blood stem cell transplants in patients with breast cancer

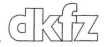

Project leaders: Priv.-Doz. Dr. Rainer Haas, Prof. Dr. Werner W. Franke

Group 3: Tumor-associated antigens and tumor targeting

Project 1: Phage-display antibody libraries: A new strategy for the identification of tumor associated antigens of the colorectal carcinoma

Project leaders: Dr. Rüdiger Ridder, Dr. Gerhard Moldenhauer

Research area III

Group 1: Blood stem cell transplants and residual tumor cells

Project 1: Therapeutic uses of adhesion molecules in the mobilization and transplantation of hematopoietic stem cells

Project leaders: Priv.-Doz. Dr. Rainer Haas, Prof. Dr. Margot Zöller

Project 2: Molecular mechanisms of the interaction of adhesion molecules in the mobilization and transplantation of hematopoietic stem cells

Project leaders: Priv.-Doz. Dr. Rainer Haas, Priv.-Doz. Dr. Reinhard, Schwartz-Albiez

Project 3: Inhibition of the leukemia-specific BCR-ABL expression and of the proliferation of Philadelphia-chromosome-positive CML cells using antisense nucleic acids and ribozymes

Project leaders: Dr. Ralf Kronenwett, Dr. Andreas Hochhaus

Group 2: Apoptosis

Project 1: Activation of the CD95 signal pathway in leukemias and solid tumors with chemotherapy and radiotherapy

Project leaders: Prof. Dr. Klaus-Michael Debatin, Prof. Dr. Peter H. Krammer

Project 2: Immune evasion of tumor cells by interference with the APO-1/Fas(CD95) receptor/ligand system in hepatocellular carcinoma

Project leaders: Priv.-Doz. Dr. Peter R. Galle, Prof. Dr. Peter H. Krammer

Project 3: Molecular basis of the signal pathway of the APO-1/Fas(CD95)-mediated apoptosis in leukemias

Project leaders: Prof. Dr. Peter H. Krammer, Prof. Dr. Klaus- Michael Debatin

Project 4: Significance of apoptosis in cells of the supporting tissue, in particular osteosarcoma cells and osteoblasts

Project leaders: Dr. Hans C. Mau, Prof. Dr. Klaus-Michael Debatin

Group 3: Tumor tolerance

Project 1: Identification of tumor-specific T-cell antigens in human cancer of the colon

Project leaders: Prof. Dr. Stefan Meuer, Dr. Ulrich Moebius

Project 2: Induction of specific immune responses against breast and ovarial cancers using immunogenic tumor cell varieties

Project leaders: Prof. Dr. Diethelm Wallwiener, Dr. Ulrich Moebius

Project 3: Blocking of the immune suppressive effect of the tumor marker neuron-specific enolase (NSE)

Project leaders: Dr. Yvonne Samstag, Priv.-Doz. Dr. Georg Sczakiel

Group 4: Tumor therapy with bispecific antibodies and recombinant ScFv constructs

Project 1: Production and preclinical evaluation of bispecific monoclonal antibodies and recombinant ScFv constructs for the induction of a T-lympho-

cyte-mediated cytotoxicity against human colorectal carcinoma

Project leaders: Dr. Gerhard Moldenhauer, Dr. Stefan Riedl

Project 2: Production and testing of recombinant human immune toxins for the treatment of lymphatic leukemias and malignant lymphomas

Project leaders: Prof. Dr. Melvyn Little, Prof. Dr. Klaus-Michael Debatin

Research Area III:

Group 1: Diagnostics

Project 1: Use of PET in recurrence diagnostics and monitoring of new therapies for malignant tumors

Project leaders: Dr. Dr. Jürgen Debus, Dr. Michael Knopp

Project 2: Use of PET in recurrence diagnostics and monitoring of new therapies for malignant tumors

Project leaders: Prof. Dr. Peter Georgi, Dr. Uwe Haberkorn

Group 2: Tumor therapy

Project 1: Stereotactically guided irradiation techniques for the head and body

Project leaders: Dr. Dr. Jürgen Debus, Prof. Dr. Wolfgang Schlegel

Project 2: Conformation radiotherapy with the help of inverse planning and intensity-modulated photon fields

Project leaders: Dr. Dr. Jürgen Debus, Prof. Dr. Wolfgang Schlegel

Project 3: Application and further development of new radiotherapy techniques using a computer-controlled multivane slit collimator in combination with the table-translation irradiation method

Project leaders: Dr. Dr. Jürgen Debus, Dr. Bernd-Michael Hesse

Project 4: Cooperation for the clinical introduction of laser-induced fluorescence diagnostics (LIFD) and photodynamic therapy (PDT) for malignant tumors with macromolecularly coupled photosensitizers

Project leaders: Dr. Johannes Gahlen, Dr. Wolfgang Maier-Borst

Research Area IV:

Project 1: Identification and characterization of carcinoma-specific surface domains in single metastasizing cells and micrometastes: Cell- and molecular-biological bases for the improvement of stem cells transplants

Project leaders: Priv.-Doz. Dr. Rainer Haas, Prof. Dr. Werner W. Franke

Project 2: Differentiation-specific expression of the plakoglobin/armadillo gene family in the skin and its tumors: New diagnostic possibilities

Project leaders: Prof. Dr. Ingrid Moll, Prof. Dr. Werner W. Franke

Project 3: Overcoming tumor resistance mechanisms by means of the covalent coupling of methotrexate to albumin

Project leaders: Dr. Gernot Hartung, Dr. Eva Frei

Project 4: Genetic modifications as markers for the diagnosis and prognosis of gastrointestinal tumors

Project leaders: Prof. Dr. Manfred Schwab, Dr. Johannes Gebert

Project 5: Cell-biological studies of the expression and location of the cell-cell-contact-mediating components desmoplakin, desmoglein, and E-cadherin and their significance for the progression of head and neck cancers

Project leaders: Dr. Franz X. Bosch, Priv.-Doz. Dr. Jürgen Kartenbeck

Project 6: Expression of the multidrug resistance proteins (MRP) in human hepatocellular carcinoma

Project leaders: Prof. Dr. Dietrich Keppler, Dr. Markus Möhler

Project 7: Rational chemotherapy of lung cancer

Project leaders: Dr. Heinrich Becker, Priv.-Doz. Dr. Christof Granzow

Project 8: Molecular-genetic studies of the significance of the genetic status of the p53 tumor suppressor gene for the progression of head and neck cancers

Project leaders: Dr. Franz X. Bosch, Priv.-Doz. Dr. Hanswalter Zentgraf

Project 9: The significance of the parathormone-related protein for tumor metastasis and growth

Project leaders: Dr. Tobias Schilling, Prof. Dr. Werner W. Franke

Project 10: Multimodal analysis of tumor-cell heterogeneity in pancreatic cancer in terms of cytogenetics, proliferation, apoptotic activity, and resistance to chemotherapy

Project leaders: Dr. Caroline Verbeke, Priv.-Doz. Dr. Hanswalter Zentgraf

Project 11: Studies with new functional-biological procedures and noninvasive determination of multidrug resistance in patients with mammary tumors and malignant lymphomas for the optimization and individualization of therapy management

Project leaders: Prof. Dr. Ludwig Strauss, Priv.-Doz. Dr. Adelheid Weiss

Project 12: Tenascin-C isoforms and dissociation products in metastases of colorectal carcinomas and their clinical relevance

Project leader: Dr. Stefan Riedl

Project 13: Navigation system for liver surgery: 3D reconstruction for the documentation of growth kinetics of liver metastases

Project leaders: Dr. Wolfram Lamadé, Priv.-Doz. Dr. Hans-Peter Meinzer

The above-described research activities of the Tumor Center are partially supplemented by studies carried out in collaboration with other tumor centers and facilities, for example, with the European Organisation for Research on Treatment of Cancer (EORT), the Swiss Institute for Applied Cancer Research (Schweizerisches Institut für Angewandte Krebsforschung – SIAK), and the Oncological Working Groups of the German Cancer Association.

For the planning and evaluation of studies in the field of clinical oncology in the Tumor Center, for scientific research projects on the topic of the epidemiology of cancer, and for assessing medical therapies and diagnostic procedures, the Tumor Center employs a biometrician, who is also consulted by many of the parties collaborating with the Tumor Center.

The documentation of tumors at the Tumor Center Heidelberg/Mannheim is kept in the form of a cancer register which has separate sections for the three clinical partners. It is not possible to keep a central register for the whole Tumor Center because of the laws on data protection.

Further Activities

According to the statutes of the Tumor Center, its aims include the continuing and further education of doctors working in oncology. Regular advanced training events are held at the Tumor

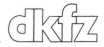

Center by the Oncological Working Groups Heidelberg or Mannheim in cooperation with the North Baden Regional Medical Chamber. These events serve to give practicing doctors access to the results of clinical tumor research and basic research on oncology as well as providing them with further education. In particular, the hospital doctors and private practitioners are made familiar with research results which have already been adopted in the form of new treatments at the hospitals of the Tumor Center. The choice of seminar topics emphasizes the significance of interdisciplinary cooperation in tumor research and treatment. The acceptance of these advanced training events among the doctors is high.

The topics of the most recent events are listed below:

Oncological Working Group Heidelberg:

1997 (01. Feb.): Multimodal Combination Therapies

1996 (03. Feb.): Current Status in the Diagnosis and Therapy of Gastrointestinal tumors

1995 (07. Oct.): Early Diagnosis – the Chance for the Cancer Patient

1995 (04. Feb.): High-Dose Therapy with Blood Stem Cell Transplantation for Solid Tumors and Diseases of the Hematological System

Oncological Working Group Mannheim:

1997 (18. Oct.): Colorectal Tumors

1996 (19. Oct.): Breast Cancer – New Trends in Diagnosis and Therapy

1995 (21. Oct.): Neoadjuvant Therapy Concepts.

Every two years special advanced courses are held in Heidelberg for fami-ly doctors. They address „Oncology for the Family Doctor – Topics Relating to Prevention, Treatment, and Aftercare". The last such event took place on Dec. 7, 1996.

In connection with the action week „Europe Against Cancer", the Tumor Center organized the initiative „Action Against Cancer – Prevention and Early Diagnosis", which was held in the week 7-14 October 1995. A brochure for doctors with the title „Früherkennung" (Early diagnosis) was published within the previously mentioned series of the Tumor Center, and on Saturday 7th October a further education event was held under the banner „Early Diagnosis – The Chance for the Cancer Patient". A campaign was organized to inform citizens about the causes of cancer, its prevention, and the opportunities for early diagnosis: a leaflet drawing attention to means of prevention, warning signs upon which a doctor should be consulted, and examinations for early diagnosis, was distributed to about 100 000 households in the Heidelberg region. This leaflet also invited members of the public to attend a program of talks and advise to be held from Monday, Oct. 9th to Saturday, Oct. 14th. On each day, the talks concentrated on a particular type of cancer: On Monday – lung cancer; on Tuesday – breast cancer; on Wednesday – cancer of the digestive tract; on Thursday – leukemias and lymphomas; on Friday – prostate cancer; and on Saturday – both skin cancer and cancers of the head and neck. The talks of the medical professionals were followed by extremely interested audiences. Many of those in attendance were sufferers or the relatives of cancer patients, who wanted to obtain further information and learn, for instance, about the hereditary risks involved. After the presentation, there was always a lively discussion and question-and-answer session. In the foyer of the communication center of the Deutsches Krebsforschungszentrum, in which the event took place, the visitors could take advantage of an information program about healthy eating, suitable sports activities, cancer prevention, and the work of self-help organizations. On Tuesday, the day specializing in breast cancer, women were taught about self-examination for breast tumors; on Wednesday, when the topic was tumors of the digestive tract, the health insurance company Barmer, which had generously sponsored the action week, offered individual dietary advice at their information stand. The verdict of the visitors: „You should hold this event three times a year".

Finances

The clinical oncology is financed from the budget of the hospitals. The research activities of the Tumor Center are supported, on the basis of the above-described external refereeing, by funds provided by the Federal Ministry of Education, Science, Research, and Technology (90 percent) and by the Ministry for Science, Research, and Art of the State of Baden-Württemberg (10 percent), which are channeled through the budget of the Deutsches Krebsforschungszentrum. The running of the coordination and administrative office and its activities is financed by the four contractual partners. The continual updating and extension of the series of brochures published by the Tumor Center is made possible in part by donations.

233

The Association for Clinical-Biomedical Research

The Association for Clinical-Biomedical Research (Verbund Klinisch-Biomedizinische Forschung, KBF) was founded in 1992 by five members of the Hermann von Helmholtz Association of National Research Centers (HGF, formerly AGF), which focuses on research related to health. The founding members in alphabetical order are the: DKFZ - Stiftung Deutsches Krebsforschungszentrum, Heidelberg (German Cancer Research Center), GBF - Gesellschaft für Biotechnologische Forschung mbH, Braunschweig (Center for Biotechnological Research), GSF - GSF-Forschungszentrum für Umwelt und Gesundheit GmbH, München (Research Center for Environment and Health), KFA - Forschungszentrum Jülich GmbH, Jülich (Jülich Research Center), and MDC - Stiftung Max-Delbrück-Centrum für Molekulare Medizin, Berlin-Buch (Max Delbrück Center for Molecular Medicine).

In the following years, three more HGF members were admitted: the Karlsruhe Research Center (Forschungszentrum Karlsruhe, FZK) in Karlsruhe, the Institute for Aviation and Space Medicine of the German Aviation and Space Research Institute (Institut für Luft- und Raumfahrtmedizin der Deutschen Forschungsanstalt für Luft- und Raumfahrt, DLR) in Cologne, and the Heavy Ion Research Center (Gesellschaft für Schwerionenforschung mbH, GSI) in Darmstadt. The following research facilities became associated members: the German Institute of Human Nutrition (Deutsches Institut für Ernährungsforschung, DIfE) in Potsdam-Reh-

brücke, the Borstel Research Center (Forschungszentrum Borstel, FZB) in Borstel, the Heinrich Pette Institute for Experimental Virology and Immunology (Heinrich-Pette-Institut für Experimentelle Virologie und Immunologie, HPI) in Hamburg, the Tumor Biology Clinic (Klinik für Tumorbiologie, KTB) in Freiburg, and the Central Institute for Mental Health (Zentralinstitut für Seelische Gesundheit, ZI) in Mannheim. Thus, the association now encompasses 13 research institutes.

The aim of the association is to contribute to the improvement of clinically oriented biomedical research by optimizing the quality of relevant research endeavors and specifically supporting joint projects with clinical partners.

The association has two organs, the Board and the Coordinating Committee, which control its work in close cooperation with each other.

The Board consists of the scientific directors of the participating facilities and two members from business.

The Coordinating Committee is appointed by the Board and consists of prominent scientific representatives of the respective institutes. Their number depends on the proportion of health-related research in the overall scientific activities of the institute. Currently, the Coordinating Committee consists of 17 members. The Board and the Coordinating Committee usually meet jointly to discuss questions relating to the organization and subject matter of the association.

Quality optimization is sought mainly by an appropriate appointment policy and an evaluation of the research performed at the member facilities.

The participating research institutes have agreed to admit to their appointment commissions two external members named by the Association. It is thereby hoped that, on the basis of a broad expertise, the candidates best qualified for leading positions will be chosen.

The members of the association attach great importance to the regular evaluation of their research work by internal and external - as a rule internationally staffed - expert commissions. The association endeavors to harmonize the appraisal procedures in the member institutes and to ensure that the best scientists in a particular research area comment on the work done or, if required, give recommendations concerning a reorientation of the work. These evaluations can have a profound influence on the structure and orientation of existing focuses of research. Representatives of the association always take part in inspections of the member institutes.

Furthermore, the association tries to undertake a certain coordination of future research efforts, aiming, in particular, to prevent large overlap of the scientific activities.

In addition to the above-mentioned organizational measures aimed at quality optimization, the association wants to make a contribution to clinical research by specifically supporting cooperation projects between groups from the member institutes and clinical partners - preferably university hospitals - and by providing funds for working visits of scientifically active clinicians to member institutes. For the duration of their research activity at member institutes, it is planned to compensate the hospitals for the loss of their medical skills.

The association reports on the work done in annual meetings. These meetings are connected with scientific symposia in which the most prominent scientists from Germany and abroad take part. The first such symposium was held in the fall of 1993 at the Deutsches Krebsforschungszentrum in Heidelberg on the topic of „Gene Diagnosis and Gene Therapy".

Further symposia took place in 1994, under the heading „Genetic Instability" at the GSF Research Center for Environment and Health; in 1995, on the topic of „Complex Genetic Diseases", at the Max Delbrück Center for Molecular Medicine; and in 1996, on the topic „Molecular Targets for Drug Development", at the GBF Center for Biotechnological Research.

Organs
of the Foundation

As provided by § 7 of its Statutes and Articles, the Foundation has the following organs:

- the Board of Trustees with the Scientific Committee,
- the Management Board, and
- the Scientific Council.

The Board of Trustees

As stipulated by § 8 of the Statutes and Articles of the Foundation, the Board of Trustees supervises the legality, expediency and economy of the management of the Foundation's activities. It decides upon the Foundation's general research objectives and important issues of research policy as well as its financial affairs. In addition, it determines management principles and the principles governing performance evaluation. It also sets up the financial plans, which cover a period of several years, including any expansion and investment programs. As a rule, the Board of Trustees convenes twice a year.

In 1994, the Board of Trustees took the following decisions:

- Approval of the appointment of Dr. Peter Angel as head of the temporary division „Signal Transduction and Growth Control".
- Approval of the establishment of the temporary division „Theoretical Bioinformatics".
- Approval of the establishment of the division „Medical Physics", and of the appointment of Prof. Dr. Wolfgang Schlegel as its head.
- Approval of the establishment of the division „Molecular Genome Analy-

sis", and of the appointment of Dr. habil. Annemarie Poustka as its head.
- Approval of the conversion of the temporary division „Organization of Complex Genomes" into a permanent one.

Furthermore, the results of the external evaluations of the Research Programs „Cancer Risk Factors and Prevention" and „Radiological Diagnostics and Therapy" were discussed.

In 1995, the Board of Trustees was concerned, among other things, with the following issues:

- Approval of the report „Entwicklung und Perspektiven des Deutschen Krebsforschungszentrums" (Development and Prospects of the Deutschen Krebsforschungszentrum).
- Approval of the thematical reorientation of the Research Program „Bioinformatics" and its renaming to „Genome Research and Bioinformatics".
- Approval of the establishment of the temporary division „Functional Analysis of Viral Oncoproteins".
- Appointment of the head of Dr. Martin Vingron to division „Theoretical Bioinformatics".
- Appointment of Dr. Dirk Schadendorf to head of the clinical cooperation unit „Dermato-Oncology".

In addition, the Board of Trustees discussed the results of the external evaluations of the following Research Programs:

- „Applied Tumor Virology"
- „Cell Differentiation and Carcinogenesis"
- „Tumor Cell Regulation"
- „Diagnostics and Experimental Therapy".

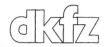

In 1996, the decisions taken by the Board of Trustees included the following:

– Appointment of the new Administrative Member of the Management Board, Dr. Josef Puchta.

– Approval of the establishment of the clinical cooperation unit „Radiotherapy", and of the appointment of Dr. Dr. Jürgen Debus as its head.

– Approval of the appointment of the coordinator of the Research Program „Genome Research and Bioinformatics", Priv.-Doz. Dr. Sandor Suhai.

– Approval of the establishment of the division „Experimental Pathology".

– Approval of the establishment of the division „Molecular Mechanisms of Carcinogenesis and Tumor Defense".

– Approval of the establishment of the division „Medical Physics and Biophysics".

– Approval of the establishment of the temporary division „Mechanisms of Viral Oncogenesis".

– Approval of the establishment of a new central facility, „Biostatistics".

Furthermore, the Board of Trustees discussed the results of the external evaluation of the Research Program „Tumor Immunology".

The task of the Scientific Comittee, as stipulated by § 10 of the Statutes and Articles of the Foundation, is to prepare the decisions of the Board of Trustees in all scientific matters. It is responsible, in particular, for the continuous evaluation of results through scientific assessments. Alongside doing the groundwork for decision-making for the Board of Trustees, the Scientific Comittee appoints expert commissions composed of leading international scientists for external evaluations.

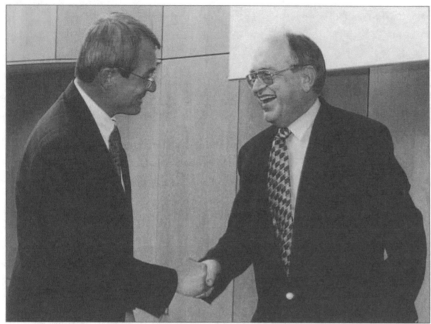

Fig. 113
The Administrative Member of the Management Board, Dr. Reinhard Grunwald, receives his farewell in April 1996 from Prof. Dr. Werner Franke, Chairman of the Scientific Council

The Management Board

As stipulated by § 14.1 of the Statutes and Articles, the Foundation is directed by the Management Board. This consists of at least one scientific and one administrative member (§ 15.1). The chairman is the scientific representative of the Foundation. The Board of Trustees appoints the members of the Management Board after consultation with the Scientific Council (§ 15.2).

Since May 1, 1983, Prof. Dr. med. Dr. h.c. mult. Harald zur Hausen has directed the Management Board as its chairman and is also its scientific member. In May 1993, he was re-appointed for a third five-year term. Dr. jur. Reinhard Grunwald, who had been the administrative member of the Management Board since 1984, was elected during his third period of office to the position of General Secretary of the German Research Association (DFG -

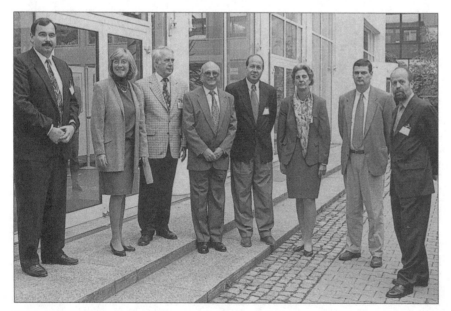

Fig. 114
Shortly after taking up his duties: Dr. Josef Puchta, Administrative Member of the Management Board of the Deutsches Krebsforschungszentrum (left) with participants of the 6th Heidelberg-Rehovot conference on Management Instruments and Experience: The Mayor of Heidelberg, Beate Weber; Dr. Bernd Martin, Max Planck Institute for Nuclear Physics; Yaakob Naan, Weizmann Institute, Rehovot; Moshe Vigdor, Hebrew University, Jerusalem; Romana Gräfin vom Hagen, University of Heidelberg; Dr. Israel German, Ben Gurion University, Beer Sheva, Dr. Wolfgang Henkel, Deutsches Krebsforschungszentrum

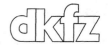

Deutsche Forschungsgemeinschaft). He, thus, resigned from the Management Board in 1996. Dr. rer. pol. Josef Puchta was named as his successor on August I, 1996 for a period of five years.

In a multi-disciplinary, complex, and necessarily decentralized research institution the traditional management functions of planning, decision-making, and supervision, are less hierarchically structured. Scientific management is primarily based on encouraging and promoting ideas, coordinating processes, and balancing multiple interests.

Thus, in its main task of defining the scientific program of the Deutsches Krebsforschungszentrum, the Management Board focuses on deciding which research projects to initiate and which to terminate, how to distribute the Center's resources according to performance, and how to further improve operating processes. The collaboration with the Foundation's committees and its sponsors and the cooperation with scientific partners in Germany and abroad are important aspects of the work of the Management Board. Another important recent concern has been the further development of the electronic network linking the Center to the international, particularly European, and national scientific communities.

The work of the Management Board is considerably supported by advisory committees. In the past, the Management Board has delegated the following tasks to permanent commissions: evaluation of the performance of the departments following internal inspection by the members of the extended Management Board; selection of scientists for awards, bonuses, promotions, and tenure; assessment of all applications; and supervision of all work subject to the German Gene Technology Law.

Other tasks are delegated to ad hoc commissions. The Management Board is supported in its work by the units reporting directly to the Board and by the administration.

The Scientific Council

The task of the Scientific Council is to advise the Board of Trustees and the Management Board in all relevant scientific issues. In a number of important matters, decisions of the Management Board require the consent of the Scientific Council.

The Scientific Council deals, in particular, with research projects and programs, appointments, the utilization of research results, the evaluation of performance, the advancement of scientific information exchange, the collaboration with universities and other research facilities, budget planning, and investment programs.

The Scientific Council consists of 16 members, comprising the coordinators of the eight research programs and an equal number of elected representatives from the scientific staff.

As a rule, the Scientific Council convenes once a month. A number of expert commissions and a permanently staffed office support the Council in its work and in the preparation of decisions.

The current, seventh 3-year term of office of the Scientific Council ends in February 1988. Preparations for new elections will therefore have to be started by the end of 1997.

Members of the Scientific Council
(February 1995 – January 1998)

Prof. Dr. Werner W. Franke (Chairman)
Priv.-Doz. Dr. Jürgen Kartenbeck
Research Program Cell Differentiation and
 Carcinogenesis

Prof. Dr. Friedrich Marks
Dr. Petra Boukamp
Research Program Tumor Cell Regulation

Prof. Dr. Helmut Bartsch
Dr. Nikolaus Becker
Research Program Cancer Risk Factors and Prevention

Prof. Dr. Thomas Boehm
Prof. Dr. Melvyn Little
Research Program Diagnostics and Experimental
Therapy

Prof. Dr. Gerhard van Kaick
Prof. Dr. Wolfgang Schlegel
Research Program Radiological Diagnostics and
Therapy

Prof. Dr. Jean Rommelaere
Priv.-Doz. Dr. Elisabeth Schwarz (Deputy Chairperson)
Research Program Applied Tumor Virology

Prof. Dr. Peter H. Krammer
Dr. Gerhard Moldenhauer
Research Program Tumor Immunology

Priv.-Doz. Dr. Sandor Suhai
Priv.-Doz. Dr. Hans-Peter Meinzer
Research Program Genome Research and
Bioinformatics

Dipl.-Math. Siegfried Herz
Secretary of the Scientific Council

Members of the Scientific Council
(February 1998)

Prof. Dr. Werner W. Franke (Chairman)
Prof. Dr. Eberhard Spiess
Research Program Cell Differentiation and
Carcinogenesis

Prof. Dr. Friedrich Marks
Priv.-Doz. Dr. Petra Boukamp
Research Program Tumor Cell Regulation

Prof. Dr. Helmut Bartsch
Dr. Barbara Bertram
Research Program Cancer Risk Factors and Prevention

Prof. Dr. Margot Zöller
Prof. Dr. Melvyn Little
Research Program Diagnostics and Experimental
Therapy

Prof. Dr. Gerhard van Kaick
Priv.-Doz. Dr. Dr. Jürgen Debus
Research Program Radiological Diagnostics and
Therapy

Prof. Dr. Jean Rommelaere
Priv.-Doz. Dr. Elisabeth Schwarz (Deputy Chairperson)
Research Program Applied Tumor Virology

Prof. Dr. Peter H. Krammer
Priv.-Doz. Dr. Bruno Kyewski
Research Program Tumor Immunology

Priv.-Doz. Dr. Sandor Suhai
Prof. Dr. Jörg Langowski
Research Program Genome Research and
Bioinformatics

Dipl.-Math. Siegfried Herz
Secretary of the Scientific Council

14

Staff Council

The reduction in personnel and the effect of this on the working conditions of the staff at the Deutsches Krebsforschungszentrum are concerns of ever greater importance for the Staff Council. Not only are efforts directed towards the protection of employees' rights within the Center: equally important is the need to draw the attention of those responsible at Federal and State level to the - from the viewpoint of the Staff Council - misguided cost-cutting policies in research. The Staff Council supports the demands that the efficiency of government-funded research should be promoted through flexibility in the allocations and through competition between the research institutes. However, because of the immense significance of research for our future, this should not be allowed to cause further job losses and reduced funding.

The Staff Council of the Deutsches Krebsforschungszentrum is actively supporting these aims and is intensively involved in the work of the Association of Works and Staff Councils of Non-University Research Facilities (AGBR) of the Hermann von Helmholtz Association of National Research Centers. This is evidenced by statements and announcements in which the Works and Staff Councils critically review the Federal Government's research policy.

Since the policy is to give priority to financing research projects, most staff have only temporary employment contracts. This means that more and more staff in research institutes are lacking social security and facing potential unemployment at the end of their contract.

It is the opinion of the Staff Council that permanent employment should remain a mutually held principle of our society. According to the principle of social partnership, the government has a responsibility to the employed population. We observe that in the present context irresponsible deviations from this fundamental principle are occurring.

Two problems need to be critically examined

There are a large number of doctoral students working at the Deutsches Krebsforschungszentrum. The increase in their number has partially served to compensate for the reduction in established positions. Doctoral students work in the same manner as research staff. They are fully involved in the research program and with hourly rates of pay of DM 24.82 ($ 14.26) are cheap labor. The neglect of the support of young scientists is entirely the responsibility of the politicians. Through their decisions to economize on research funding, they are jeorpardizing the scientific basis for the future of research in Germany. The slashing of the University Special Program III to almost zero, which enabled additional doctoral students to be financed, simply emphasizes the wrong course that is being taken by research policy, the true aim of which should be to improve the structure of research in Germany.

The special support of women has also been one of the victims of the economies. There is hardly any mention of women's support any more, let alone any decisive action. The Deutsches Krebsforschungszentrum, despite the intense demands of the women's initiative for the external appointment of a women's representative, has not as yet taken advantage of the existing opportunities for the support of women. The activities of the women's initiative have gained acceptance, but they are not able to fully replace the work of a women's representative. The women's initiative carried out a survey among women: showed, among other things, that women are poorly paid and that their attempts to plan their lives so as to accommodate both family and career are severely hampered by temporary employment contracts.

Brigitte Hobrecker

Members of the Staff Council
(Status: June 1997)

Dr. Folker Amelung,
Member of the Board

Dr. Holger Friesel

Hanspeter Götz

Siegfried Herz

Brigitte Hobrecker, Chair

Annekathrin Kollenda

Jutta Müller-Osterholt

Dr. Hartmut Richter

Heinrich Schmitt, Vice-chair

Rolf Schmitt, Member of the Board

Ingeborg Vogt

Ulrike Wagner

Peter Zöpfgen

15

Administration

The administrative activities during the early 1990s were determined largely by the introduction of the new research structure at the Center. Subsequently, since 1993, the opportunities for administrative initiative have been significantly influenced by the stagnation and partial decline in the financial support received from public sources. Further improvements in the efficiency of the services offered by the administration (through, among other things, improved opportunities for the staff to gain qualifications), testing the cost-effectiveness of using external staff for some administrative tasks (outsourcing), intensified efforts to obtain external sponsorship, and also measures relating to the commercial exploitation of research results (participation in the BioRegio competition of the Federal Ministry of Education, Science, Research, and Technolo-

gy): were the main aims of the administration. The major activities thereby were:

– A continuation of the reorganization of the data processing in the administration;

– Administration of personnel and positions, salaries, and travel expenses;

– Introduction of measures to increase the flexibility of the staffing structure with the view to improving overall performance, together with the introduction of greater possibilities for part-time work on the basis of individual wishes;

– A restructuring of the accounting department to the system of double-entry book keeping. This is expected to be completed at the beginning of the financial year 1998 and will

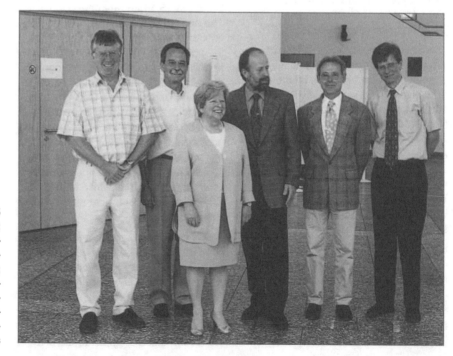

Fig. 115
Heads of the Administrative Divisions: Winfried Schwarz, Finance and Accounting; Rudi Lange, Technical Services; Elfriede Egenlauf, General Administration; Dr. Wolfgang Henkel, Head of Administration; Klaus Pregartner, Personnel and Social Affairs; Dr. Rolf Zimmermann, Procurement/Materials. Not pictured: Gerhard Sommer, House Services

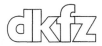

then be brought into line with the practices at the other other facilities of the Helmholtz Association of German Research Centers. The reorganization is accompanied by a restructuring of the applications within the departments responsible for finance, accounting, and procurement, the aim being to improve the financial reporting and information structures. The future applications will be supported by standard SAP software and will form the basis for an effective controlling:

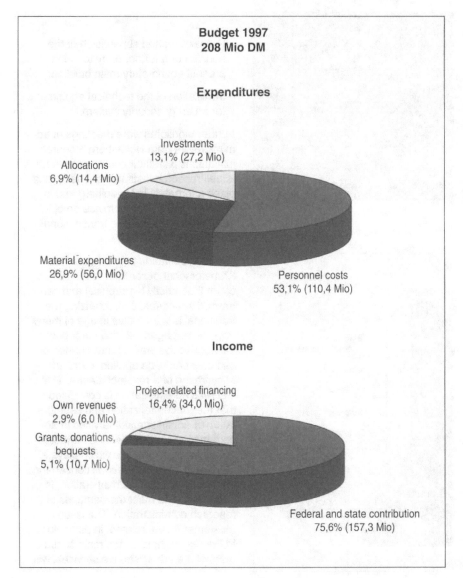

Budget 1997
208 Mio DM

Expenditures

Investments
13,1% (27,2 Mio)

Allocations
6,9% (14,4 Mio)

Material expenditures
26,9% (56,0 Mio)

Personnel costs
53,1% (110,4 Mio)

Income

Project-related financing
16,4% (34,0 Mio)

Own revenues
2,9% (6,0 Mio)

Grants, donations, bequests
5,1% (10,7 Mio)

Federal and state contribution
75,6% (157,3 Mio)

- The integration into one unit, both organizationally and in terms of their premises, of the previously separate stores for technical goods, office supplies, laboratory equipment, and also the goods entry point;

- Further development of the data-processing support for decentralized procurement;

- The purchase of further guest appartments for accommodating, in particular, visiting scientists from abroad;

- Involvement in the procurement and installation of major equipment (among other things, a positron emission tomograph, a linear accelerator, a whole-body MR system, and a computer tomograph);

- Exchange of experience and cooperation with the University of Heidelberg and with the University Hospitals, with a view to more economical procurement of external services;

- More intensive attempts to acquire external support (e.g., from the European Union, the Association for Clinical-Biomedical Research, and the German Research Association);

- Extensive renovation of the buildings (for example, renovation of the inner courtyard; cleaning of the concrete; installation of a new main ventilation plant);

- Supervision of the building measures for the clinical-bioscientific cooperation units with the University of Heidelberg;

- Major renovation of the sixth floor: of the main building and continuation of the renovation and modernization deemed necessary by the trade inspectorate for safety and health reasons;

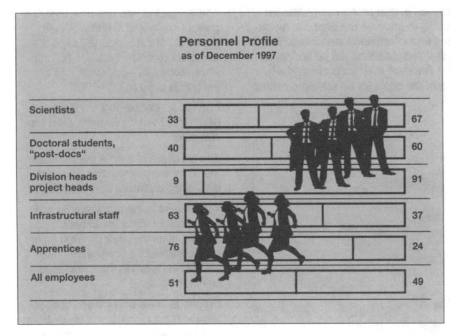

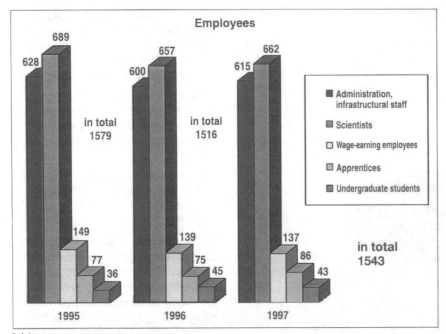

Aerial photo of the Neuenheimer Feld in Heidelberg with the main building of the Deutsches Krebsforschungszentrum in the center. Behind it on the right: building of the Applied Tumor Virology Research Program; behind it on the left: Zentrum für Molekulare Biologie Heidelberg of the University of Heidelberg

– Preparation and supervision of the addition of a further story to the at present seven-story main building;

– Installation of the technical equipment for an entry security system.

Further highlights were meetings of administrators from Heidelberg research institutions with their counterparts from Israeli research institutions. These take place alternately in Heidelberg and in Rehovot, Israel. They provide an opportunity to continue the transnational exchange of experience.

The administration of the Deutsches Krebsforschungszentrum takes into account that strictly hierarchical and centralized structures, characterizing the traditional adminstrative image of many government agencies and other public services to the present day, cannot, or can only partly, be applied to the administration of a research center. The Center's administration is convinced that the „decentralization and segmentation of administrative services in accordance with customer and market requirements", a principle which plays a major role in considerations concerning the reform of public administration, is better suited to meet the demands of a research administration. The issue of „customer focus" related, in particular, to the researchers as the main consumers of the administrative services, will

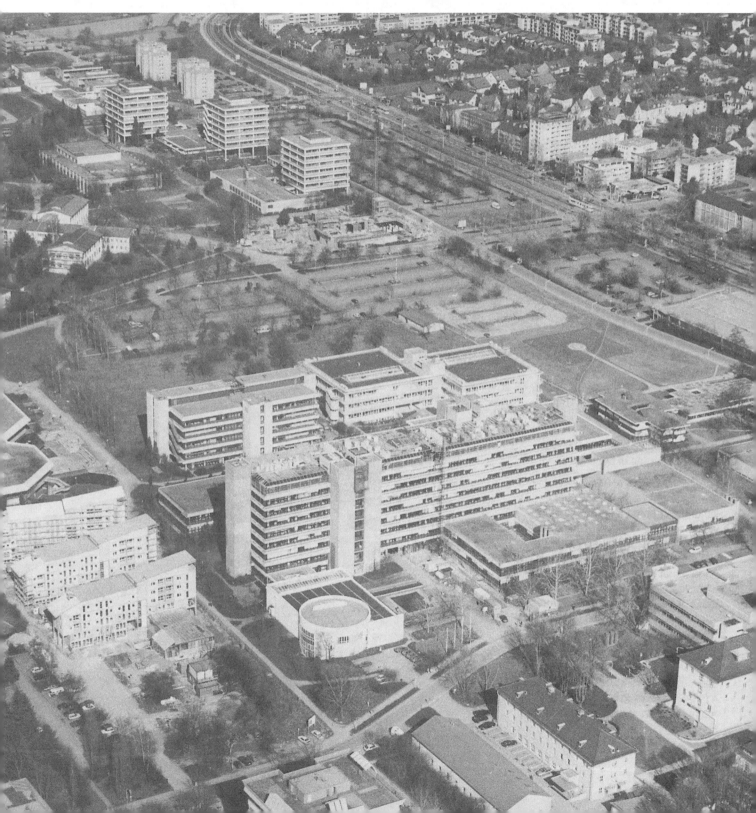

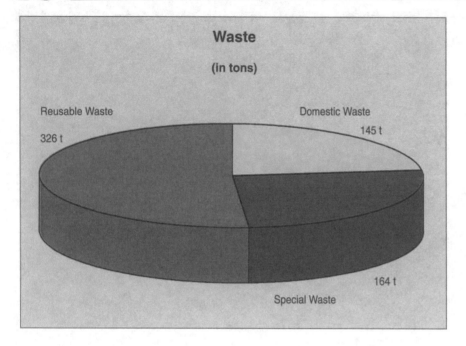

Waste

(in tons)

Reusable Waste
326 t

Domestic Waste
145 t

164 t

Special Waste

in the future gain even more importance in all areas of administration.

A decentralization of administrative processes at the Deutsches Krebsforschungszentrum can provide the individual scientist with a broader scope for
action when managing his or her administrative requests. However, it is important that the responsibility for administrative actions is clearly defined and
that scientists only take over immediate
administrative tasks when there is good
reason for this.

The administration thus concentrates
its efforts primarily on offering qualified
services when required, thereby leaving
it to the scientist to choose the best
mode of action in the individual situation.

16

Teaching, Vocational Training, and Continuing Education

Teaching

Scientists from the Deutsches Krebsforschungszentrum are actively involved in teaching by offering a wide range of practical courses for advanced students, seminars, colloquia, and lectures. Every semester, they give more than 100 courses and lectures, primarily at the University of Heidelberg, but also at the Universities of Karlsruhe, Tübingen, and Kaiserslautern, as well as at various professional colleges.

During the years 1994, 1995, and 1996, there were 637 doctoral and diploma students involved in the research work of the Deutsches Krebsforschungszentrum. During this period, they produced 262 diploma, doctoral, and "Habilitation" theses recorded in the annual list of publications "Veröffentlichungen" from the Deutsches Krebsforschungszentrum.

The Center also engages in continuing education efforts, e.g., by offering further education and special training for doctors, held mainly by representatives of the Research Program Radiological Diagnostics and Therapy. Thus, the Center organizes regular ultrasound courses at the basic, advanced and advanced levels.

In order to support highly-qualified young scientists, the Center finances five positions for young scientists and a further ten to 15 positions based on team-oriented project proposals from its special funds, i.e., from donations to the Deutsches Krebsforschungszentrum. Thus, young scientists can spend up to three years working in research projects submitted on a competitive basis by researchers from the Center. Another endeavor to promote the up-coming generation of scientists is the Center's trainee program. Students from the Study Foundation of the German People (Studienstiftung des Deutschen Volkes) are given the opportunity to gain practical experience in cancer research during a stay of up to eight weeks, and a similar program is offered to students from Stanford University (Krupp Foundation).

The Deutsches Krebsforschungszentrum regularly invites winners of the competition „Jugend forscht" (Youth doing research). They may stay for up to one week in a division whose research activities they find particurly interesting for thematical or methodological reasons.

In addition, the Center continually organizes events aimed at introducing scientists from all over the world into new techniques and methods.

The colloquia held at the Deutsches Krebsforschungszentrum also serve as an instrument for introducing new scientific ideas and stimulating the scientific discussion among researchers working within and outside the boundaries of the Center. During the years 1994 to 1996, almost 700 lectures on special topics were delivered by lecturers from 32 countries. The series of colloquia organized by the Deutsches Krebsforschungszentrum is part of a joint program entitled "Bioscientific Lectures" by the University of Heidelberg, the Max Planck Institutes located in Heidelberg, and the European Molecular Biology Laboratory (EMBL). Lecture announcements by the above institutes are collected and updated weekly by the Center's press office.

Vocational Training

For 20 years now the Deutsches Krebsforschungszentrum has offered apprenticeships as specified in the vocational training law and in collaboration with the professional colleges of Baden Württemberg. This training of apprentices has become an established feature of the Center and is highly regarded by the industry of the Rhein-Neckar Region.

The spectrum of training available places particular emphasis on careers in laboratory work.

It now encompasses the following:

Laboratory professions 82 %
  69 %: Biology laboratory assistant

  13 %: Medical assistant, Chemical laboratory assistant, Radiation protection engineer (diploma of the professional college), Animal keeper (specializing in the care of domestic and experimental animals)

Technical professions 4 %:
  Precision engineer, Joiner

Administrative professions 14%:
  Business management (diploma of the professional college, specializing in state-run institutions), Commercial clerk in office communication.

The Deutsches Krebsforschungszentrum accept many young people from the local region, far more than will actually be offered later employment at the Center. It thereby aims to provide as many poeple leaving school as possible with useful and modern vocational training. The number of permanent jobs in relation to the number of apprentices has remained at a constant level of about 10 % since 1990 and is, thus, far above the typical levels in industry.

Through the end of 1996, more than 600 apprentices had successfully qualified, with a high standard of training being maintained throughout. Despite the fact that the Center is unable to offer positions to many of the qualified apprentices, these young people generally find good positions either in the region or further afield. Vocational training at the Deutsches Krebsforschungszentrum is clearly an attractive option, as witnessed by the relatively large number of applicants. The low birthrate years, however, has caused the number of applicants to decline somewhat and currently the number is around 350. The Deutsches Krebsforschungszentrum offers 25 apprenticeships each year. Thus between 10 and 15 people leaving school apply for each available place.

In the future ever greater demands will be placed on vocational training. Today the young people working in the various departments, regardless of whether they are being trained in laboratory or managerial skills, are already learning sophisticated modern techniques that will prepare them for the challenges of the future. During their training the apprentices spend periods in several of the different Research Programs in order to experience the broad and continually changing spectrum of activities of a research institute. An important aim of the training should be to develop the personal abilities and competencies of the apprentice, including, for example, readiness to accept responsibility and ability to learn and cooperate. A run-of-the-mill training program is no longer sufficient to meet the complex demands of a research institute such as the Deutsches Krebsforschungszentrum. It is automatically expected of the

trainees and the staff that they work flexibly and can perform a variety of tasks. This assumes, alongside excellent specialist knowledge, a number of key abilities which relate, in particular, to the personality profile. These include readiness to tackle problems, high performance, endurance, but also creativity, ability to make decisions, and consciousness of responsibilities. For apprentices these qualifications are particularly important. In the Deutsches Krebsforschungszentrum the various research laboratories teach theories and methods which extend far beyond the statutory syllabus. The apprentices directly take part in research work. The intention thereby is to motivate them through responsibility. In order to realize this concept the teaching staff must be ready to support the apprentices and allow them to take responsibility for their own actions. The apprentices discover that continuous readiness to learn and the ability to translate theory into practice are features of the qualifications needed in modern technical works. By taking on greater responsibility the apprentices find that they have more opportunity for decision-making and more independence; thus, their job satisfaction also increases.

The practical training in the laboratories is complemented by regular practical and theoretical instruction in the training laboratory, leading to an appropriate synthesis of theoretical knowledge and practical skills.

The content of the Center's training goes well beyond statutory requirements. This is evidenced by the high proportion of apprentices who qualify early and by the high quality of their final results. Over the last 6 years, 31 of the 77 biology laboratory assistants

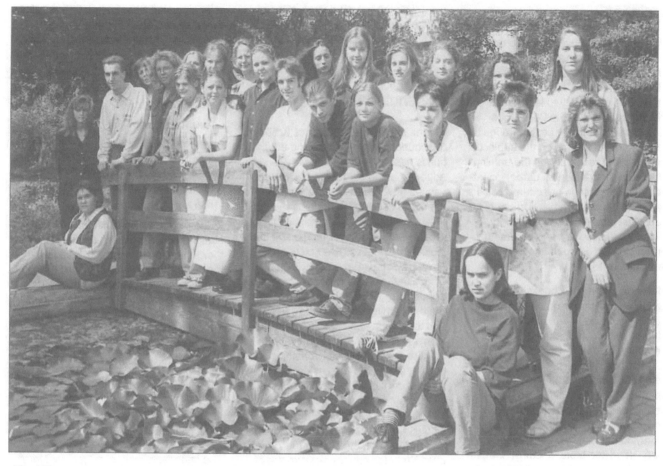

Fig. 116
Apprentices at the Deutsches Krebsforschungszentrum in 1996 with their instructors Dr. Nesta Ehler, head of the working group (third from the left in the background), Tatjana Kirchhoff-Muranyi, Sybille Zottmann, and Karin Ruppert (from the right, middle row)

were able to finish their period of training 6 months early on account of their good performance.

It is not uncommon for a newly qualifying biology laboratory assistant from the Deutsches Krebsforschungszentrum to obtain the best result among those awarded by the professional association.

In 1996, in recognition of their excellent achievements, five apprentice biology laboratory assistants were proposed by the Chamber of Industry and Commerce of the Rhein-Neckar Region as recipients of a grant for the support of special talent under the programm "Professional Training of the Federal Ministry of Education, Science, Research, and Technology".

The training program at the Deutsches Krebsforschungszentrum Heidelberg is the responsibility of three full-time staff members. Their expertise has also gained recognition outside the Center.

Trainees

During the last two years more than 500 students from schools in the region have sought information about the main areas of work in a scientific laboratory. One possibility to learn about the training program of the Deutsches Krebsforschungszentrum is through the regular school forums on the subject of „training and research". In the training laboratory at the Center, career-oriented practical classes are offered twice a year. For security reasons, many of the specialist laboratories are no longer allowed to be used for demonstrating professional work to young people (potential trainees).

More than 60 high-school students are taking part in career-oriented practical training courses in our specialist laboratories. Individual wishes of the students are taken into account as much as possible in selecting the specialist field which they encounter. The time spent on the practical course is an important component in helping young people to choose a career. Furthermore, 50 students from technical colleges, studying biotechnology, computer science, electronics, and industrial chemistry, have in recent years spent their practical semester working at the Center.

Students of biology and medicine are applying in increasing numbers to spend their university vacations doing practical work at the Center. The most popular disciplines are molecular biology, biochemistry, immunology, and genetics.

The large number of trainees who undertake unpaid work at the Center demonstrates the high expectations placed on the practical work in the research laboratories in terms of the guidance it offers in choosing a career.

Continuing Education

For the staff of the Deutsches Krebsforschungszentrum continuing education is essential, since skills and knowledge are being overtaken by new advances faster than ever before. The spectrum of scientific endeavors and their aims has changed significantly in recent years. The ever-increasing complexity of the tasks of the Research Center places great demands on its staff. But the success of the Center depends strongly on the people who work there. Learning is itself a form of work and the willing ness of individuals to learn is an expression of their commitment to the Deutsches Krebsforschungszentrum. The systematic program of continuing education is thus an investment which, in the long term, is as valuable to the staff as it is to the Center. On the basis of a terms-of-service agreement, the staff of the Deutsches Krebsforschungszentrum are offered a wide-ranging continuing education program, which has so far been extended every year. On the one hand, it contains the courses that have proved they worth in previous years, and, on the other, it takes into account the changing needs and wishes of the staff by including, at the suggestion of the various organizational units, both subjects of general interest and specialist courses.

These aspects are reflected in the annually appearing program of continuing education and in the decisions about releasing staff from their duties in order that they can attend courses. The Center's continuing education activities include:

– specific measures to provide the staff with knowledge tailored to their individual needs

– measures to provide groups from various organizational units with the necessary training for coping with the constantly changing demands, and

– events aimed at improving cooperation and communication.

In the past year, approximately 1300 staff members took part in internal further education events; 337 staff took the opportunity to attend external events. These, it should be noted, do not include scientific lectures or meetings of the various research divisions or project groups.

The continuing education department is also intensifying its program of instruction for the more than 250 doctoral and diploma students, since their knowledge and skills play a decisive role in the overall performance and success of the Center.

The interdisciplinary seminars that form part of the graduate support program offer, for example, an introduction to the subject of laboratory animals including practical work or to biostatistics. They are very well attended by the young scientists, as are the events on more general topics, such as the preparation of scientific manuscripts or presentation techniques.

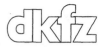

Advisor for Graduate Students

Very many students express interest in carrying out their diploma or doctoral projects at the Deutsches Krebsforschungszentrum. The number of applicants is between three and five times higher than the number of places available. The majority of applicants come from the University of Heidelberg, but there are also many from other German universities and a few from abroad.

The administrative statistics indicate that there were approximately 250 doctoral students at the end of 1996. About two-thirds of these were supported by the Center's own funds and the majority of the remainder by external grants. With a 60% contingent, men continue to form the larger group. The average age of the doctoral students is 29.3 years, the men with their average of 29.7 years being significantly older than the women at 28.6 years. In terms of academic discipline, the largest contingent are the biologists, who comprise about 60% of all doctoral students. The others include – in roughly equal numbers – medical students, physicists, chemists, pharmacologists, mathematicians, and computer scientists. This distribution reflects the stongly multidisciplinary nature of the Center. About 85% percent of the doctoral students graduate from one of the various faculties of the University of Heidelberg.

Since 1990, the doctoral and diploma students at the Deutsches Krebsforschungszentrum have benefited from the presence of a Graduate Student Advisor. Three major responsibilites are associated with this position:

– To advise applicants for diploma and doctoral work and put them in touch with the potential supervisors best corresponding to their own wishes and abilities;
– To organize the graduate program;
– To offer advice and support to students who have problems.

Advice to Applicants

The advice received from the Graduate Student Advisor has been well received in virtually all cases, since it is personal and, thus, effective. It has been possible to answer many questions in the preliminary stages of an application.

The Graduate Program

The Graduate Program operates on the basis of voluntary participation. Courses aimed at improving communications skills and the writing of scientific results have been particularly well received. There has also been great interest in the courses designed to improve methodological and theoretical skills and those offering insights into modern investigative techniques, subjects which appear to be somewhat neglected during a typical university education.

These aspects are thus given special attention, and this is achieved in collaboration with the working group for training and continuing education. But general scientific and cancer-research related subjects are not left unattended either. These subjects are covered in the lecture series on foundations and progress of cancer research, given by the divisional heads and senior scientists.

In a special event held at the beginning of each year, the doctoral and diploma students present their own research results. Additional incentives for participating are the travel grants that are awarded for exceptional results and for the best presentations.

Information events are organized with a view of establishing contact with industry. These give students insights into the employment practices in research, production, and marketing fields and help them to identify appropriate careers opportunities.

The students themselves have also undertaken various initiatives:

Working groups have been formed to discuss ethical questions that arise in the methods and applications of modern biology. These efforts resulted in panel discussions and lecture series that extended far beyond the confines of the Center and were accorded great acclaim. In the meantime a book containing the edited lectures from these events has been published. It bears the title "Gentechnik, Ethik und Gesellschaft" ("Gene technology, ethics, and society") and was published by Springer Verlag in Heidelberg. Another initiative was the organization of a graduate forum. Its aim was to strengthen the scientific and personal contacts among the doctoral students during a two- to three-day stay at a location well away from Heidelberg; here, without any "supervision", talks and discussions were held for and by the students.

The funding of the doctoral students represents a major problem. It is an undisputed fact that their energy and commitment make an essential contribution to the research achievements of the

Deutsches Krebsforschungszentrum. In relation to this, they receive very little financial recognition. With the support of the staff council, doctoral students started an initiative aiming to improve their financial situation. The new model was a compromise, which, from the point of view of the students, is still less than satisfactory. But the restrictions imposed on the sponsor and the currently weak economic climate mean that even the present proposals are being called into question. This situation is a problem not only for the Center; it also has a more wide-ranging impact on society. The inadequate support of the next generation is clouding the future for all of us. Although this problem has been recognized, much too little is being done to tackle it.

Wherever people work on the same premises and in close contact, there are bound to be occasional interpersonal problems. The doctoral students often find themselves in an inferior and confused position. In such cases the active support of an outside individual such as the graduate student advisor has proved to be immensely helpful.

Advisor for Graduate Students:

Prof. Dr. Eberhard Spiess

The Karl Heinrich Bauer Course Laboratory

Financed with the help of the Association for the Furtherance of Cancer Research in Germany, the Karl Heinrich Bauer Course Laboratory has provided teaching facilities since the end of 1992.

With a total floor-space of 250 qm, it allows courses on scientific methods to be offered to up to 25 participants. A main laboratory with laboratory benches is supplemented by a cell-culture laboratory, a refrigeration room, an equipment room, a radionuclide room, a darkroom, and a washing-up room. For carrying out experiments, the laboratory contains a full set of basic scientific equipment, which allows a wide-ranging application of cell- and molecular-biological techniques. The standard equipment includes sterile workbenches, incubators with controllable gas atmosphere, spectral photometers, ultracentrifuges, and refrigerated centrifuges; further accessories are automatic pipettes, water baths, ice-shavings machines, microbalances, and, for example, equipment which can be used to implement all common electrophoretic separation methods.

The main users of the laboratory are the scientists of the Deutsches Krebsforschungszentrum, who, as part of their often considerable teaching duties for the University of Heidelberg, take advantage of the facility for holding practical classes. Since the laboratory is authorized as a genetic engineering facility of security level 1, has permission for the use of radioactive substances, and is excellently equipped with modern apparatus, the scientists

who use it can demonstrate the practical routines needed in their own research to their students. The laboratory space is also available, to a more limited extent, for the teaching duties of members of the medical and natural sciences faculties of the University of Heidelberg.

The practical facilities are also used for international courses on experimental methods. A frequent purpose of such courses is to teach the participants special methods which make use of apparatus that is lent by the manufacturer. The manufacturer may also be involved in holding the course. A further advantage when carrying out such courses is

Fig. 117

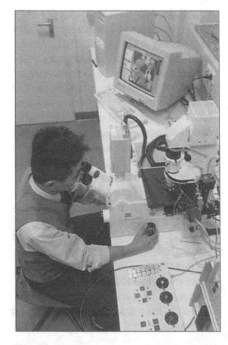

252

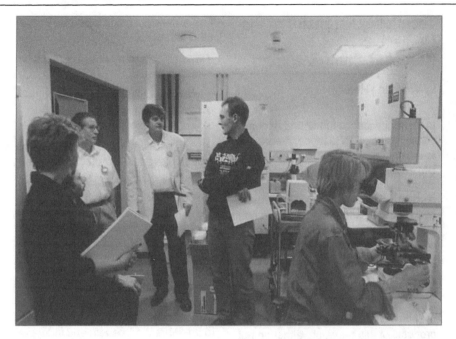

that the laboratory has direct access to the Communications Center of the Krebsforschungszentrum, which houses a lecture theater and seminar rooms.

The high level of demand means that the practical rooms are booked out during the semester and also heavily used in the vacations. Free slots are rented out to companies, which offer application-oriented courses in the use of their own new products to an international spectrum of customers.

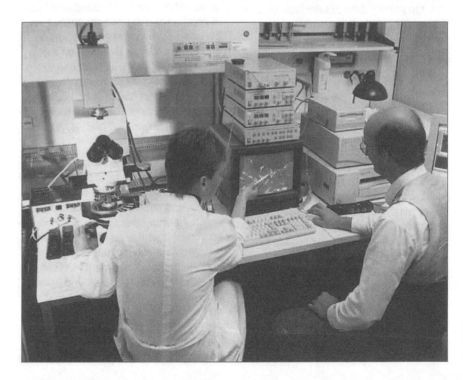

Figs. 117, 118, 119
Discussions and work in progress in the K.-H. Bauer Course Laboratory

17

Current Topics

Technology Transfer at the Deutsches Krebsforschungszentrum

by Wolfgang Henkel

In Germany, public funding of nonuniversity facilities for science, research, and development currently amounts to DM 13 billion annually. This support is motivated by the desire to provide a secure future for all citizens. The expectation is that, by supporting fundamental research (both pure and target oriented) and also applied research, results can be obtained that are of benefit to society and to the process of economic development. The patenting of ideas, the generation of useful know-how, and the issuing of licenses are valuable byproducts of this research: although not the top priority they are nonetheless an important indication of the success of government research funding.

Thus, the Deutsches Krebsforschungszentrum has for many years supported the efforts of the Federal Government to identify industrial applications of research results. It is true that the Deutsches Krebsforschungszentrum, as a facility for fundamental research, must necessarily give first priority to the publication of research results and to the communication of information and material within the constructs of scientific exchange. However, it also endeavors to achieve the protection of ideas and know-how whenever this can be usefully integrated into the work of the center. This is the case, in particular,

– when there are good prospects of economic exploitation because a commercial partner already exists or there are good chances of a success-

ful cooperation being achieved in the near future;

– when it is thereby possible to secure key positions;

– when the utilization of research results can thereby be accelerated, e.g., in developing therapies;

– when economic utilization can only be achieved by a protection of rights.

With this policy, the Deutsches Krebsforschungszentrum attempts to make the results gained from government funded research available for the benefit of the general public. It seeks openings for commercial exploitation and encourages its research results to be seen in this context, also with a view to finding new ways of financing future research work. Simultaneously, it seeks to preserve the freedom and independence of its fundamental research and to constantly delineate the boundary between commercial exploitation on the one hand and free research on the other. This is a difficult tightrope to walk, and one that demands great sensitivity. Success can only be achieved through a continual dialog between scientists, administrative parties, and industrial partners.

In order to fulfill these aims, the Deutsches Krebsforschungszentrum has for a long time been working closely with small, medium, and large companies within the framework of various cooperation and patent agreements. Information events involving patent attorneys and the patent departments of German research facilities have served in the past mainly to inform doctoral students and postdoctoral scientists about patent application procedures and the steps required to start up a company. A meeting held in spring of 1995 together

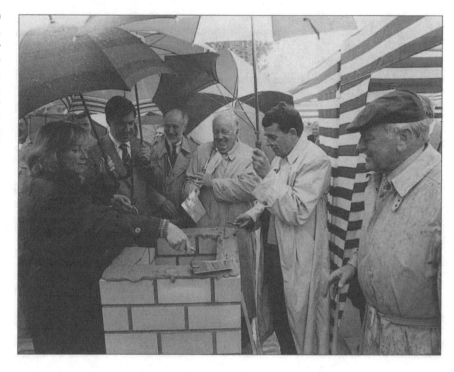

Fig. 120
The Mayor of Heidelberg, Beate Weber, Baden Württemberg's Minister of Economics Dr. Walter Döring, building contractor Roland Ernst, and the Managing Director of „Technologiepark Heidelberg GmbH" Dr. Klaus Plate, laid the foundation stone of a new building „Biopark" in the Heidelberg Technology Park on May 6, 1997

with the Heidelberg Chamber of Industry and Commerce served to establish contacts between science and industry; these are maintained by the quarterly „industry days" of the Heidelberg Technology Park, which have been held in the Center since then. The Deutsches Krebsforschungszentrum is a member of the association „Rhein-Neckar-Dreieck", which promotes communication and cooperation in this region between industry, scientific institutions, and the relevant public bodies. Furthermore, the Deutsches Krebsforschungszentrum had a decisive influence on the region's entry for the competition „Bioregio", organized by the Federal Ministry for Education, Science, Research, and Technology (BMBF), in which the Rhein-Neckar region was chosen as one of the three winning regions.

In terms of organization, the promotion of technology transfer at the Deutsches Krebsforschungszentrum is handled by a department of the Management Board. The department comprises a technology-transfer advisor who is a qualified scientist with several years' experience in industry and also the working group patents/licenses in the administration. These specialists are available to advise the staff of the Center in matters of patenting and to receive details of new inventions and register them for the Deutsches Krebsforschungszentrum. The further processing is taken care of by a firm of patent attorneys, which, on the initiative of the Deutsches Krebsforschungszentrum, opened a branch office in Heidelberg in 1997. This firm also supports the Deutsches Krebs-

forschungszentrum in its efforts to exploit the patents.

Following what is known as the MPG model (a scheme for rewarding inventors that was developed by the Max Planck Society), inventors at the Deutsches Krebsforschungszentrum receive as an incentive 30 percent of the net license income from an invention as an employee's reward. A further 30 percent go to the inventor's scientific group in order to strengthen the research activities in the Center, and the remaining 40 percent are assigned to the central funds.

As early as the 1980s the Deutsches Krebsforschungszentrum was already assisting young scientists in their efforts to exploit research results in their own companies: The new companies were

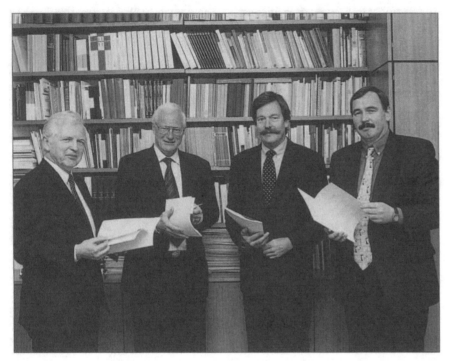

Fig. 121
Signing of a licensing agreement with the company Klinge Pharma GmbH of Munich for the use of patents on the chemotherapy of solid tumors (the coupling of cancer drugs to the carrier substance human serum albumin). From left to right: Prof. Dr. Harald zur Hausen, Scientific Member of the Management Board, Wolfgang Schoch and Dr. Wolfgang Tinhof, the two Managing Directors of Klinge Pharma GmbH, and Dr. Josef Puchta, Administrative Member of the Board

allowed easier access to research results and mutual assistance with personnel was offered for special laboratory techniques. These efforts have been intensified recently through initiatives to found Steinbeis Centers and through measures to support the starting up of joint ventures between economists and scientists. Furthermore, within the framework of the Bioregio concept of the Rhein-Neckar region, the Deutsches Krebsforschungszentrum has recently started to offer potential founders of new companies both theoretical and material support, the latter according to the stipulations of the sponsors, which are recorded in the memorandum on the support of the foundation of new companies from existing organizations and also in the guidelines of the BMBF of August 1996.

The Deutsches Krebsforschungszentrum welcomes all measures of sponsors which aim, through the provision of additional means – where appropriate linked to a specific purpose -, to facilitate the registration of patents and ensure the protection of rights. This creates the opportunity, in the preliminary stages of a commercial exploitation and without needing to tap research funds, to produce a pool of patent rights, the economic benefits of which often only materialize several years later.

Dr. Wolfgang Henkel
Head of Administration

Since March 1997 Dr. Ruth Herzog heads the newly established Office of Technology Transfer

Measurability of Research Quality? The Journal Impact Factor and Citation Analysis

by Rolf-Peter Kraft

In Germany, as in other countries, the reduced availability of research funds, an expert evaluation system that is overtaxed, and the obviousness of rank lists have led to an increased use of bibliometric methods to measure research quality. To assess the relevance of research conducted by scientists (in addition to other evaluation procedures) the publication history of the authors is used as a criterion with increasing frequency. The basis for most of these evaluations are citation studies that use the Science Citation Index (SCI) and other sources.

In the meantime the SCI is consulted in Germany when filling professorial positions, distributing research funds based on performance in publicly financed research facilities as well as in comparable facilities in private industry, or qualifying scientists to act as university lecturers. It is also used when presenting the annual or performance reports of research institutions and university clinics as well as when courting high ranking scientific journals. The index is used in broad areas of basic research, including biomedicine, in whose disciplines publications play an important role in fostering the exchange of scientific ideas.

Two almost arbitrarily selected press reports from the months of November 1996 through January 1997 permit one to suspect if not recognize the „boom" in the quantitative evaluation possibilities of research results. The German Press Agency reported on 11/28/96: The budget of the Federal Ministry for Research will „be reduced by almost 900 million to a total of 14.8 billion marks. This represents an excessive reduction of 5.6 percent…New political objectives (according to Rüttgers) in the form of more competitively oriented sponsorship of research are being established." And: „For subsidies, Bonn demands more performance from researchers…The HWWA (one of the economically oriented research institutes in the Federal Republic of Germany) and the work that it conducts appears to be endangered…The experts (of the Scientific Council) note that collaborative arrangements with academic institutions as well as publications in prestigious scientific journals are lacking there" (*Frankfurter Rundschau* on 1/7/97). The last citation directly leads to the topic at hand. The Science (as does the Social Science) Citation Index provides the numbers for evaluating journals in the natural (as well as social and economic) sciences.

The Science Citation Index

The Science Citation Index, founded in 1963, is one of the most comprehensive available databases of scientific literature. Currently, approximately 650,000 references to publications in the natural sciences, mathematics, and biomedicine are found therein each year. In addition to a list of sources and abstracts, it also contains the cited references from the appendix of the publications in question. The original idea behind this unique and specialized index in the natural sciences was the realization that scientific authors usually cite those studies that contain ideas or results that are used, developed further or disproved. The number of ascertainable citations in the database (or in the printed version) for a particular publication is viewed as an indication of the response it has garnered or the effect it has had among scientific colleagues.

The SCI encompasses a core of approximately 3,500 scientific journals. They contain more than 12 million citations each year. Exclusively so-called peer-review journals are included in the database; these journals only publish articles that have first successfully passed review by proven experts in the field. Especially prestigious journals (such as *Science*) usually reject up to 85 percent of the submitted articles on the basis of their quality guidelines. In this manner a sound, qualitative selection of publications usually occurs and this results in a corresponding selection of the contributions that are included in the SCI.

The Journal Impact Factor

An important byproduct of the Science Citation Index that has appeared since 1976 is the publication Journal Citation Reports (JCR). As in the case of the main index itself, it is published by the Institute for Scientific Information (ISI), a successful nonprofit organization in Philadelphia, Pennsylvania, USA. The founder of the institute is Eugene Garfield, chemist and librarian, and simultaneously forerunner and pioneer in the field of citation research and practice.

The Science Citation Index indicates which author is citing another author in a specific article. In the Journal Citation Reports this information is classified ac-

```
              Journal Citation Reports (JCR) on CD-ROM -- 1995 Science Edition
                        Journal Rankings Sorted by Impact Factor


        Journal                           1995    Impact  Immed.   1995     Cited
Rank    Abbreviation          ISSN    Total Cites  Factor  Index   Articles Half-Life
--------------------------------------------------------------------------------------
   1  *CLIN RES              0009-9279     1651    58.286             0        5.7
   2  *ANNU REV IMMUNOL      0732-0582     9088    49.509  3.333     24        4.4
   3  *ANNU REV BIOCHEM      0066-4154    17825    44.414  3.167     30        7.4
   4  *CELL                  0092-8674   139106    40.481  7.373    475        4.6
   5  *ABSTR PAP AM CHEM S   0065-7727       66    31.000  0.000      7
   6  *ANNU REV CELL BIOL    0743-4634     5223    30.548                      5.1
   7  *PHARMACOL REV         0031-6997     6013    30.387  1.800     15        5.8
   8  *ANNU REV NEUROSCI     0147-006X     5552    29.083  3.600     20        5.3
   9  *NAT GENET             1061-4036    15056    28.543  7.161    180        2.0
  10  *NATURE                0028-0836   257287    27.074  6.043    945        6.2
  11  *IMMUNOL TODAY         0167-5699    12127    25.228  2.752    101        3.6
  12  *NEW ENGL J MED        0028-4793   103033    22.412  4.913    413        6.4
  13  *MICROBIOL REV         0146-0749     6439    22.098  1.552     29        5.7
  14  *SCIENCE               0036-8075   203375    21.911  4.738   1037        5.6
  15  *PHYSIOL REV           0031-9333     9132    20.545  1.357     28        8.1
  16  *TRENDS NEUROSCI       0166-2236    11190    19.972  3.111     81        4.8
  17  *ENDOCR REV            0163-769X     6097    19.921  2.613     31        5.1
  18  *REV MOD PHYS          0034-6861    10112    19.407  1.235     17      > 10.0
  19  *ADV IMMUNOL           0065-2776     3333    19.000  1.810     21        6.2
  20  *GENE DEV              0890-9369    23474    18.793  2.762    248        3.6
  21  *TRENDS PHARMACOL SCI  0165-6147     9391    17.556  2.220     50        4.4
  22  *LANCET                0099-5355    89957    17.490  3.929    490        6.3
  23  *TRENDS BIOCHEM SCI    0968-0004    11769    17.217  2.898    108        3.9
  24  *NEURON                0896-6273    22885    16.619  2.395    271        3.7
  25  *BEHAV BRAIN SCI       0140-525X     2579    15.625  0.600     20        7.5
  26  *CA-CANCER J CLIN      0007-9235     1639    15.500  7.857     21        3.0
  27  *IMMUNITY              1074-7613     1653    15.354  2.730    141        1.3
  28  *J EXP MED             0022-1007    55708    15.126  2.516    461        5.0
  29  *CHEM REV              0009-2665    14913    14.513  0.966     88        6.5
  30  *STRUCT BOND           0081-5993     1145    14.000  1.667      6      > 10.0
```

Fig. 122
Extract from the Journal Citation Reports 1995, section Journal Rankings by Impact Factor, which gives the frequency of citations of the original articles published in a particular journal and the resulting impact factor for that journal

cording to specific journals. In this manner one can tell which journal was cited most frequently. Since the number of citations depends on the number of articles published in a particular journal (the greater the number of published articles, the more frequently they can be cited elsewhere), Garfield calculates the so-called „impact factor". In German, this can best be translated as the „influence factor" (Einflußfaktor) or the „journal range" (Zeitschriften-Reichweite). It is calculated as the quotient of the number of citations that refer to articles in a journal and the number of arti-

cles that were published in this journal. For example, if 1,000 citations were registered as referring to articles in a specific journal and this journal, itself, published 100 articles, the impact factor of this journal is 10. The ranking shown in Figure 122 for the reproduced Table of Journals forms the basis for evaluating scientific journals. The relative number expressed as the impact factor for each particular journal, analogous to the citation frequency of an author, serves as an indication of the respect or reputation that a journal has in its field.

The impact factor for a journal in the year 1995 includes those citations that were counted in 1995 and that referred to journal articles published in the previous two years (1993 and 1994) divided by the number of articles that appeared in the same journal during 1993 and 1994. This definition is based on the (not always applicable) assumption that the typical article is cited most frequently during the two years following its publication. The relatively short time period assures that newly appearing journals can quickly be included in the ranking without significantly affecting the validity of the number in a negative manner.

The immediacy index provides information about the quickness with which articles in a journal, on average, are cited or about the time delay since an article has been published. It only includes citations that refer to articles published in the same year. Journals that have a high immediacy index generally attract the attention of authors who are especially interested in rapidly making their research results known to others.

Especially for evaluations in the field of library science, the so-called half-life of a journal (Fig. 122) is of interest. It refers to the age structure of the citations of a given periodical and describes that time period, from the perspective of the current year, in which 50 percent of all the citations of this journal are to be found. It approximately represents the loss of value that a journal exhibits over time. Within certain limits, the half-life can correlate with the scientific field of the journal.

Of special significance for authors are the lists of the scientific disciplines of journals arranged according to impact factors. They enable one to see at a

```
                Journal Citation Reports (JCR) on CD-ROM -- 1995 Science Edition
                        Journal Rankings Sorted by Impact Factor
                              (Filtered by CELL BIOLOGY)


       Journal                            1995      Impact  Immed.   1995     Cited
Rank   Abbreviation          ISSN      Total Cites   Factor  Index  Articles  Half-Life
----------------------------------------------------------------------------------------
   1   *CELL                0092-8674    139106     40.481  7.373    475      4.6
   2   *ANNU REV CELL BIOL  0743-4634      5223     30.548                    5.1
   3   *EMBO J              0261-4189     59817     13.505  2.281    638      4.6
   4   *TRENDS CELL BIOL    0962-8924      2704     12.748  2.104     77      2.3
   5   *J CELL BIOL         0021-9525     65782     12.480  2.078    514      6.0
   6   *MOL CELL BIOL       0270-7306     55869     10.498  2.206    751      4.4
   7   *MOL BIOL CELL       1059-1524      3997      9.376  1.246    134      2.7
   8   *NAT STRUCT BIOL     1072-8368      1458      8.738  2.293    140      1.3
   9   *STRUCTURE           0969-2126      1409      8.082  1.462    143      1.5
  10   *ONCOGENE            0950-9232     16403      7.991  1.041    608      3.2
  11   *CURR OPIN STRUC BIOL 0959-440X     2487      7.376  0.942     86      2.6
  12   *INT REV CYTOL       0074-7696      3762      5.292  0.276     29      9.3
  13   *CRIT REV ONCOGENESIS 0893-9675      443      4.940  0.500      4      2.8
  14   *J CELL SCI          0021-9533     11757      4.827  0.820    377      4.0
  15   *MATRIX BIOL         0945-053X       880      4.375  0.167     36      3.5
  16   *CELL DEATH DIFFER   1350-9047        97      4.250  0.813     32
  17   *CELL GROWTH DIFFER  1044-9523      2663      4.179  0.486    179      3.1
  18   *J BIOENERG BIOMEMBR 0145-479X      1823      4.102  0.390     59      3.9
  19   *AM J RESP CELL MOL  1044-1549      3986      4.014  0.571    170      3.4
  20   *DNA CELL BIOL       1044-5498      3335      3.788  0.342    111      5.0
  21   *EXP CELL RES        0014-4827     13084      3.525  0.410    400      7.3
  22   *RECEPTOR CHANNEL    1060-6823       234      3.516  0.438     16      1.9
```

Fig. 123
Extract from Journal Citation Reports 1995, section Subject Category Listing by Impact Factor, for some of the cell biology journals

Fig. 124
Extract from Journal Citation Reports 1995, section Subject Category Listing by Impact Factor, for the journals on medical computing

```
                Journal Citation Reports (JCR) on CD-ROM -- 1995 Science Edition
                        Journal Rankings Sorted by Impact Factor
                           (Filtered by MEDICAL INFORMATICS)


       Journal                            1995      Impact  Immed.   1995     Cited
Rank   Abbreviation          ISSN      Total Cites   Factor  Index  Articles  Half-Life
----------------------------------------------------------------------------------------
   1   MED DECIS MAKING     0272-989X       785      2.082  0.317     41      6.0
   2   ACAD MED             1040-2446      1380      1.090  0.214    248      3.4
   3   STAT MED             0277-6715      2043      1.084  0.241    191      5.5
   4   ARTIF INTELL MED     0933-3657        92      0.850  0.040     25
   5   INT J TECHNOL ASSESS 0266-4623       400      0.726  0.083     60      5.1
   6   M D COMPUT           0724-6811       192      0.704  0.640     25      4.2
   7   INT J BIOMED COMPUT  0020-7101       321      0.667  0.088     91      4.0
   8   METHOD INFORM MED    0026-1270       367      0.631  0.543     46      4.8
   9   MED BIOL ENG COMPUT  0025-696X      1325      0.551  0.179    145      8.3
  10   MED EDUC             0308-0110       673      0.543  0.146    103      6.7
  11   BIOMED TECH          0013-5585       167      0.478  0.180     50      5.3
  12   IEEE ENG MED BIOL    0739-5175       156      0.352  0.011     91      4.8
  13   MED INFORM           0307-7640       118      0.344  0.000     14      5.4
  14   COMPUT METH PROG BIO 0010-468X       594      0.264  0.000     91      9.9
  15   J MED ENG TECHNOL    0309-1902        98      0.200  0.000     16
  16   INT J CLIN MONIT COM 0167-9945        91      0.185  0.000     23
  17   J AM MED INFORM ASSN 1067-5027         9      0.027  0.028     36
```

glance the high ranking periodicals of a specific scientific field and answer one of the questions most frequently asked of the Science Citation Index: what significance do the journals in which a certain author or a research group publishes have? Figure 123 shows an extract of journals in cell biology with the associated impact factors; it begins with the journal „Cell" which has an average citation frequency of 40 per article within two years. In contrast, the list for medical informatics (Fig. 124) begins (with the title „Medical Decision Making") at an impact factor of two. This discrepancy indicates in an exemplary manner the completely different citation practices (and publication rates) within individual scientific disciplines, even within the framework of the biological sciences. Therefore, it is impossible to compare the citation rates of journals from different disciplines (as well as of authors from different scientific fields). Comparisons on the basis of a journal's impact factor and the personal citation frequency are exclusively allowed and valid within the limits of a particular scientific discipline.

Citation Analysis

The second question that is frequently asked of the indices is: What rank does an author (from a bibliometric viewpoint) occupy in his discipline? As mentioned, the main work, The Science Citation Index, should be used to answer this question. Simply adding the impact factors of all the journals in which an author has been published hardly proves adequate for such an evaluation. The author profited (or suffered) from the good reputation (or the poor reputation) of the other authors who also published in the same scientific journal. On the other hand, the number of citations of his publications by others as indicated in the SCI volume (citation section) or the database version proves to be an adequate measure for this purpose (compare Fig. 125). The SCI gives the author's name in capital letters and beneath this in bold letters his cited publications that fall within the time frame of the index. The listing for each publication begins with the year of publication, the name of the journal in international abbreviated form, volume and page number; the names of the citing authors or publications follow in normal letters. Citations in books are not included in the index.

The extract shown for the author, J. F. Holland, and his citations in Figure 125 received a value of 18. His ten publications between the years 1989 to 1993 are cited 18 times. This includes one citation by the author himself and a double citation by one of his scientific colleagues.

The following will indicate some of the weaknesses and traps inherent in this procedure. This contains the implicit question to what extent is the expressed respect for another author that is given in the form of a citation (publication, research results) to be equated with scientific significance or quality. If these are to be regarded as equivalent, it would be a mandatory prerequisite for citations to be made purely on a factual or scientific basis. However, publishing scientists know that the citing of other publications, as a social act, is not only determined by purely factual or scientific concerns.

Scientists cite themselves or under certain circumstances form so-called citation cooperatives that exclude other au-

```
HOLLAND JE
80 4TH INT C EXP SOILS     1   302
   CHENG Y      SOIL SCI SO   57 1542 93
HOLLAND JF
89 AUST J EXP AGR    29   843
   FELTON WL     AUST J EX A    34  229 94
   LAWRENCE PA   SOIL TILL R    28  347 94
91 REV SCI INSTRUM    62   69
   BURLINGA.AL   ANALYT CHEM    66 R634 94 R
   COULSON LD    APPL SPECTR    48 1125 94
   DODONOV AF    ACS SYMP S    549  108 94 R
   HOLLAND JF      "          549  157 94 R
   MIRGOROD.OA   ANALYT CHEM    66   99 94
   WOLLNIK H     INT J MASS    131  387 94
92 AUST J AGR RES    43   123
   GARSIDE AL    AUST J EX A    34  647 94
93 CANCER MED    p1
   JAIN RK       SCI AM        271   58 94
   LUK GD        ALIM PHARM      7  661 93
   ZUHOWSKI EG   J CHROMAT B   655  147 94 N
93 CANCER BIOL    p1
   OLIVERO OA    CANCER RES     54 6235 94
93 CANCER MED    p618
   GUTHEIL JC    J BIOL CHEM   269 7976 94
93 CANCER MED    p1182
   BEAUREGA.P    TR MED REV      8  184 94 R
93 CANCER MED    v1
   OVERBEEK F    EUR J NUCL     21  997 94 R
93 J CLIN ONCOL    1   75
   FENNELLY D    SEMIN ONCOL    21   21 94
93 41TH P ANN C AM SOC  A 14
   BURLINGA.AL   ANALYT CHEM    66 R634 94 R
HOLLAND JG
58 SCIENCE   128   61
   SEE SSCI FOR 1 ADDITIONAL CITATION
   TAKAHASH.M    BEHAV PROC     32  133 94
```

Fig. 125
Extract from the Science Citation Index 1994 showing some of the entries for the author J. F. Holland

thors in order to further certain schools of thought. Such groups pose the potential danger of selecting and, thereby, benefiting those individuals who are most well-known. Completely new areas of research require an inordinately long time before they are taken up by others and are cited. Young scientists generally cannot demonstrate a comparable citation frequency to that of authors with academic careers that have lasted many years. Finally, reviews (summarizing research reports) and methodical studies have an unusually high chance of being cited.

Several of these difficult to assess factors can be excluded by the methodical improvement known as the science impact index (SII) which was developed by Siegfried Lehrl. The SII excludes re-

views, self-citations, and multiple citations by other authors (as an indication of a citation cooperative) within one year. According to the SII, the citation value of Holland in the chosen example (Fig. 125) is not 18 but is instead 16. Showing consideration for young authors, in comparative studies the publication time-frame (underlying the citation rate) can be limited to the active time of all the considered publishing authors. In this manner the SII contributes to an objective statistical acquisition of data and an optimized comparability of citation rates.

Furthermore, the continuing development of citation studies permits the establishment of standards for specific fields of scientific endeavor. In 1991 Lehrl determined the average field-specific citation frequency per year for West German authors in medical disciplines. They ranged (in the non-clinical area) from 1.7 for individuals in the field of nuclear medicine to 10.1 for immunologists.

Generally, one can state that the reliability of citation studies significantly in-

Fig. 126
Model of the relationship between the quantitative (publication rate) and qualitative aspects of research capacity (from S. Lehrl)

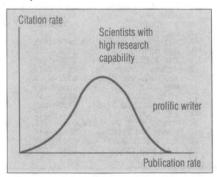

creases with the number of scientists and publications that are included (or with the size of the corresponding „scientific community") and to this extent has gained widespread acceptance. In small, specialized fields of study, falsifying influences can have a much more noticeable effect, because of the small size of the database. As representative of the two opposite extremes, one can name the fields of molecular biology and genetics on the one hand and medical informatics on the other hand. Under the named preconditions, the validity of citation analysis is much greater than the simple publication rate (compare Fig. 126).

The basic prerequisite for attaining high citation rates is naturally publishing in English, the worldwide recognized scientific language in the natural sciences and biomedicine. Articles that are published in German, for example in biomedical basic research, are a priori clearly at a disadvantage.

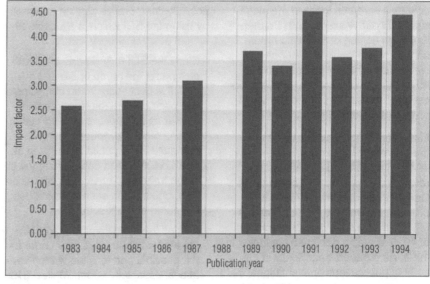

Fig. 127
Average impact factor of the scientific journals (1983-1994) in which scientists from the Deutsches Krebsforschungszentrum have published their results. Note: The Krebsforschungszentrum is a multidisciplinary research facility which involves disciplines with typically high impact factor journals (for example, cell biology) and disciplines with lower impact factor journals (for example, medical computing)

Citation Analysis in Practice

In Anglo-American countries the discussed quantitative procedures have been accepted for roughly 20 years. They complete the evaluation of scientists and research groups by committees of experts (peer reviews) as well as the assessment according to the relative amounts of acquired additional funding.

The Scientific Council in Bern has for several years used this procedure to evaluate the performance standard of their own Swiss research endeavors. The Federal Research Report issued by the German Federal Minister for Science and Technology mentions this procedure in positive terms for the first

time in 1993. At the Deutsches Krebsforschungszentrum appropriate analyses are used in addition to (or as part of) peer reviews conducted as part of an evaluation by experts. Using the journal impact factor in 1994/95, a study was conducted that examined the publication behavior of authors at the Cancer Center over time. It indicated that at the center there existed a clear trend to publish in high ranking journals (compare Fig. 127). Within the Helmholtz Association of German Research Centers, additional facilities have begun using citation analyses in their evaluation procedures.

Furthermore, citation studies can be conducted to comparatively evaluate the performance of research facilities or

even to assess the competence in a specific scientific discipline at the level of entire (federal) states. The research group of the ISI continuously publishes smaller and more comprehensive analyses, rankings of authors or current, highly-cited, so-called „hot papers" in the journal Science Watch. It also publishes specialized products such as the Topical Citation Report or the National Science Indicators. Studies on the basis of the SCI are conducted in Germany by the German Central Library for Medicine in Cologne and the Institute for Scientific and Technical Research (IWT) at the University of Bielefeld among other institutions. The results of the IWT, especially with regard to the effectiveness and the influence of German research institutions, appear regularly as a research index in the magazine, *Bild der Wissenschaft* (German language edition of Scientific American). Also the journals, *Science* and *Nature,* consistently present remarkable findings. Most of the named publications are available in the Central Library of the Center.

In the library, the Science Citation Index is available in printed form from 1945 until 1994 and as a database (available to all PCs connected to the Center's intranet) from 1988 to the present day. Journal Citation Reports (JCR) are available in printed form as of 1976 and as a database beginning in 1994. As required, specifically in the case of publications or evaluations, every staff member has access to appropriate information. In doubtful cases consulting the JCR with its impact factors can prove advisable for an author since it is known that 90 percent of all citations in biomedicine are concentrated in 10 percent of all the journals. More than 40 percent of the published articles included in the SCI do not receive more than one citation. In biomedicine (including basic research), one should strive to have articles published in journals with an impact factor of more than three. Values that range from one to three represent average recognition levels. Issues relevant to exceptional disciplines have been discussed. These fields can be seen in the specialty field lists of the JCR.

The Central Library supports staff members with advice and assistance in compiling personal citation analyses and naturally (if necessary) in seeking out suitable journals with high impact factors before submitting articles for publication. A few tips are given below that pertain to compiling personal or possibly comparative citation analyses by using the SCI which is available at almost every university library:

– Since the SCI only reports cited articles under the name of the first author, it is necessary when compiling a complete citation rate for an author, insofar as he appears as a co-author among other individuals, to use the complete list of published articles as one's basis. When determining the citation frequency of each individual article, one must in each instance use the name of the first author.

– Names that contain an umlaut (Möller, etc.) must be looked for under all the possible and feasible written variations, especially under „Moller" (US written convention) and „Moeller".

– In the case of double names (e.g., Alsen-Hinrichs), it can occur that the second component of the name is simply omitted or is combined with the first component. To avoid missing relevant information, both of these written conventions must be considered.

– First names are written with initials. Hans-Günter becomes „HG". To be on the safe side, the variation „H" should also be considered. Hyphens that are commonly used in German are omitted.

– Several authors having the same name (e.g., D. Meyer, H. Schulz) can be differentiated by using the scientific discipline, the address and, when nothing else helps, the list of published articles.

A final comment: As impossible as it is for ambitious scientists to avoid the dictum of „publish or perish", they will in the future very much (also on the „European continent") have to deal with the journal impact factor and citation analysis. However, these quantitative methods cannot replace traditional qualitative and subjective procedures such as peer reviews or evaluations by recognized experts. They are intended to supplement conventional procedures and as needed - between comprehensive evaluations - to provide „momentary snapshots" of the recognition that individual scientists or research groups have attained among their scientific colleagues. Not least important is the fact that using the discussed procedures requires that scientific articles be published in English which in turn contributes to the competitiveness of German biomedical research on an international, worldwide level.

Rolf-Peter Kraft, M. A.
Central Library

Selected publications

Science Citation Index: an international multidisciplinary index to the literature of science, medicine, agriculture, technology, and the behavioral sciences. ISI Press, Philadelphia (1945 ff.)

Science Citation Index, annual: Journal Citation Reports; a bibliographic analysis of science journals in the ISI data base. ISI Press, Philadelphia (1976 ff.)

Garfield, E.: Citation indexing: its theory and application in science, technology, and humanities. Wiley, New York (1979)

Bundesbericht Forschung 1993, Hrsg.: Bundesministerium für Forschung und Technologie, Bonn (1993)

Lehrl, S.: Der Science Impact Index als Maß der Durchsetzung sowie der Forscherqualität und -kapazität von Wissenschaftlern. Anwendung und Güteeigenschaften. Media Point Verlagsgesellschaft, Nürnberg (1991)

Kahl, M.: Zitatenanalyse mit den Journal Citation Reports des Institute for Scientific Information. Bibliothek, Forsch. u. Praxis 19, 30-63 (1995)

Korwitz, U.: Welchen "Rang" hat ein Wissenschaftler? Nachr. f. Dok. 46, 267-272 (1995)

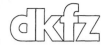

Evaluation of Scientific Work – Criteria and Structures

by Harald zur Hausen

Where financial resources come predominantly from the tax payer, their expenditure – also on research – must be accompanied by proof that they are being usefully employed. But what is „useful" in research and what is not? And who is able to exercise control and document performance?

In the following I shall attempt, using the example of the Deutsches Krebsforschungszentrum, to address these questions, although I do not claim that all of the points possess general validity.

As a National Research Center, the Deutsches Krebsforschungszentrum has a definite research responsibility: through its investigations of the causes of cancer, their mechanisms, and of prevention, diagnostics, and treatment, to make a contribution to solving the problems of cancer. This task puts certain restrictions on the freedom of the scientists working here, although it is the policy of the Center that these restrictions should not be viewed too narrowly. It is particularly research at the periphery of a particular discipline that has often proved to be the most fruitful, even though its relevance to the main task may not always be immediately obvious.

How can one assess whether research is consistent with the primary aims? Furthermore, how can one identify criteria which accurately represent the scientific performance and, indeed, the performance in relation to the expenditure involved?

In science at least there are generally accepted standards: The first criterion is the list of publications, an indication of whether a scientist was able to publish his or her results in scientific journals with their strict „peer review" system (anonymous evaluation by independent experts). Generally speaking, the harsher its refereeing system, the better the reputation of the journal. The impact of a particular paper on the field as a whole can be quantified by the number of citations which it receives in the years following its publication.

In a strict sense, this is of course not an objective criterion: the importance of a new and original idea or a completely new experimental result will not always be understood immediately and may even be overlooked by the scientific community. This risk is clearly larger when the work is published in a lesser-known journal – and perhaps only in German.

Another criterion for success is the acquisition of external funding. In cancer research, such resources stem predominantly from the German Research Association (Deutsche Forschungsgemeinschaft, DFG), the German Cancer Aid (Deutsche Krebshilfe), the European Union, the Federal and State Ministries, private foundations, and from industry, and are generally granted on a competitive basis to the best applicants. The greater the competition, the stricter are the selection criteria, and thus the higher the prestige associated with an award. Not all such funds are awarded competitively: for example, when a research program is of interest to the pharmaceutical industry, the latter may spontaneously offer financial support if the results promise to be commercially useful.

Another point relates to the successful establishment and leadership of a research group. In general, scientific achievement is the result of teamwork, i.e., the collaboration of scientists among one another and with the technical staff. This requires both the planning of experiments and the provision of detailed scientific advice. The successful completion of doctorates and of „habilitation" theses are valuable indicators of a good team, but even more important are the team spirit and the enthusiasm with which the group members pursue their joint aims. This, again, is not an unambiguous and objective criterion, but nonetheless has an influence as an additional factor in the full evaluation.

Finally, it should be said that a scientist ought to be able to present a comprehensible and justifiable concept for the work he or she is pursuing. This should display, on the one hand, an awareness of the problem at hand, and, on the other, sensible ideas about how to tackle it within the constraints of the available or expected financial means.

Young scientists at the start of their careers will have to be granted a certain advantage, and their original ideas cannot be judged against a background of previous achievements alone.

The evaluation measures described above are the basis of a multifaceted system of evaluation at the Deutsches Krebsforschungszentrum which is carried out at three levels: the external evaluation of the Research Programs, the internal divisional presentation, and the annual performance-related award of resources.

For the past 14 years external evaluations at the Deutsches Krebsforschungszentrum have taken place every 5 years, originally of its individual institutes and, since their dissolution, of the various Research Programs. For this purpose the scientists prepare extensive documentation in English describing their previous work, future plans, utilization of resources, and sources of external funding. This material is presented to the assessors well in advance. The assessors themselves number between eight and twelve and are all experts of international repute, principally from English-speaking countries. They are selected by an independent committee, the Scientific Committee of the Board of Trustees, and they come to Heidelberg to spend 2,5 days studying and familiarizing themselves with the performance of the relevant Research Program. They conclude their assessment with a written report detailing the strengths and weaknesses of the program; this together with a number of specific recommendations goes to the Management Board and to the Scientific Committee. The groups concerned have the opportunity to respond to the report, which usually, after further discussion by internal bodies, leads to changes that largely correspond to the recommendations made.

The internal divisional presentations, which likewise have a 14-year history, follow a quite different procedure: originally with a frequency of every 2 years, due to the increased number of divisions, they now usually affect each division only every 3 years. These „inspections" always involve the Scientific Member of the Management Board, and the members of the Scientific Council are also invited to participate. Particularly important is the participation of 4 scientists from the Center, who, together

with the Management Board, decide upon the performance-related distribution of resources. The inspections require this group, approximately every 14 days, to spend one afternoon informing themselves about the work and aims of a particular division. It is an intention of the internal presentations that the young scientists should also have a chance to speak. Apart from the list of papers published since the last inspection, a list of personnel, and information about external funding, no other written documentation is required and thus the effort involved for the division is not excessive. No written report is produced following these inspections: Sufficient opportunity for criticism is provided by the subsequent discussion, and individual conversations with the heads of division are the basis for any suggested changes.

External assessments and internal presentations are only useful if they have consequences. These may include, for example, special support of groups judged to be working well and even the founding of new divisions as a positive signal and, at the other end of the spectrum, curtailing of staffing, materials, and investment resources, reduction in space available, or even – in the most negative case – the closure of a division. All these measures have been taken at one time or another as a consequence of this evaluation procedure.

When carrying out the recommendations arising from both the external evaluation and the internal inspection, a special role is played by the small group of scientific representatives of the Center who, together with the Scientific Member of the Management Board, are responsible for determining the standards for the annual distribution

of performance-related resources. This involves a detailed discussion for every division and every research group of how well it satisfies the above-mentioned criteria, and also considers its publications list for the previous year. The result is the assignment of one of five evaluation grades to each group or division. The lowest grade leads to a significant reduction in the amount of support received, and the highest to an analogous increase. This comparative evaluation is not made public, but each group may obtain its result.

The measures described here may not always be sufficient to guarantee a just evaluation of each individual case. Every such procedure is sure to have certain weaknesses. However, when individual evaluations take place every year, this makes it easier to correct any isolated injustices, the consequences of which are then less severe.

The extensive and costly system of evaluation that the Deutsches Krebsforschungszentrum employs has had a number of consequences for the Center that go far beyond the assessment of individual projects. It has strengthened the staff members' conciousness of their performance and thereby led to a healthy self-confidence; it has also resulted in an objectively definable improvement in performance and, above all, has promoted the national and international reputation of the Center. The assessment of the research by top scientists from abroad, who, despite occasional, and even harsh, criticism, have to date almost always gone away with a very positive impression of the activities of the Center, has in the event turned out to be one of the most significant measures leading to the international acclaim of the Center's performance.

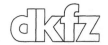

Who can contribute more to the recognition of scientific achievement in cancer research than internationally renowned scientists from this field?

Assessment and evaluation are not static processes: they need to be consistently continued (and also monitored by the Center's management and governing bodies). In their dynamics they offer the best guarantee of the useful employment of resources, and also an assurance and improvement of the quality of scientific work. At the Deutsches Krebsforschungszentrum they provide the basis for fulfilling its mission of discovering the causes of cancer and the factors that induce it, of preventing the occurrence of cancer, and of contributing to the welfare of cancer patients.

Prof. Dr. Dr. h.c. mult. Harald zur Hausen
Chairman and Scientific Member
of the Management Board

18

Press and Public Relations

The Media

In the field of public relations, the years 1994, 1995, and 1996 were characterized by a sustained interest of journalists in the work of the Deutsches Krebsforschungszentrum, particularly in questions related to genome research, genetic research, and cancer chemoprevention – a newly established field of research at the Center. During this time, about 700 interviews with scientists, background talks, and shootings for TV productions were organized. In addition, about 2 500 inquiries from journalists and about the same number coming from the general public and institutions received. Some journalists were referred to interview partners from the Deutsches Krebsforschungszentrum and elsewhere; others were sent printed material or given information on relevant sources. The Office of Press and Public Relations issued 155 press releases informing about scientific advances, structural and staff changes, scientific symposia, and prizes awarded. All these activities found a strong echo in the press: Adding up the copies of all newspapers and magazines which reported on the Deutsches Krebsforschungszentrum, one finds a total of 100 to 120 million copies each year.

Among the eight press conferences organized in the period covered, those held in 1995 and 1996 focusing on research into the human genome had special priority. In 1995, on June 11 and 12, about 50 science and medical journalists from all over Germany were given the opportunity to learn about projects in genome research and matters relating to a participation of the Deutsches Krebsforschungszentrum in a federal support program for genome research. The press seminar ended with a discussion with Dr. Jürgen Rüttgers, Federal Minister of Education, Science, Research, and Technology, on aspects of the promotion of genome research in Germany and its international integration. Furthermore, Dr. Rüttgers and the journalists were given presentations of several projects on the premises.

More in-depth information on genome research was presented at the International Human Genome Meeting of the Human Genome Organization (HUGO) held from March 21 to 24 1996 in Heidelberg, where the Press and Public Relations Office was in charge of the international press activities. On the occasion of this meeting, three press conferences were held for representatives of the national and international media. Alongside the accompanying press releases, the press office also prepared a series of seven background papers on the different aspects of genome research which were discussed at this meeting by participants from all over the world. For this conference alone, 80 interviews and discussions between journalists and scientists were arranged. Topics of the press conferences were „Ziele und Inhalte der Genomforschung" (Objectives and Contents of Genome Research), „Gesellschaft und Gene - Determiniert die Genforschung die Zukunft unserer Gesellschaft?" (Society and genes – Will Genetic Research Determine the Future of Our Society?) and „Krankheit und Gene" (Disease and Genes). More than 80 journalists made use of the facilities provided for them and attended the conference.

One of the highlights of the media coverage was the international sympo-

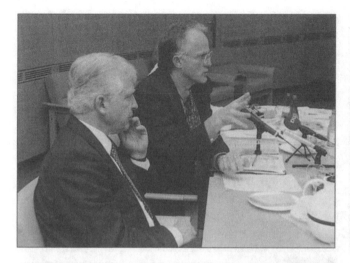
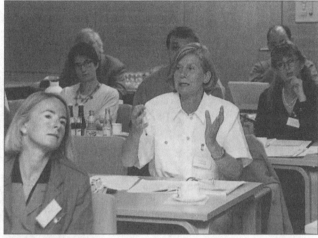
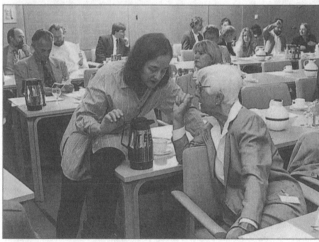
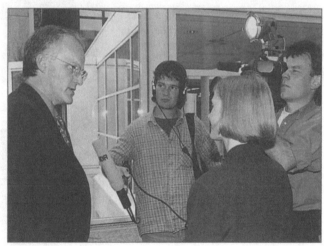

Figs. 128, 129, 130, 131
In 1995, a two-day information event on the topic of genome research was organized for journalists. At the accompanying press conference dealing with the promotion of genome research in Germany and its international integration, Federal Research Minister Dr. Jürgen Rüttgers talked about his plans and ideas

sium on „Krebschemoprävention: Molekulare Grundlagen, Mechanismen und Studien" (Cancer chemoprevention: Molecular Bases, Mechanisms, and Studies) from September 9 – 11, 1996, which was accompanied by a press conference on September 10. More than 100 press folders with written material were supplied and also sent out on request. The interest shown in the topic of chemoprevention is also linked to the European study „Krebs

und Ernährung" (Cancer and Diet) - a study carried out by the Deutsches Krebsforschungszentrum in Heidelberg investigating possible connections between dietary habits and the occurrence of cancer.

In 1993, the Deutsches Krebsforschungszentrum established the Wolfgang Rieger Grant intended to support a sound media coverage of scientific issues and at the same time to provide

267

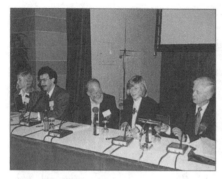

Fig. 132
Opening of the 1996 Human Genome
Meeting in Heidelberg. In the center: the
Mayor of Heidelberg, Beate Weber

Figs. 133, 134
Opening press conference (from left to
right): Prof. Dr. Gert-Jan van Ommen,
Vice-President of HUGO Europe, Prof. Ha-
rald zur Hausen, Chairman of the Manage-
ment Board of the Deutsches Krebsfor-
schungszentrum, Hilke Stamatiadis-
Smidt, Head of the Division of Press and
Public Relations, Prof. Bernd Sutherland,
President of the Human Genome Organ-
ization, and Prof. Kay E. Davies, who
chaired of the scientific organization
committee for the Heidelberg meeting

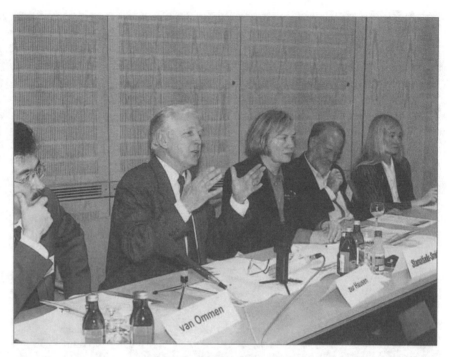

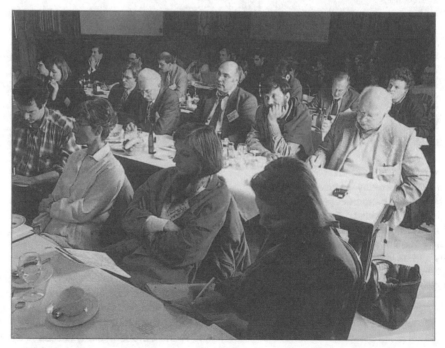

further training for science and medical
journalists. Recipients visit the Center's
laboratories for a period of one to four
weeks and are given a chance to acquire knowledge on molecular-biological techniques and methods. The grant
is awarded within the framework of the
„European Initiative for Communicators
of Science (EICOS)"- a program of the
Max Planck Society. In 1994, the grant
was awarded for the first time to two
foreign journalists from Hungary and
Spain. In 1995, two journalists from

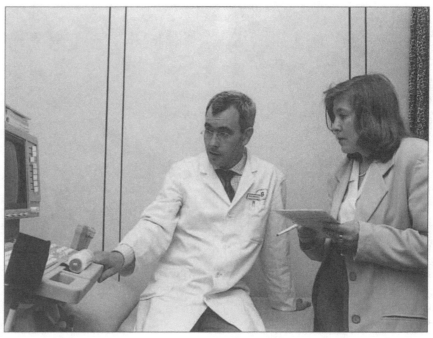

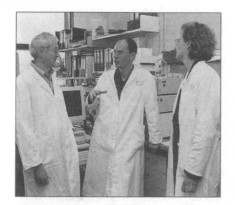

Fig. 135
The work of the Division of Toxicology and Cancer Risk Factors was of particular interest to Holger Hank from the radio station Deutsche Welle in Cologne (center). Here he discusses scientific issues with Dr. Norbert Frank and Dr. Clarissa Gerhäuser during his fellowship stay in 1997

Fig. 136
Dr. Yekaterina Kalikinskaya, science journalist from Moscow, in conversation with Dr. Stefan Delorme, Division of Oncological Diagnostics and Therapy

Fig. 137
The science journalists Dan Stoica from Bucharest (right) and Susanne Lilli Bräm-Leemann from Zürich (seated) seen during their research visit at the Division of Immunogenetics headed by Prof. Dr. Bernard Mechler (center)

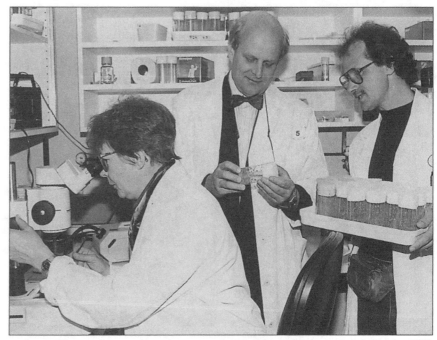

Switzerland and Romania visited the Center's laboratories to do research and receive further training. In 1996, the grant went to two female science journalists from Russia and Germany. The recipients considered their stay as extremely useful for the news coverage in their respective home countries. Another important aspect is that the jour-

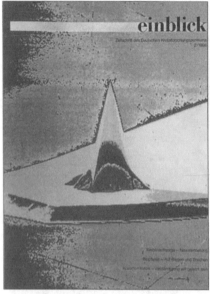

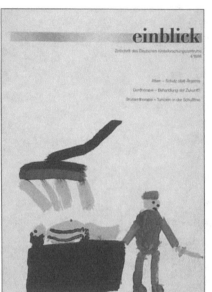

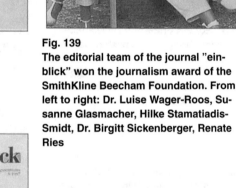

Figs. 138a, b, c, d
Cover pages of the journal "einblick"

Fig. 139
The editorial team of the journal "einblick" won the journalism award of the SmithKline Beecham Foundation. From left to right: Dr. Luise Wager-Roos, Susanne Glasmacher, Hilke Stamatiadis-Smidt, Dr. Birgitt Sickenberger, Renate Ries

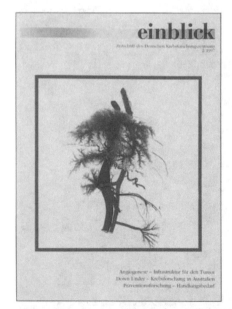

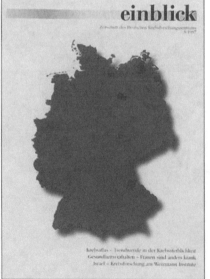

nalists are given the opportunity to come into contact with scientists from a wide variety of research areas.

The Journal „einblick"

In 1995, the Center's journal „einblick" won the journalism award of the SmithKline Beecham Foundation in Göttingen. Particularly acclaimed was the manner in which „einblick" translates results of basic medical research into a language and form that can readily be understood by the general public. The prize was awarded on the basis of

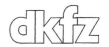

the issue „einblick – Gene und Krebs" (English version: einblick - Genes and Cancer), a project supported by the European Union, which was carried out in cooperation with the Imperial Cancer Research Fund (ICRF) in London. For the first time ever this prize was awarded to a publication of a government financed institution.

In the period of this report, 11 issues of „einblick" appeared. The demand for subscriptions is exceptionally high, making it necessary to constantly increase the number of copies produced. In 1996, on the occasion of the journal's tenth anniversary, a double issue - the issue 1/1997 - was produced. This issue was devoted primarily to the transfer of research results obtained at the Center into clinical practice and industrial exploitation. Also on this occasion of the journal's anniver-

Fig. 140

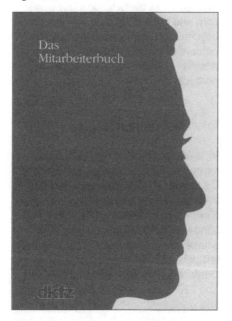

Fig. 141

As a means of internal communication, the press office issues a monthly eight page newsletter comprising news and information of interest to the staff

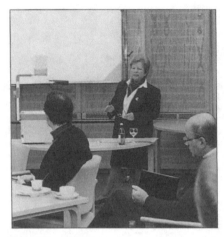
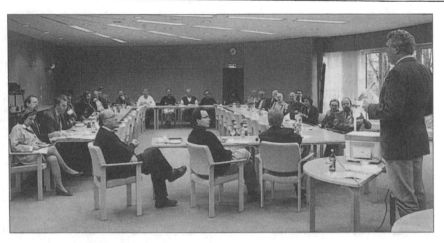

Figs. 142 a, 142 b
Elfriede Egenlaut (left) and Priv.-Doz. Dr. Hans-Peter Meinzer lecture at a "jour fixe". Elfriede Egenlaut talks about possibilities of project-related financing, Dr. Meinzer about the foundation of a Steinbeis Center for Medical Computing

sary, „einblick" carried out a survey among its readers through a questionnaire enclosed in issue 4/1996. The questionnaire was returned in time by 1024 readers, i.e., 14 percent of the journal's subscribers. 72 percent of the respondents read „einblick" out of private interest, 62 percent for professional reasons (multiple answers were possible). 60 percent of the readers are men, of which three quarters have a university degree. One half of the female subscribers attended university. All other types of further education were represented equally. Two thirds of the participants indicated in the questionnaire that they have a basic or advanced (professional) knowledge of medicine and/or the natural sciences. Nearly every fifth subscriber is or was a cancer sufferer, and more than half of the respondents have a cancer patient in their family. 90 percent rated the readability of the articles as good or even very good. At the same time, 96

percent said that „einblick" teaches them new things. 18 percent of the readers work in research, 13 percent at educational establishments, 11 percent are journalists, 11 percent treat cancer patients, 8 percent work in the psychosocial field, 7 percent provide information about cancer for the public, 4 percent work in administration, and the remainder did not give any details. 4 percent are currently employed at the Center, another 4 percent worked there in the past; 3 percent are cooperation partners of the Center, while 46 percent indicate that they have no connections with it. 50 percent of the respondents are between 20 and 50 years old, the other half is over 50. As many as 75 percent of the readers pass the journal on to family members, friends, acquaintances, or colleagues. 97 percent consider the activities pursued in cancer research as justified, 85 percent would even like to see them intensified. The subscribers are most interested in fun-

damental oncological research. With 80 percent readership, the articles on this topic are read the most, followed by articles on new therapies and diagnostic methods, risk factors, cancer prevention, and early diagnosis. Articles on psychosocial assistance are read by 55 percent of the respondents, those on alternative treatment methods by 46 percent.

Internal Communication

In 1995, much effort was devoted to improving communication within the Deutsches Krebsforschungszentrum. With the help of trainees and in cooperation with the Center's Division of Personnel and Social Affairs, a booklet whose title translates as „Das Mitarbeiterbuch – Leben und Arbeiten im Deutschen Krebsfor-schungszentrum: The DKFZ from A to Z" was conceived and published. Its aim is to provide

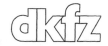

Fig. 143
Tapestries by Yolande von Plato

Fig. 144
As part of a series of events entitled "Art and Science", Gisela Debatin presented her figurines from Fayence

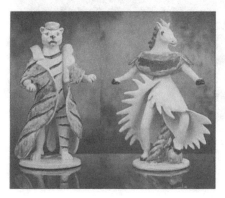

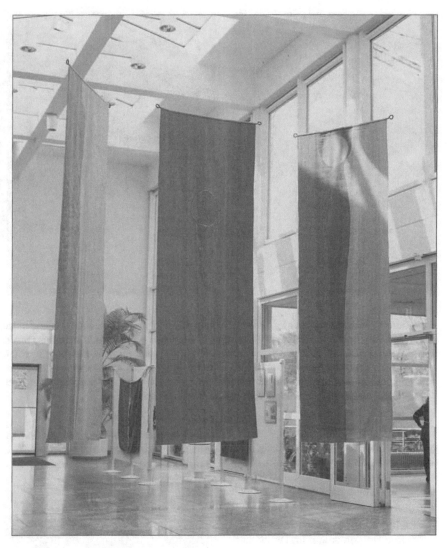

staff members with readily understandable information in an appealing layout, thus making it easier, particularly for new staff members, to access the Center's services or to inform themselves about regulations, responsibilities, etc. A loose-leaf enclosure, which is updated regularly, lists in-house contact persons with their room and telephone numbers. In addition, the internal newsletter „dkfz intern" was conceived and first published at the end of 1995. „dkfz intern" generally comprises eight pages, which are produced via desktop publishing. It is issued monthly and contains news and information from the areas of science and administration which could be relevant for the staff. Currently, „dkfz intern" has a circulation of 2 100. It is distributed to every staff member and also to interested retired staff of the Center.

Alongside these tools of internal communication, the Center's Press and Public Relations Division compiles a list of „Biowissenschaftliche Vorträge im Heidelberger Raum" (Bioscientific Lectures in the Heidelberg Area). This list is updated every two weeks, and, since 1996, has also been available via Internet (www.dkfz-heidelberg.de/kid/kol-

loq.htm). Also about every two weeks, a press digest („Pressespiegel") featuring topics of current public interest is published. It contains press clippings from the following categories: news coverage of the Deutsches Krebsforschungszentrum, local news, research policy, research and health, cancer, environment, and smoking. The press di-

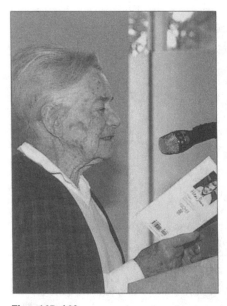 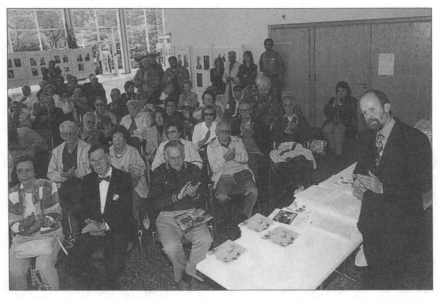

Figs. 145, 146
Hilde Domin read from her poetry on the occasion of a visit by former Jewish fellow citizens of Heidelberg at the exhibition „Entlassen – die vertriebenen Heidelberger Dozenten" („Dismissed – the exiled Heidelberg professors"). Dr. Wolfgang Henkel (on the right of the picture) gave an overview of the exhibition's history and content. When this exhibition had been shown first in Rehovot, Israel, visitors were struck by how the injustice and discrimination was hidden behind the banalities of daily life. The exhibition will remind and encourage the young generation to stand up for the civil rights of the individual, and to maintain the integrity of the German Constitution, which was created after the fall of the Third Reich

Fig. 147
The art teacher Ludwig Schmeisser from the Heidelberg Bunsen-Gymnasium presents the drafts submitted by his pupils for the artistic decoration of the patients' area at the Deutsches Krebsforschungszentrum

gest is compiled by analyzing daily, weekly, and monthly newspapers, magazines, and articles on cancer which are provided by a press clipping service.

Furthermore, the working group „Arbeits- und Betriebskultur im Deutschen Krebsforschungszentrum" (Working Climate and Corporate Culture at the Deutsches Krebsforschungszentrum) was founded in 1994. Since then, the working group has assessed the situation and tackled the question of how to improve the working climate. The resulting concept involving staff members in key positions and „multipliers" includes specific proposals for appro-

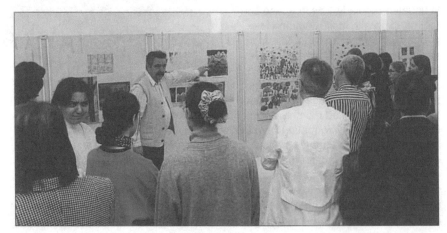

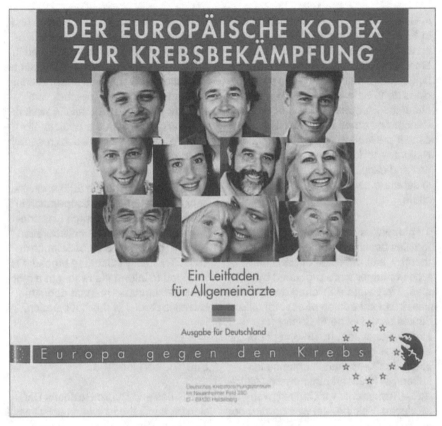

Fig. 148
A European project to inform practicing doctors in Germany about the possibilities for prevention and early diagnosis of cancer

priate measures was worked out and was scheduled to be discussed within the Center and implemented in 1997. During the conceptional phase, the press office and the staff department already launched several initiatives. Thus, since 1996, there has been a monthly „jour fixe" for the heads of department to meet and discuss topics of general interest or current affairs. The measures proposed by the working group relate to questions of employee guidance, communication, and aspects concerning the working environment.

The art exhibitions which have been organized by the press office since 1981 also form part of the internal communication. They are also aimed at furthering contacts between Heidelberg citizens, cooperation partners, and former and present staff members of the Deutsches Krebsforschungszentrum. At the same time, young artists are given the opportunity to present their work to a large audience. The years 1994, 1995, and 1996 saw 15 such exhibitions, some of which were characterized by a focus on contemporary history or science.

One of the highlights was the exhibition „Entlassen - die vertriebenen Heidelberger Dozenten" (Dismissed – The Exiled Heidelberg Professors), which was initiated by Dr. Wolfgang Henkel and presented on the occasion of a visit by former Jewish fellow citizens of Heidelberg in the framework of Heidelberg's 800-year jubiliee in 1996. This exhibition illustrated the harm done by the persecution of Jewish scientists at Heidelberg University. It was based on investigations conducted by the Heidelberg historian Dr. Dorothee Mußgnug. „Heilen mit schweren Teilchen" (Healing with Heavy Particles) was the topic of a touring exhibition of the European Center for Nuclear Research (CERN) that was shown at the Deutsches Krebsforschungszentrum in the same year. A photo exhibition documented the humanitarian commitment of a female physician working for the organization „Ärzte für die Dritte Welt" (Physicians for the Third World) in Calcutta.

In 1996, the Deutsches Krebsforschungszentrum also continued its cooperation with the Bunsen Gymnasium in Heidelberg, which was started several years ago. In their art lessons, pupils designed a concept for the painting and artistic decoration of hallways and rooms frequented by cancer patients for diagnostic and therapeutic purposes. In March 1997, the drafts submitted by pupils of all ages were presented in the foyer to staff members of the Deutsches Krebsforschungszentrum.

Internet

On its home page (www.dkfz-heidelberg.de), the Deutsches Krebsforschungszentrum describes its aims and gives details about the research focuses in the various divisions. The press releases issued by the Center are also available on the Internet (www.dkfz-heidelberg.de/presse/). In order to better respond to the growing demand for cancer information by the general public, the Deutsches Krebsforschungszentrum asked the US National Cancer Institute (NCI) for a licence to distribute selected information from the American cancer information system PDQ (Physician Data Query). Basic information about the various types of tumors, their diagnosis, and standard therapy is being translated into German and should be available on the Internet in 1997. These texts will provide initial information, e.g., for those citizens who fail to reach the telephone Cancer Information Service (KID) at peak times.

Publications

The brochure „Die zehn Regeln zur Bekämpfung des Krebses und ihre wissenschaftlichen Grundlagen" (The Ten Rules for Fighting Cancer and Their Scientific Background), of which 40 000 copies were published for the general public with European Union funds, went out of print in a very short time. Thereafter, financial support was solicited from the European Union for another brochure aimed at informing general practitioners. This project was carried out in cooperation with 5 other European partners from France, Great Britain, Ireland, and Italy. On the occasion of the „European Week Against Cancer"

in October 1995, general practitioners in 13 European countries were provided with a total of 500 000 copies of this brochure, which was translated into 10 languages. The booklet gives physicians up-to-date scientific information about the European Codex for Fighting Cancer and about the possibilities for cancer prevention and early diagnosis. National activities in the field of prevention and early diagnosis are described in separate national parts of the brochure.

12 pamphlets for patients and their families dealing with the diagnosis, therapy, and aftercare of particular types of tumor were produced by KID staff. They were published and distributed in a total edition of several million copies by the Federal Center for Health Education. In 1996, a set of brochures of a new type entitled „Betroffen? – Behandlungsmöglichkeiten bei Krebserkrankungen" (Afflicted? – Treatments for Cancer) was produced. This project was carried out jointly by the Deutsches Krebsforschungszentrum, the Cancer Information Service KID, the Charité in Berlin, the company Lilly Deutschland GmbH, the Institute and Outpatient Clinic for Psychosomatic Medicine, Psychotherapy, and Medical Psychology in Munich, the Psychosocial Advisory Center in Trier, the Robert Rössle Clinic in Berlin, and the hospital „Mutterhaus der Borromäerinnen" in Trier. The project entitled „Sprechende Medizin" (Speaking Medicine) is aimed at intensifying communication between practicing doctors and patients and their relatives in the field of oncology and at providing the specialist background needed for this purpose. In addition, KID has started a complete revision of

the book „Thema Krebs - Fragen und Antworten" (Subject Cancer – Questions and Answers), first published in 1993. The revised edition will again be published by Springer-Verlag, Heidelberg and New York. Together with freelance science journalists, work is underway to produce a book intelligible to nonspecialists about research on the human genome.

A brochure marking the 20th anniversary of German-Israeli cooperation in the field of cancer research was conceived and produced in collaboration with the Israeli Ministry of Science in 1997. The richly illustrated brochure is intended to inform the reader in a readily understandable manner about the scientific results of this cooperation.

Information Booths

The Press and Public Relations Division presents the individual activities of the Deutsches Krebsforschungszentrum by organizing information booths at selected conferences. In 1994 and 1995, the Center was represented at the Hanover Fair, where it presented information about genetic engineering and about two projects relating to new approaches in cancer therapy. Information booths were also organized, e.g., at the 1994 and 1996 German Cancer Conferences in Hamburg and Berlin, at the „Interhospital" Fair, and at the 1995 X-Ray Conference in Würzburg. In addition, the Cancer Information Service (KID) was represented with information booths at eight events in various places, including Heidelberg, Mannheim, Hamburg, Berlin, Wiesbaden, and Bielefeld.

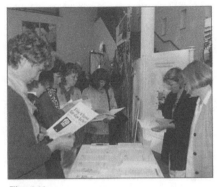

Fig. 149
Patients receiving information at the booth of the Cancer Information Service KID at a Patients' Day.

Fig. 150
Dr. h.c. Diemut Theato (center) and Dr. Renate Heinisch, Members of the European Parliament, accompanied by Werner Pfisterer, Member of the Baden-Württemberg State Parliament, learned about new methods of irradiation from Otto Pastyr, engineer in the Division of Medical Physics, and Dr. Dr. Jürgen Debus, senior physician in the clinical cooperation unit "Radiotherapeutic Oncology"

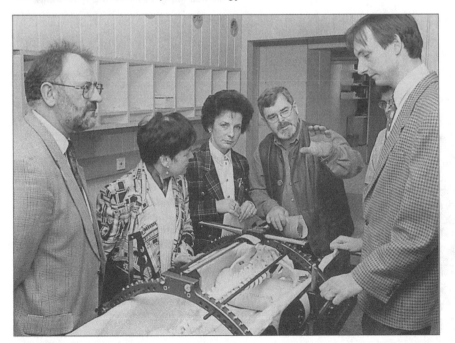

Organization of Events

In 1994, the Press and Public Relations Division prepared and organized a meeting of scientists holding key positions at the Deutsches Krebsforschungszentrum at Reisensburg castle. Their task was to plan the Center's research program for the next five years. In 1994, 1995, and 1996, the press office also supported the organization of 39 scientific symposia and events, of which the following deserve special mention: the Human Genome Meeting in March 1996, organized in cooperation with the European Office of HUGO in London, and the 1997 Jubilee Symposium on the occasion of the 20th anniversary of the cooperation between the Deutsches Krebsforschungszentrum and scientific institutions in Israel. In addition, the press office supervised and undertook the public relations activities for the following prize presentations: the Meyenburg Prize, the Walther and Christine Richtzenhain Prize, the Dr. Emil Salzer Prize, and the Ernst von Leyden Prize (see the chapter „Evaluation of Results and Main Research Objectives").

Visitors' Service

The visitors' service within the Press and Public Relations Division endeavors to offer groups and individuals visiting programs tailored to their particular interests. In the years 1994 to 1996, about 3 000 visitors were given the opportunity to learn about specific aspects of the research program of the Deutsches Krebsforschungszentrum in lectures, discussions or first hand in the Center's laboratories, and to meet scientists from various disciplines. For instance, 10 Pupils' Forums entitled „Krebsforschung heute - Wissenschaftler im Gespräch mit Schülern" (Cancer Research Today – Scientists in Dialog with Pupils), which were specifically geared to high-school pupils, were organized. These forums comprise not only lectures on topical and interesting areas (such as AIDS and research into cancer prevention), but also a two hour visit to the laboratories or discussions with the scientists about their training and their day-to-day work in research. The Pupils' Forums were complemented by a series of events under the banner „Ohne Rauch geht's auch" (No

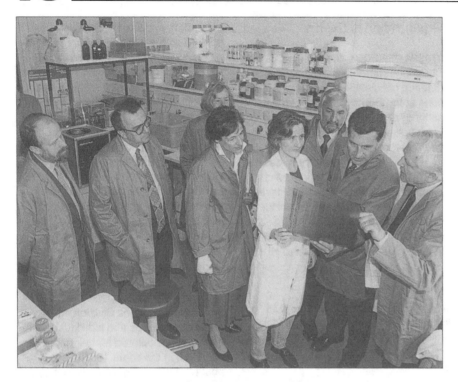

Fig. 151
Information visit by members of the parliamentary group of the CDU in the Baden-Württemberg State Parliament and the State Press Association. Prof. zur Hausen explains special features of a viral genome to the chairman of the parliamentary group, Günther H. Oettinger

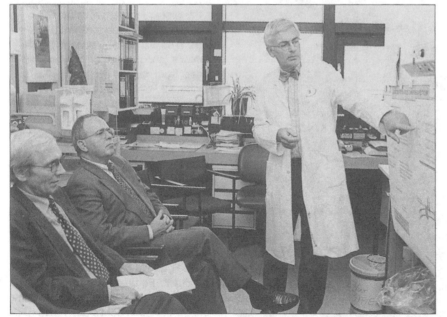

Fig. 152
State Secretary Dr. Fritz Schaumann of the Federal Ministry of Education, Science, Research, and Technology, accompanied by Dr. Michael Hackenbroch, assistant secretary at the ministry, learns from Prof. Dr. Manfred Wießler, head of the Division of Molecular Toxicology, about a new method to improve chemotherapeutic cancer treatment, which is being developed in cooperation with the company Asta Medica until it is approved for clinical use

Smoke - More Fun). Organized in schools in the city of Heidelberg and the surrounding area, these events were aimed at supporting the schools' endeavors to educate pupils about the long-term harmful effects of smoking. They usually comprised three lectures or dialog based presentations of the scientific-medical knowledge of the effects of smoking. In 1995, seven such events took place in cooperation with 6 high schools for pupils aged 10-18.

Special information forums for patients and former patients, the majority of which are organized in self-help groups, present new developments in oncology or current standards in diagnosis and therapy for various tumor forms. The six Patients' Forums organized in the years 1994, 1995, and 1996 met with exceptional interest among the target audience. Members of self-help groups outside Heidelberg traveled for up to two hours by bus to attend the forums. The Deutsches Krebsforschungszentrum considers these forums as a model that could inspire other medical institutions, in particular the Tumor Centers.

In 1995 and 1996, four events for biology and physics teachers, hospital nursing staff, and medico-technical assistants were organized.

In terms of numbers, the press office has primarily taken care of visiting groups from the Heidelberg area, organizing special information events to cater for their particular professional or personal interests. In this way, the local people recognize the significance of this national research center for life in this region.

Among the groups and individuals who visited the Center were Edelgard Bul-

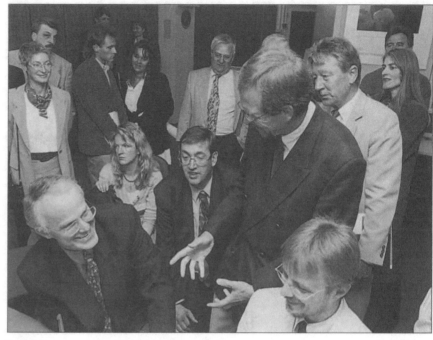

Fig. 153
Federal Research Minister Dr. Jürgen Rüttgers, accompanied by the Member of Parliament Dr. Karl A. Lamers and a group of science journalists, discusses the possibilities associated with the three-dimensional radiotherapy planning developed at the Center with Prof. Dr. Wolfgang Schlegel, Head of the Division of Medical Physics

Fig. 154
Visit by Prof. Dr. Gustavo Kouri, President of the Pedro Kuori Institute in Havanna, Cuba, accompanied by Jörge Fuchs of the German Academic Exchange Service. On the right of the picture: Priv.-Doz. Dr. Valerie Bosch

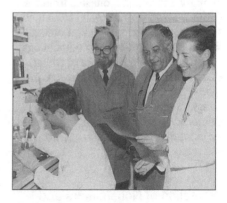

mahn, Gudrun Schaich-Walch, and Dr. Karl Lamers, Members of the Bundestag; Dr. h.c. Diemut Theato and Dr. Renate Heimisch, Members of the European Parliament; Helga Solinger, Minister of Employment, Health, Family, and Social Affairs of the State of Baden-Württemberg; Werner Pfisterer, Member of the Landtag of Baden-Württemberg; Dr. Jürgen Rüttgers, Federal Research Minister; Josef Dreier and Dr. Fritz Schaumann, Parlia-

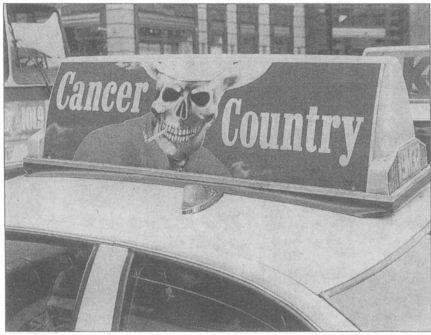

Fig. 155
The movement for the protection of non-smokers is gaining ever more ground in the US; in Germany, the "Coalition Against Smoking" is fighting for a pan-European ban on the advertising of tobacco products

mentary Secretaries; officials from the Federal Science and Health Ministries; science attachés from foreign embassies in Bonn; high-ranking delegations from the People's Republic of China, Russia, Japan, India, and Mexico. In November 1996, Princess Dr. Chulabhorn Mahidol of Thailand visited the Center for the second time, in particular to learn about research into cancer risk factors.

Protection of Nonsmokers and Tobacco Prevention

At a meeting on 26th November 1996, attended by scientists, doctors, and public relations experts, the „Heidelberg declaration on tobacco prevention for children and young people in Germany" was elaborated under the guidance of the Deutsches Krebsforschungszentrum, among other things, as a means of supporting a law to protect nonsmokers. This declaration was made widely known in parliamentary and executive circles and was also received with great interest by the media. On the same day, Prof. Dr. Klaus Hurrelmann from Bielefeld spoke at the Center about the current state of knowledge concerning tobacco prevention among children and young people. This was part of an event attended by more than 300 teachers, parents, and ex-

perts from the field of public health. The Deutsches Krebsforschungszentrum continues to be involved in the „Koalition gegen das Rauchen" („Coalition Against Smoking"), which was founded in 1992 and now has more than 100 members. The third meeting of the Coalition in 1994 addressed the topic of „Armut und Rauchen in Deutschland" (Poverty and Smoking in Germany) and the 1995 event was a symposium „Ärzte gegen das Rauchen? Ärzte gegen das Rauchen!" (Doctors against Smoking) dealing with the special cancer prevention tasks of doctors in private practice. The publicity activities for both events were undertaken by the Deutsches Krebsforschungszentrum. In 1996 the Coalition held its symposium on the topic of legislation to protect nonsmokers. In order to extend our present knowledge about ways of informing children and young people of the dangers of smoking and about the influence of the family way of life, a survey was made in 1996 in Heidelberg and the Rhein-Neckar region, in which 3852 children between 9 and 11 years of age were asked about their attitudes to health and their life style. The basis for this survey was a model questionnaire of the American Health Foundation (President: Prof. Ernest Wynder). It is intended that the results yielded in the USA survey should be compared with the results of the Heidelberg survey. The results will give guidance for target-group specific education and help in drawing up recommendations for institutions concerned with health information. The Coalition Against Smoking is represented in the European Network for Smoking Prevention by a member of staff from the Press and Public Relations Division of the Deutsches Krebsforschungszentrum. This network replaced the Anti-Tobacco Working Group of the European Union in 1996. Another member of staff from the Center's press office was appointed in the same year as the German representative on the Advisory Board of the European Network, Young People and Tobacco.

The active support of trainees in the field of scientific journalism and public relations plays an essential role in making possible the wide spectrum of activities. In the years 1994 to 1996, there were again 28 trainees working in the department. These included, among others, 18 biologists, a biochemist, a physicist, an economist, and a graphic designer. The trainees, whose major activity is assisting with the production of the journal „einblick", become involved in the day-to-day work of the department and support its staff particularly by gathering information, in journalistic tasks, and in looking after journalists. The usual stay for a trainee is between three and six months and, thereafter, these people often rapidly find a position in the press and public relations department of another institution, or in journalism.

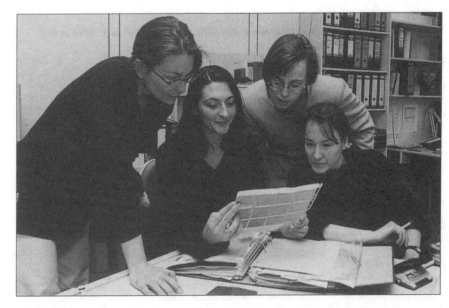

Fig. 156
Trainees usually spend three months at the Office of Press and Public Relations, gaining practical editorial experience. Without their additional help, the regular publication of the journal "einblick" would hardly be possible. The editors Dr. Claudia Walther and Monika Mölders (from left to right, back row) discuss the selection of photos for one of the issues with the trainees Christine Hesse and Kerstin Ansorge (from left to right, front row)

The Telephone Cancer Information Service (KID: Krebsinformationsdienst)

A new and effective concept in health care is the availability of individual information on the telephone. An example of the successful implementation of this scheme in Germany is the Cancer Information Service (KID: Krebsinformationsdienst) at the Deutsches Krebsforschungszentrum.

KID was founded in 1986 with the aim of providing information to help people overcome both their disease and the day-to-day problems that it entails. KID thereby attempts to reduce the fears and prejudices and to support the patients' own activities. Over the years it has become a bridge between the scientific world of the specialists and the general public. To provide comprehensible, up-to-date, and complete factual information in this sensitive area of medicine, on the one hand, and, on the other hand, to facilitate access to the institutes throughout Germany that offer care and support - these are the tasks which KID has set itself in its work.

KID is financed as a project of the Federal Ministry of Health. Since 1989 it has also received support through an annual contribution from the State of Baden-Württemberg. KID has been operating since 1986 in the Deutsches Krebsforschungszentrum and is integrated in the Tumor Center Heidelberg/Mannheim.

The year 1996 was KID's tenth year. The Deutsches Krebsforschungszentrum took this opportunity to host a gathering of all the institutions that cooperate with KID and also representatives of the Federal Government, the State, hospitals, practicing doctors,

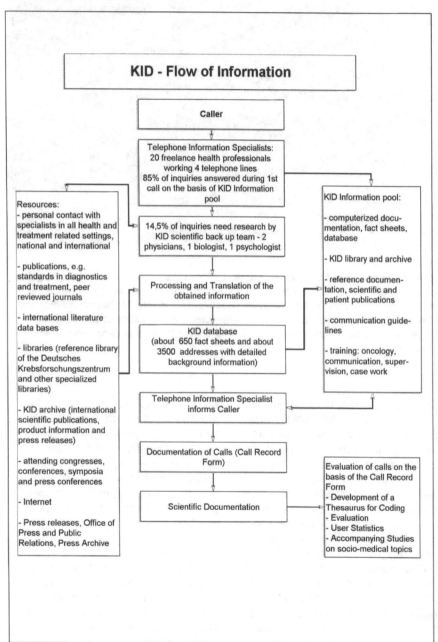

Fig. 157
The sequence of search steps involved in answering the question of a caller to the Cancer Information Service

KID - Flow of Information

Caller

Telephone Information Specialists:
20 freelance health professionals
working 4 telephone lines
85% of inquiries answered during 1st
call on the basis of KID Information
pool

Resources:
- personal contact with specialists in all health and treatment related settings, national and international

- publications, e.g. standards in diagnostics and treatment, peer reviewed journals

- international literature data bases

- libraries (reference library of the Deutsches Krebsforschungszentrum and other specialized libraries)

- KID archive (international scientific publications, product information and press releases)

- attending congresses, conferences, symposia and press conferences

- Internet

- Press releases, Office of Press and Public Relations, Press Archive

14,5% of inquiries need research by KID scientific back up team - 2 physicians, 1 biologist, 1 psychologist

Processing and Translation of the obtained information

KID database
(about 650 fact sheets and about 3500 addresses with detailed background information)

Telephone Information Specialist informs Caller

Documentation of Calls (Call Record Form)

Scientific Documentation

KID Information pool:

- computerized documentation, fact sheets, database

- KID library and archive

- reference documentation, scientific and patient publications

- communication guidelines

- training: oncology, communication, supervision, case work

Evaluation of calls on the basis of the Call Record Form
- Development of a Thesaurus for Coding
- Evaluation
- User Statistics
- Accompanying Studies on socio-medical topics

self-help groups, and the media. All these parties have assessed the performance of KID in educating and informing the public; their joint conclusion is that KID is an indispensable instrument for ensuring access to the various sources of cancer care available within the health system.

Information for Conquering Disease

A large number of studies have shown that information can be supportive in the process of overcoming disease. Patients who felt themselves to be insufficiently informed were more liable to complain of experiencing discrimination and neglect on account of their cancer in their daily life and their jobs.

Efficient communication involves personal interaction, with consideration of the other person's affiliation to social groups that may have specific forms of speech and behavior. The closer the relationship between the provider of the information and the recipient in terms of their dialogue, the easier it becomes for them to understand one another. Particularly information which relates to complex life situations can scarcely be communicated as objective knowledge without considering its relation to the individual situation of the person or group concerned and without the possibility of a dialogue. Attempts that ignore this simply don't get through.

KID Provides Individual Information

In this sense KID serves an important function as a supporting measure: The particular strengths of this service lie in

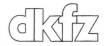

the personal information and in being able to react to needs expressed in a conversation. The medium chosen for this purpose, i.e., the telephone, offers the necessary potential for direct communication and an individual response to the enquirer, who may, if he or she wishes, remain anonymous. KID considers itself as a „turntable" for up-to-the-minute information in the field of oncology; KID does not dispense advice and does not express its own opinion. Rather, it passes on the latest scientific knowledge and, indeed, also a picture of topics that are still scientifically controversial. In this way, it aims to create a basis which enables the caller to arrive at his or her own decisions, both through self-determination and through two-way communication with the responsible doctor. It is not the aim of KID to replace communication with the doctor; it tries, instead, in the initial stages of such discussions, to assist in clarifying the questions to be addressed.

The Service:

– is known through the media, which publish the telephone number;
– supplements reports in the media about cancer by providing background information;
– evaluates and interprets this information for the individual caller;
– draws attention to pamphlets published by the various organizations and/or evaluates these;
– can be a part of intervention campaigns which attempt to achieve increased use of early diagnosis measures and to draw attention to target-group-oriented information about cancer prevention or cancer causes,

or to the possibility of taking part in clinical studies;
– supports the communication between doctor and patient by helping in advance with the structuring of questions addressed to the doctor, by interpreting and explaining the information given by the doctor, and by supporting the caller in the event that he or she wants to ask for a second opinion;
– explains the tasks and aims of cancer research with information about the latest research results;

– draws attention to the existing services provided for care, treatment, and aftercare;
– collects addresses and data from throughout the country concerning cancer-related institutions and provision of care, making these accessible to every citizen;
– gives feed-back on the needs of the callers, on their level of knowledge about cancer, on their opinions and activities, etc., to organizations that are active in elucidating the subject of cancer for the public.

Fig. 158
The President of the German Bundestag, Prof. Rita Süßmuth, opened the international congress on "Future Aspects of Cancer Information in Europe" in September 1997. From the left: Prof. Michael Wannenmacher, Chairman of the Tumor Center Heidelberg/Mannheim; Dr. Josef Puchta, Administrative Member of the Board of the Deutsches Krebsforschungszentrum; Prof. Sabine von Kleist, Vice-president of the German Cancer Aid; Beate Weber, Mayor of the City of Heidelberg; Prof. Rita Süßmuth, President of the German Bundestag; Lilly Christensen, Member of the Board of the Association of European Cancer Leagues; Prof. Peter Drings, General Secretary of the German Cancer Society

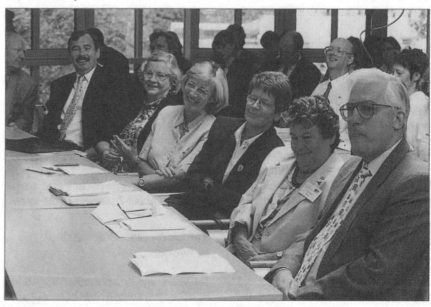

18

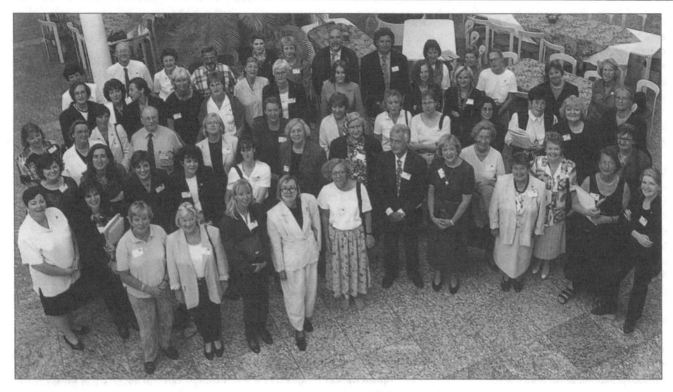

Fig. 159
Heidelberg was the meeting site for representatives of cancer information services from 38 European and overseas nations

To further publicize the activities of KID, its staff members gave approximately 20 presentations at congresses and other events during the years 1995 and 1996. They were also represented at eight such events with an information stand. KID staff have given talks at the International Cancer Congress, the German Cancer Congress, The World Conference for Cancer Organisations, and the Congress of the Organisation of European Cancer Research Institutes (OECI), among other things, on studies of the subject „Cancer and Age".

Who, then, are the callers? Over 45 percent of the callers are patients and 40 percent are close relatives of suffer-

ers. Two-thirds of the callers are women. But doctors and other health professionals also make use of KID: about 7 percent of the inquiries come from this source. The remaining callers are other interested citizens who themselves are not directly or indirectly affected, but whom KID is also eager to help with information about cancer prevention. This source of calls also accounts for about 7 percent of the total.

European and International Networks

Ten years ago KID issued an invitation to representatives, in particular of can-

cer leagues, from other European countries. This was to be the beginning of what has today become a European network of cancer telephone services. The broadest aim of this network is, and must be, to give every citizen of every country the same chance in reaching decisions and determining their own fate in relation to cancer, supported by a repository of internationally gathered knowledge, and also to contribute to reducing the incidence of cancer by providing information about risk factors.

Over the last decade there has been something of a boom in Europe in terms of newly created cancer informa-

284

tion services. KID has provided individual start-up help for services in Austria, Switzerland, and Turkey. It cooperates particularly closely with the German-language cancer information services in Austria and Switzerland. In the annual „tri-national" meeting, the details of this cooperation are discussed and developed. A major topic has been the design and analysis of documentation forms and, on the basis of these, the design of a common form to be used in joint analyses. At present the services are carrying out a comparative analysis of inquiries about therapies with unproven effectiveness. The development and results of this cooperation are also presented at the meetings of the European cancer information services, which provide an opportunity for the now more than 36 telephone cancer services in Europe to exchange their experiences. This year's meeting will take place in Heidelberg from the 7th to the 9th of September 1997 with the support of the European Union. It will carry the banner „Future Aspects of Cancer Communication in Europe." One has thus come full circle from the very first meeting, which was initiated exactly 10 years ago by KID in Heidelberg and in which representatives of the then six European and two non-European cancer information services took part.

Over the last few years attempts have been underway to introduce cancer information services in other non-European countries. In 1996, within the framework of the World Conference for Cancer Organisations in Melbourne, Australia, a worldwide network was initiated under the patronage of the Union Internationale Contre le Cancer (UICC) with the collaboration of KID.

In March 1966, the "International Partner Award" of the National Cancer Institute, US Cancer Information Service, was given to Hilke Stamatiadis-Smidt, head of KID, in San Francisco. KID was awarded the prize for its exemplary activities aimed at establishing an international cancer communications network for the benefit of the general public.

In 1997, the Annelies Schleich Grant was created with the support of the company Lilly Deutschland GmbH. It supports an arrangement between the Deutsches Krebsforschungszentrum and the National Cancer Institute of the USA in Bethesda, Washington, in which each year one staff member of the German Cancer Information Service and one staff member of the American Cancer Information Service can each spend four weeks in the other country. The aim is to facilitate the international communication of contemporary knowledge on cancer research and the fight against cancer and, particularly through an exchange of experiences, to contribute to a continuous improvement of the information given to the general public. The grant is named after Dr. Annelies Schleich, who died in 1990 and who was head of the department „Invasion and Metastasis" at the Deutsches Krebsforschungszentrum and also managing director of the former Institute for Cell Research. After her retirement, she supported KID from its very first day onwards by offering callers the benefit of her wide knowledge as a doctor and cancer researcher.

Acceptance

Since a telephone service can react directly to the individual need for information, its acceptance among the popula-

tion is unusually high. In a sample survey of 297 callers to the German Cancer Information Service, 91 percent expressed satisfaction with the information given by KID. In contrast, only 47 percent were satisfied with pamphlets and other information material. The work of a telephone service can be flexibly adapted to the potential of existing information channels and their ability to serve the needs that arise.

In the 11 years of its work, KID has given nearly 120 000 callers individual information. From Monday to Friday, from 8 a.m. to 8 p.m., anybody can call under the number 06221/410121. A great many more attempts to contact KID - calls which could not be taken - were registered on a counter, and indicate how great the demand is and how urgent the need to increase the capacity of the service.

Three times a week - on Tuesdays, Wednesdays, and Thursdays, from 6 p.m. to 8 p.m. - KID offers, in addition, information in Turkish. The intention here is to provide Germany's largest minority group, which is particularly handicapped by special cultural, social, and language barriers, with better opportunities to take advantage of the health services available in Germany.

Publications

In order to give as many people as possible access to the large information pool of KID, despite the limited capacity of its staff, KID has produced the book „Thema Krebs - Fragen und Antworten" (Subject cancer - questions and answers), published in 1993 by Springer-Verlag and soon to appear in a new edition. For the Federal Center for Health Information, KID has so far pro-

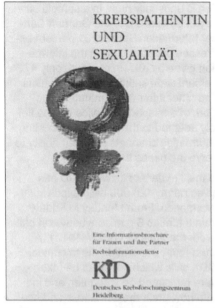

Fig. 160
The first edition of a new series of pamphlets from the Deutsches Krebsfor-schungszentrum. A further pamphlet for male cancer sufferers, „Krebspatient und Sexualität", will follow

Fig. 161
This set of pamphlets on the topic of „Speaking medicine – Patient and doctor in dialog" is the result of a cooperation project and is intended to help both doctors and patients

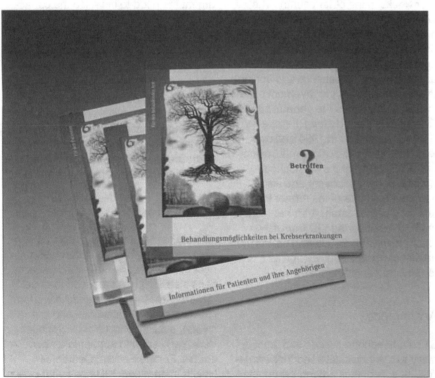

duced an additional 12 pamphlets on various tumor locations, which have been distributed in large numbers since 1990, and four comprehensive patient-oriented KID brochures. Two other pamphlets on the topic of sexuality and cancer are „Krebspatientin und Sexualität" and „Krebspatient und Sexualität", intended to help female and male cancer sufferers, respectively. Their printing was supported by the Meyenburg Foundation. In the period covered, KID has also produced, in collaboration with the company Lilly Deutschland GmbH, a doctor-patient pamphlet aimed at improving communication between doctor and patient. Its title translates as „Speaking medicine - Patient and doctor in dialog - Afflicted? Treatments for cancer" and it was conceived in association with hospital doctors and psychologists. This pamphlet will appear in 1997 and be supplied to doctors' practices throughout Germany.

From Basic Research to the Citizen

Twenty staff members from different professions in health care - psychologists, doctors, nurses, biologists, and others - man up to four telephone lines simultaneously in a shift system. Most of these people have been involved from the very beginning. The members of staff take part in a comprehensive annual training program, in which scientists and clinicians from all disciplines impart basic oncological knowledge, which is extended and deepened through continuous further training about new developments.

The training of the staff also includes communication seminars and regular psychological supervision, which offer

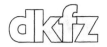

the opportunity to review difficult and troubling conversations and to further improve the competence in a conversation.

Approximately a quarter of the inquiries received by KID can be answered immediately with the help of its own information pool. New questions, which relate, for example, to the very latest research data or to new procedures with as yet unknown effectiveness, are passed on to the research team, a small team of scientists from the fields of medicine, biology, and psychology, whose task it is to research and make available answers in a readily understandable form. These members of staff have access to numerous sources of information on oncological matters: international oncological literature, diagnostic and therapy recommendations of various tumor centers, the extensive collection of documents and articles that is kept at KID, numerous libraries (in particular the scientific library of the Deutsches Krebsforschungszentrum), international literature databases, the Internet, and also personal contacts to clinicians and scientists in Germany and elsewhere. Specialist knowledge is always available, due, in particular, to the close proximity and structural coupling to the Deutsches Krebsforschungszentrum and the clinics of the Tumor Center Heidelberg/Mannheim. However, KID does not pursue a policy of „self-promoting" information; rather, it operates on the principle of comprehensive nationwide and integrative information. By passing on addresses nationwide, KID assists the caller in finding the necessary care and treatment as close as possible to his or her home. The information given is based on the state-of-the-art in oncological preven-

tion, diagnostics, treatment, clinical research, and basic research.

Important basic information in text form, and also approximately 3000 addresses and details about what the various cancer-related institutes can offer - from tumor centers through aftercare clinics to psycho-social advice centers - are kept in a database which is continuously extended and brought up to date. This database has been specifically designed to meet the needs of the service and runs on networked personal computers, making the information directly available on the telephonist's screen. All telephone conversations are documented on forms, which provide the basis for the statistical analysis and for associated research projects. Numerous studies have accompanied the work of the Cancer Information Service during the 11 years of its existence. An example is the 1996 study of the KID callers' knowledge and beliefs about risk factors, prevention, and early diagnosis, a study sponsored by the European Union within the „Europe Against Cancer" initiative.

Readjustment After Clinical Treatment

The questions addressed to the Cancer Information Service are extremely diverse. The main topic is therapy (62 percent); this is followed by aftercare, diagnostics, and cancer risk factors. If the question concerns a particular type of cancer, in the case of men the most frequent are cancer of the intestine, prostate cancer, and bronchial carcinomas; for women, breast cancer features in more than 45 percent of the cases. On the other hand, the rarer tumor types are over-represented in terms of

the number of questions relating to them. The most common occasion for calling KID is after completion of a first treatment, i.e., following release from hospital. An important function of the service is evidently to help patients and their relatives in this phase of readjustment and new orientation.

Integrated in the Federal Government's full program for fighting cancer and in the corresponding European program „Europe Against Cancer", KID has shown itself to be an innovative model for the communication of scientific matters to the public. The strong resonance which KID has found supports the conception of the service as an independent central point of contact, as a new and necessary link between experts and the general public, and as a valuable supplement to the information provided by health information bodies and the media.

Meetings, Workshops, and Symposia

For many years now, the Deutsches Krebsforschungszentrum has organized an intensive information exchange between scientists in Germany and abroad.

The following events, which took place between 1994 and 1996, deserve special mention:

3rd Colloquium on Cellular Signal Transduction „Cell Cycle Signalling"
Colloquium of the Deutsches Krebsforschungszentrum

January 14, 1994

„Transport in the Liver"
Falk Symposium No. 74, Falk Foundation e.V., Freiburg, in cooperation with the Deutsches Krebsforschungszentrum

January 27–28, 1994

„Gesunde Schule – Lebensraum Schule" (The Healthy School – School Environment) – Concepts and Models for the Future
Specialist conference for primary school principals in Heidelberg and the Rhein-Neckar Region
Organized by the Heidelberg Public Health Center, the Agency for Environmental Protection and Sanitation of the City of Heidelberg, and the Deutsches Krebsforschungszentrum

March 17, 1994

„Health Effect of Internally Deposited Radionuclides"
International Seminar of the Commission of the European Community, the US Department of Energy, and the Federal Agency for Radiation Protection in cooperation with the Deutsches Krebsforschungszentrum

April 18–22, 1994

5th X Chromosome Workshop of the Deutsches Krebsforschungszentrum

April 24-27, 1994

„EURONEU 2" Human Neuroblastoma, Recent Advances in Clinical & Genetic Analysis
Conference of the Deutsches Krebsforschungszentrum in the framework of the BIOMED 1 Program of the European Union

June 9–10, 1994

7th Heidelberg Cytometry Symposium
Meeting of the Society for Cytometry in cooperation with the Deutsches Krebsforschungszentrum

October 20–22, 1994

4th Colloquium on Cellular Signal Transduction – Liquid Mediators, Signal Transduction and Transport
Colloquium of the Deutsches Krebsforschungszentrum

January 20, 1995

German-Taiwanese Workshop on the topic of „Tumorprävention" (Tumor Prevention)
Workshop of the German Research Association (DFG) and the Deutsches Krebsforschungszentrum

February 23–24, 1995

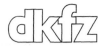

Technology Conference „Biotechnik"
(Biotechnology) of the Chamber of In-
dustry and Commerce of the Rhein-
Neckar Region in cooperation with the
Deutsches Krebsforschungszentrum

March 27, 1995

8th Symposium of the „Sektion experimentelle Krebsforschung (SEK)" (Section for experimental cancer research)
of the German Cancer Society in cooperation with the Deutsches Krebsforschungszentrum and the Institute of
Pathology of the University of Munich

March 29–31, 1995

„Cell Interactions in Malignancy, Development and Differentiation"

International Conference of the German
Cell and Tissue Culture Society and the
German Section of the European Tissue Culture Society in cooperation with
the Deutsches Krebsforschungszentrum

April 2–5, 1995

„Praktische Aspekte bei der
Durchführung von krebsepidemiologi-
schen Studien, insbesondere Fall-Kon-
trollstudien, in der Bundesrepublik
Deutschland" (Practical Aspects of
Cancer Epidemiology Studies in Ger-
many, with Particular Emphasis on
Case Control Studies)

Workshop of the Deutsches Krebsforschungszentrum in cooperation with the
German Society for Medical Documentation and Statistics, and the German
Society for Social Medicine and Prevention

April 27–28, 1995

„Grundlagen der dreidimensionalen
Strahlentherapieplanung" (Fundamen-
tals of Three-dimensional Radiation
Therapy Planning)

Workshop of the Deutsches Krebsforschungszentrum

April 27–29, 1995

„Molecular Dynamic Simulations on
Biopolymers"

Workshop of the Deutsches Krebsforschungszentrum

September 6, 1995

4th International Symposium on Nu-
cleo-Cytoplasmatic Transport

Symposium of the Deutsches Krebsforschungszentrum in cooperation with
the German Research Association
(DFG)

October 1–4, 1995

1st Euroconference „Viral Oncogenesis
and Cell Cycle Control"

Conference of the Deutsches Krebsforschungszentrum

October 5–7, 1995

8th Heidelberg Cytometry Symposium

Meeting of the Cytometry Society in
cooperation with the Deutsches Krebsforschungszentrum

October 19–21, 1995

„Molekulare Mechanismen
intrazellulärer Transportprozesse" (Molecular mechanisms of intracellular
transport processes)

Scientific Colloquium of the Deutsches
Krebsforschungszentrum

January 15, 1996

„Risk Factors for Adult Leukaemias and
Lymphomas"

Symposium of the Deutsches Krebsforschungszentrum

January 15–16, 1996

„Computational Analysis of Eukaryotic
Transcriptional Regulatory Elements"

Symposium of the Deutsches Krebsforschungszentrum

January 18–20, 1996

5th Colloquium on Signal Transduction
„Transcriptional Regulation"

Colloquium of the Deutsches Krebsforschungszentrum

January 19, 1996

„Klinische und epidemiologische Krebs-
register" (Clinical and Epidemiological
Cancer Registers)

Seminar of the Deutsches Krebsfor-
schungszentrum in cooperation with the
University of Heidelberg, the German
Society for Medical Informatics, Biome-
try, and Epidemiology, the Professional
Association of Medical Computer Sci-
entists and the German Association of
Medical Documentation Specialists

February 6–7, 1996

„Aktuelle Trends in der Virologie" (Current Trends in Virology)

Symposium of the Deutsches Krebsforschungszentrum

March 19, 1996

International HUGO Conference
(Human Genome Project)

HUGO Europe in cooperation with the
Deutsches Krebsforschungszentrum

March 22–24, 1996

„Theoretical and Computational Genome Research"

International Symposium of the Deutsches Krebsforschungszentrum

March 25–27, 1996

Meeting on Cancer Chemoprevention
„Molecular Basis, Mechanisms and
Trials" of the Deutsches Krebsfor-
schungszentrum

September 9–11, 1996

9th Heidelberg Cytometry Symposium

Meeting of the Cytometry Society in
cooperation with the Deutsches Krebsforschungszentrum

October 17–19, 1996

„Dioxins and Furans: Epidemiologic Assessment of Cancer Risks and Other
Human Health Effects"

Symposium of the Deutsches Krebsforschungszentrum in cooperation with
the German Research Association
(DFG), the National Institute of Environmental Health Sciences, USA, and the
Federal Agency for the Environment,
Berlin

November 7–8, 1996

20

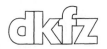

Statutes and Articles of the Foundation Deutsches Krebsforschungszentrum

Approved and published by the Ministry for Science and Arts of Baden-Württemberg in its function as supervising body with the act issued on 12 July 1991 under the file number II 730.11/32 in the Legal Gazette for Baden-Württemberg of 12 July 1991, followed by a correction on 30 September 1991 (Legal Gazette for Baden-Württemberg, No. 23, p. 595)

I. General Provisions

Section 1
Legal Form, Seat

The Deutsches Krebsforschungszentrum, a foundation under public law of the Land Baden-Württemberg, has its seat in Heidelberg.

Section 2
Purpose of the Foundation

(1) It is the purpose of the Foundation to engage in cancer research.

(2) The Foundation may undertake other tasks in this connection, inter alia further education and advanced training, and especially the promotion of young scientists.

(3) The research results are to be published.

Section 3
Non-Profit Institution

(1) As a non-profit institution the Foundation shall exclusively and directly serve the public interest, in particular scientific interests according to fiscal regulations.

(2) Any profits made may only be used for the purposes laid down in the Statutes and Articles. The Foundation may not grant benefits to any person by expenditures which run counter to the purposes of the Foundation or by disproportionately high awards.

Section 4
Assets of the Foundation

The assets of the Foundation shall consist of the goods and titles which have been or are being created or acquired with the aid of the funds placed at its disposal by the Federal Republic of Germany, hereinafter referred to as the Federal Republic, the German Land Baden-Württemberg, hereinafter referred to as the Land, or by third parties. The assets of the Foundation shall be used for the purposes laid down in section 2.

Section 5
Financing of the Foundation

(1) The Federal Republic and the Land will provide for the necessary expenditures of the Foundation in as far as this is not covered by income from other sources or by own or foreign means – with the exception of donations and investment returns therefrom – by allowances according to further agreement.

(2) The means to be provided acccording to paragraph 1 will be allocated to the Foundation according to the provisions of the budgetary law within the framework of the approved budgets of the Foundation and the budgets of the Federal Republic and the Land.

Section 6
Budget of the Foundation

(1) The budget of the Foundation must contain any receipts to be expected in the fiscal year, any probable expenses, and any probable authorizations to incur liabilities. Receipts and expenditures must be balanced.

(2) The budget will have to be approved by the authority controlling the Foundation.

(3) Grants made to the Foundation are to be recorded in an appendix to the Foundation's accounts.

II. Organs of the Foundation

Section 7
Executive Organs

The organs of the Foundation are

a) the Board of Trustees,
b) the Management Board,
c) the Scientific Council.

Section 8
Tasks of the Board of Trustees

(1) The Board of Trustees will supervise the legality, expediency, and economy of the conduct of the Foundation's transactions. It will decide on the aims of research and important research policy and financial affairs of the Foundation. It will determine the principles of management and those governing result control. It may give directives to the Management Board in special matters of research policy and finance as well as for the implementation of result control.

(2) The Board of Trustees sets up the annual budgets and the long-term financial plans including the programs for development and investment. It will decide on changes in the Statutes and Articles and on the dissolution of the Foundation as well as on other matters laid down in these Statutes.

(3) The following matters must be previously approved by the Board of Trustees:

a) the annuel and long-term research programs;

b) taking up further tasks and discontinuing previous tasks;

c) the foundation, dissolution, and amalgamation of research programs, divisions, and central facilities, the start and termination of projects, and the extension of research programs and projects;

d) the appointment and recall of the heads of divisions, of the administrative director as well as of the directors of central facilities and projects, as well as the appointment of the coordinators of the research programs;

e) the regulations for research programs and projects;

f) the regulations for elections and the rules of procedure;

g) the regulations governing appointments;

h) principles governing the utilization of the research results of the Foundation;

i) extraordinary legal transactions and measures exceeding the framework of current business operations which may exert considerable influence upon the position and activity of the Foundation; significant agreements concerning cooperation with other German undertakings and institutions, and agreements concerning cooperation with foreign undertakings and institutions; entering into contracts which impose upon the Foundation obligations exceeding a period of one year, inasfar as they are not within the scope of normal business or provided for in the approved budget;

k) drawing up, changing or terminating employment contracts in excess of or outside the tariff, granting other benefits in excess of or outside the tariff, as well as entering into contracts exceeding an amount fixed by the Board of Trustees;

l) measures of collective tariff commitments of formation and general regulations concerning remuneration and social benefits, as well as setting up directives governing the granting of reimbursement of travel and moving costs, of separation allowances, and of expenses for the use of motor vehicles.

(4) For particular types of legal transactions and measures, the Board of Trustees may give its agreement in general.

(5) In urgent cases it is sufficient to have the prior written consent of the President and the Deputy President of the Board of Trustees. The other members of the Board of Trustees are to be immediately informed by the President about the action.

Section 9
Composition of the Board of Trustees

(1) The Board of Trustees consists of, at most, eighteen honorary members.

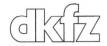

(2) Out of these

a) four members – one of them being the President – will be delegated and removed from office by the Federal Republic,

b) two members – one of them being the Deputy President – will be delegated and removed from office by the Land,

c) three scientists working for the Foundation and without a seat on the Management Board – at least one of them being head of a division – will be appointed by the Land in agreement with the Federal Republic from a list of six nominees drawn up by all members of the scientific staff. Further details will be settled by election regulations to be issued by the Management Board in consultation with the Scientific Council and with the consent of the Board of Trustees. If those appointed have seats on the Scientific Council, their membership in the Scientific Council will be terminated upon acceptance of their appointment to the Board of Trustees,

d) seven external members (mainly specialits) will be appointed by the Land in agreement with the Federation upon consultation with the Management Board and the Scientific Council,

e) two members as the representatives of the University of Heidelberg, i.e., one proposed jointly by the Faculties of Medicine and Natural Sciences as well as the Rector (President) during his term of office or a professor charged by the latter, will be appointed by the Land in agreement with the Federal Republic.

(3) The members referred to in paragraph 2, items c, d and e will be appointed for a maximum period of three years. Re-appointment is permitted. After expiration of their term of office they will remain in office until the new appointments have been made according to paragraph 2, items c, d and e. Members may be removed from office for important reasons. Members leaving before their terms of office have expired must immediately be replaced from among the non-appointed applicants from the list of nominees according to paragraph 2, item c or by a new appointment according to paragraph 2, item d. Should the list of suggestions be exhausted, the procecure according to paragraph 2, item c schall be applied. Suggestion and appointment will be valid for the remaining term of office.

Section 10
Scientific Committee of the Board of Trustees

(1) The Scientific Committee prepares the decisions of the Board of Trustees in all scientific matters within the framework of section 8.

(2) The Scientific Committee bears the responsibility for the timely evaluation of the results of research programs, divisions and projects based on scientific expertise. As a rule, they set up ad hoc commissions manned by external scientists for this purpose.

(3) The Scientific Committee of the Board of Trustees consists of the external scientific members of the latter according to section 9, paragraph 2, item d. From among its members a chairman and a deputy chairman are elected. The President and the Deputy

President of the Board of Trustees may take part int he sessions as guests. The Scientific Committee may set up standing rules which also determine the competence and procedures of the ad hoc commissions in greater detail.

Section 11
Standing Rules of The Board of Trustees and its Committees

(1) The Board of Trustees may set up standing rules which also determine the competence and procedure of the Committees in greater detail. Persons who are not members of the Board of Trustees may also hold a seat on the Committees; they will not take part in passing resolutions in Committees granted jurisdiction. A representative of the Federal Republic will assume the chair.

(2) The Board of Trustees may set up Committees to prepare its decisions as well as for certain matters to be decided by the Committee itself. At least one member each according to section 9, paragraph 2, items a through d must hold a seat on each Committee.

Section 12
Meetings of the Board of Trustees and its Committees

(1) The Boards of Trustees will be convened by the President once in six months as a rule, but at least once every calendar year.

(2) The members of the Management Board as well as the chairman of the Scientific Council and the chariman of the staff representation or their deputies are entitled to attend the meetings of the Board of Trustees and its Com-

mittees in a consulting capacity, inasfar as the Board of Trustees or the Committee do not decide otherwise.

Section 13
Resolutions of the Board of Trustees and its Committees

(1) The Board of Trustees will constitute a quorum if two-thirds of its members are present or are represented in compliance with paragraph 2. The President or his deputy must be present. Comittees holding power of decision will constitute a quorum if one member each according to section 9, paragraph 2, items a through c is present or represented.

(2) If unable to attend, the members of the Board of Trustees delegated by the Federal Republic and the Land may arrange to be represented by members of their administration, other members may be represented by a member of the Board of Trustees provided with a written limited power of attorney valid for the individual contingency.

(3) Resolutions of the Board of Trustees are passed with a majority of the valid votes cast. The President and the Deputy President have a double, transferable vote. In case of parity, the President shall have the casting vote. With important questions of research policy, in financial matters, in matters according to section 8, paragraphs 2 and 3, as well as with the appointment of the members and the release of the Management Board, resolutions may not be passed counter to the votes of members of the Board of Trustees delegated by the Federal Republic or the Land.

(4) Paragraphs 2 and 3 apply to the Committees correspondingly.

(5) In individual cases, the President, or if he is prevented, his deputy may cause resolutions to be passed in writting, by telex of by cable, insofar as no member of the Board of Trustees registers his immediate protest.

Section 14
Functions of the Management Board

(1) The Management Board directs the Foundation.

(2) The Management Board seeks the prior approval of the Scientific Council on the matters set down in section 8, paragraph 3, items a through g, as well as on

– the annual budget and long-term financial plans including the programs for development and investment;

– measures for the implementation of efficiency control of scientific work;

– measures to promote the flow of scientific information within the Foundation (work reports, colloquia, hearings);

– the co-operation with universities, other research institutions and international establishments;

– the submission of the scientific progress report to the Board of Trustees.

(3) Insofar as the Scientific Council's proposals in these matters should deviate, the Management Board will initiate a renewed joint discussion with the Scientific Council. If agreement cannot be reached, the Management Board will decide. If the Management Board makes a decision which deviates from the recommendations of the Scientific Council, it will have to supply an expla-

nation in writing to the Scientific Council and the Board of Trustees.

Section 15
Composition of the Management Board, Scope of Authority

(1) The Management Board consists of at least one scientific and one administrative member. The administrative member shall be qualified for employment in the higher administrative service. The term of office for the members of the Management Board is limited and will, as a rule, amount to five years. Reappointment is permitted. Appointments may be revoked at any time.

(2) The chairman of the Management Board and the other members will be appointed and recalled by the Board of Trustees after consultation with the Scientific Council. The Scientific Council has the right of nomination for scientific members and for the chairman.

The members of the Management Board may not at the same time be co-ordinators of research programs or be members of the Scientific Council. The President of the Board of Trustees, who in this capacity represents the Foundation, will enter into, change or terminate contracts with the members of the Management Board.

(3) The chairman of the Management Board will be the scientific representative of the Foundation. Together with the administrative member he will represent the Foundation judicially and extrajudicially. In matters of current administration the administrative member may represent the Foundation on his own.

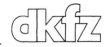

(4) The Management Board will set up standing rules which require the approval of the Board of Trustees. The standing rules will also regulate the authority according to paragraph 3, sentences 2 and 3 in the event the authorized representatives are prevented from fulfilling their function.

(5) The administrative member of the Management Board will be in charge of budget affairs in the sense of section 9 of the budget regulations of the Land Baden-Württemberg.

Section 16
Tasks of the Scientific Council

(1) The Scientific Council advises the Board of Trustees and the Management Board in all significant matters of a scientific nature. In particular, it will offer advice concerning

a) the annual and long-term research programs;

b) appointment procedures, in particular by the drawing up of appointment lists;

c) the appointment and recall of the heads of divisions as well as the directors of central facilities and projects;

d) taking up further functions and discontinuing previous functions;

e) founding, dissolving and amalgamating research programs, divisions and central facilities, starting and terminating projects, as well as extending research programs and projects;

f) issuing regulations for research programs and projects;

g) the appointments procedure;

h) principles for the utilization of the research results of the Foundation;

i) the annual budget and long-term financial plans including programs for development and investment;

k) measures for the implementation of result control of scientific work;

l) measures for the promotion of the flow of scientific information within the Foundation (work reports, colloquia, hearings);

m) the co-operation with universities, other research institutions and international establishments;

n) the scientific progress report.

In these matters the scientific Council, insofar as this is necessary according to section 14, paragraph 2, will pass resolutions about its consent with the intended decisions of the Management Board. If agreement cannot be teached, the procedure according to section 14, paragraph 3 will be applied.

(2) The Scientific-Council may demand information from the Management Board on scientific matters and matters of research policy.

Section 17
Composition and Resolutions of the Scientific Council

(1) The Scientific Council consists of

a) the coordinators of research programs,

b) an equal number of representatives of the scientific statt.

(2) The members according to paragraph 1, letter b will be elected for a period of three years by the scientific staff of the Foundation in compliance with an election order. The election

order is laid down by the Management Board in consultation with the Scientific Council and with the consent of the Board of Trustees.

(3) The Scientific Council elects from its midst a chairman and a deputy chairman.

(4) The members of the Management Board, the President of the Board of Trustees or a member of the Board of Trustees to be determined by the latter and a member of the staff representation may attend the meetings of the Scientific Council in a consultative capacity insofar as the Scientific Council does not decide otherwiese in any individual instance.

(5) The Scientific Council will constitute a quorum if two thirds of its members including the chairman or the deputy chairman are present. Resolutions require a majority of the valid votes cast.

(6) The Scientific Council in consultation with the Management Board and with the consent of the Board of Trustees will set up standing rules governing the representation of the members.

III. Research Programs, Divisions, Projects, and Central Facilities

Section 18
Research Programs and Divisions

(1) Research programs are the thematically defined and temporary collaboration of divisions.

(2) Divisions are scientifically independent research units co-operating within

research programs. There are temporally limited and unlimited divisions.

They are headed by heads of divisions who are appointed for an unlimited or limited period of time.

Being organizational units, the divisions serve the purpose of the Foundation. Within the divisions, working groups may be organized.

(3) The management of a research program consists of the heads of the divisions of that research program. It coordinates the scientific work of the divisions of that research program and makes all necessary decisions.

(4) The management of the research program nominates, with the consent of the Scientific Council and the Management Board, a coordinator from among its members. After approval from the Board of Trustees, the coordinator will be appointed by the Management Board. The term of office will amount to three years; re-appointment is possible. The tasks of the coordinators of the research programs are laid down in the standing order of the research programs, which also provides a research program committee and a research program assembly.

(5) The Management Board sets up standing rules for the divisions and the research programs after approval by the Scientific Council and the Board of Trustees.

Section 19
Projects

(1) The Foundation may carry out part of the research program in the form of projects. A project is understood to be a research activity largely structured in detail which is temporally and financially limited, bound towards a certain aim, and which exceeds the framework of a research program and which, due to its size and scientific importance, requires an independent organizational structure.

(2) The organization and implementation of projects are laid down in a project order which the Management Board will issue with the approval of the Scientific Council and the Board of Trustees.

Section 20
Central Facilities

(1) Central facilities shall serve to fulfill tasks of the entire Deutsches Krebsforschungszentrum or of several research programs and projects. They are reporting directly to the Management Board.

(2) The participation of the scientific staff in the elections to the Scientific Council and the Board of Trustees is regulated by the Management Board in the respective election orders with the approval of the Board of Trustees and the Scientific Council.

IV. Administration and Personnel Affairs

Section 21
Accounting, Auditing, and Acceptance of the Accounts

(1) Accounts must be rendered annually by the Management Board concerning the income and expenditure as well as the assets and liablities of the Foundation. Notwithstanding the legal auditing rights of the Federal Audit Office and the Audit Office of Baden-Württemberg, the annual accounts must be audited by a chartered accountant or auditing establishment. The Board of Trustees will decide who is to be entrusted with this task.

(2) At the end of the calendar year a business report and a satement of account is to be submitted to the Board of Trustees, the authority in control of the Foundation and the auditing authorities.

(3) Section 109, paragraph 3 of the budget regulations of Baden-Württemberg is applicable to the release. Organ for decision making is the Board of Trustees.

Section 22
Scientific Staff

The scientific staff as defined in these Statutes and Articles consists of all employees of the Foundation who are either university graduates or who carry out corresponding activities in the scientific field on the basis of equivalent abilities and experience and who have entered into an employment contract with the Foundation.

Section 23
Personnel Affairs

(1) Prior to the appointment of heads of divisions and the employment of scientific staff according to section 8, paragraph 3, item d, an appointment procedure is to be carried through pursuant to further regulations laid down in an appointment order to be issued by the Management Board in consultation with the Scientific Council and with the consent of the Board of Trustees.

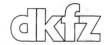

(2) Decisions concerning the legal status of civil servants employed by the Foundation will be made by the competent authorities according to the legal regulations of the Land on the basis of applications which are decided upon by the competent organs of the Foundation.

Section 24
Changes Affecting the Statutes and Articles and Dissolution of the Foundation

Resolutions concerning changes affecting the Statutes and Articles and the dissolution of the Foundation may not be passed without the votes of the members of the Board of Trustees delegated by the Federal Republic and the Land who have a double vote in such matters. The Management Board and the Scientific Council are to be previously consulted. The resolutions will not take effect until they have been approved by the authority in control of the Foundation.

Section 25
Accumulation of Assets

(1) In the event of the dissolution of the Foundation, the Foundation's assets will pass to the Federal Republic and the Land in proportion to the value of the grants made by each of them, insofar as these assets do not exceed the value of the grants awarded and any contributions made in kind at the time of dissolution. Any balance then remaining will, in agreement with the Federal Republic, be used on a non-profit basis in the sense of the paragraph titled "tax-privileged purposes" of the tax code.

Section 26
Effective Date and Transitional Provisions

(1) These Statutes and Articles will go into effect on the day following their announcement in the Law Gazette of Baden-Württemberg.

(2) With the enactment of these Statutes and Articles, the Statutes and Articles of February 7, 1983 (Law Gazette, p. 86) and July 9, 1986 (Law Gazette, p. 278) become ineffective.

(3) The membership of the acting directors of the institutes and the scientific staff members of the Scientific Council continues in the framework of their term of office until the coordinators of the research programs are appointed and new scientific staff members have been elected.

(4) The terms of office of the acting directors of the institutes will be terminated upon the enactment of these Statutes and Articles.

21

Index

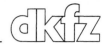

Printed in the United States
by Baker & Taylor Publisher Services